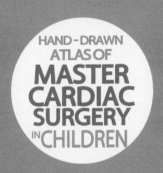

HAND-DRAWN
ATLAS OF
**MASTER
CARDIAC
SURGERY**
IN**CHILDREN**

谨以此书
纪念我们的良师挚友

翁渝国 医生

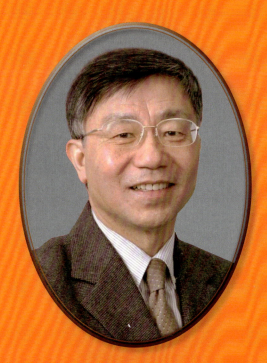

1946.09.06 — 2017.06.26

This book commemorates

Dr. Weng Yuguo,
our good teacher and friend.

汉英对照

小儿心脏外科
名家手术
手绘图解

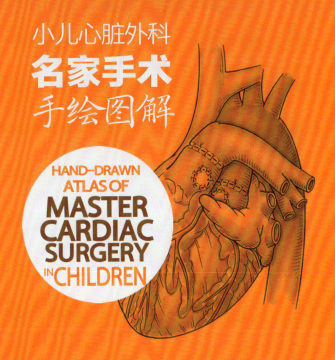

HAND-DRAWN
ATLAS OF
MASTER
CARDIAC
SURGERY
IN CHILDREN

主　编｜刘中民　翁渝国　刘锦纷

副主编｜李铁岩　华一飞

译　者｜陈水平　李清华

绘　图｜朱丽萍

人民卫生出版社
·北 京·

图书在版编目（CIP）数据

小儿心脏外科名家手术手绘图解：汉英对照 / 刘中民，翁渝国，刘锦纷主编 . —北京：人民卫生出版社，2024.8

ISBN 978-7-117-35842-2

Ⅰ. ①小⋯　Ⅱ. ①刘⋯②翁⋯③刘⋯　Ⅲ. ①小儿疾病 －心脏外科学 －图解　Ⅳ. ①R726.54–64

中国国家版本馆 CIP 数据核字（2024）第 021380 号

人卫智网　www.ipmph.com	医学教育、学术、考试、健康，购书智慧智能综合服务平台
人卫官网　www.pmph.com	人卫官方资讯发布平台

小儿心脏外科名家手术手绘图解（汉英对照）
Xiao'er Xinzang Waike Mingjia Shoushu Shouhui Tujie
（Han-Ying Duizhao）

主　　编：刘中民　翁渝国　刘锦纷
出版发行：人民卫生出版社（中继线 010-59780011）
地　　址：北京市朝阳区潘家园南里 19 号
邮　　编：100021
E - mail：pmph @ pmph.com
购书热线：010-59787592　010-59787584　010-65264830
印　　刷：北京盛通印刷股份有限公司印刷
经　　销：新华书店
开　　本：889 × 1194　1/16　　印张：49.5
字　　数：1114 千字
版　　次：2024 年 8 月第 1 版
印　　次：2024 年 9 月第 1 次印刷
标准书号：ISBN 978-7-117-35842-2
定　　价：498.00 元

打击盗版举报电话：010-59787491　E-mail：WQ @ pmph.com
质量问题联系电话：010-59787234　E-mail：zhiliang @ pmph.com
数字融合服务电话：4001118166　　E-mail：zengzhi @ pmph.com

痛失敬爱的翁医生

The loss of our beloved Dr. Weng

1986 年春，奥格斯堡的 Struck 教授给我电话，说他有一位非常优秀的外科同事因为巴伐利亚州政府不能再延长他的居留权，必须要回中国，问我是否有办法帮忙。我当时正在组建德国心脏中心（柏林），需要有经验的外科医生。由于我的同事多是年轻人，不太有经验，我必须亲自动手术。因此，Struck 教授的电话来得恰逢其时。柏林那时仍被封锁，但西柏林是没问题的。在给卫生和建设部的 Ara 博士打过电话后，我马上开始办理翁医生和他夫人及女儿到柏林的手续。1986 年秋，他到达了我院。

我很快发现，他是一位非常有经验的外科医生，于是很快升他为我的副手。他不仅会全部的心脏外科手术，还对新生儿先天性心脏病、胸腔外科、大血管以及其他器官疾病皆有所能。据我所知，他之所能全学自于中国，很多的经验来自当"赤脚医生"的经历。没有他的勤奋和才华，我的工作会很困难。德国心脏中心（柏林）（Deutschen Herzzentrum Berlin, DHZB）也不可能发展成为欧洲最大、手术量最多的中心，手术包括一些复杂手术，如

In the spring of 1986, Professor Struck called from Augsburg to ask if I could accommodate one of his colleagues, an excellent surgeon, who otherwise had to go back to China because his right of abode could not be extended by the Bayern government. At that time, I was setting up the German Heart Center (Berlin) and needed experienced surgeons. Since most of my colleagues were young and inexperienced, I had to perform all the operations myself. Therefore, Professor Struck's phone call came at the right time. Berlin was still cordoned off, but West Berlin was fine. After a call to Dr. Ara at the Ministry of Health and Construction, I immediately started to go through the formalities for Dr. Weng, his wife, and his daughter to go to Berlin. In the autumn of 1986, Dr. Weng arrived at our hospital.

Dr. Weng was soon found to be a very experienced surgeon and was promoted to be my assistant. He specialized not only in all cardiac surgeries, but also in infantile and congenital atrial septal defect, thoracic surgeries, as well as macrovascular and other organ diseases. As far as I know, he had developed his expertise in China, which mainly came from his experiences as a "barefoot doctor". Without his diligence and talent, my work would not have progressed so smoothly, and the German Heart Center (Berlin)(Deutschen Herzzentrum Berlin, DHZB) could not have developed into the largest center with the largest number of

冠心病手术、小儿先天性心脏病手术、主动脉手术、各种器官移植和人工心脏辅助装置的安装。除此以外，如遇新的或罕见病例，我会请教翁医生，经常需要他的帮忙。一直以来，我对他的团结合作与忠诚非常信任。在他的协助下，我才有勇气不拒绝那些疑难病例，而是尽我们最大的努力医治病患。这样，患者在被其他心脏中心拒绝后，仍然会对 DHZB 抱有一线希望。也因此，无数的尝试和首次进行的手术获得成功。直到今天我仍能见到数年前由翁医生主刀的那位患者，而当时若没有他那双"能手"，那位患者早已经离我们远去了。正因为如此，德国心脏中心成为了世界顶尖的医院。

他的伟大还在于帮助他的祖国中国和德国建立了合作交流的纽带。德国心脏中心与刘中民院长所在的上海市东方医院的合作始于 2000 年（那也正是翁医生走完人生最后旅程的地方）。2001 年 5 月，时任上海市副市长周禹鹏先生亲自到柏林为双方合作揭牌，从此开启了我们与中国医院合作的新里程。超过 1 000 名中国医生和其他部门的工作人员曾数月甚至多年在我院工作进修，给院里增添了很多色彩。经过翁医生以及我的助手 Norbert Franz 和 Meizhu 的共同努力，中国成为我们最大的友好国家。有时我到一个手术室，发现那里工作的都是中国人，而且手术医生、助手、护士都用中文交流。

operations in Europe, covering complex operations such as surgery for coronary heart disease, surgery for pediatric congenital heart disease, aortic surgery, various organ transplants and the installation of artificial heart assist devices. I used to consult Dr. Weng for some novel or rare cases, and I always trusted his teamwork, cooperation and loyalty. With his assistance, I had the courage not to turn down those difficult cases but rather try our best to treat them. In this way, patients would still have a gleam of hope in DHZB after being rejected by other heart centers. It was also with his assistance that countless attempts and trials had been proved to be successful. To this day, I can still see the patient, who would have already passed away but for the superb operation performed by Dr. Weng a few years ago. Because of this, the German Heart Center has become one of the top hospitals in the world.

His greatness also lies in helping to establish ties between his motherland China and Germany. The cooperation between the German Heart Center and Shanghai East Hospital, where Director Liu Zhongmin works, began in 2000. Shanghai East Hospital is also the place where Dr. Weng completed his last journey. In May 2001, Mr. Zhou Yupeng, then vice mayor of Shanghai, personally came to Berlin to launch a bilateral cooperation, and since then, we have embarked on a new journey of cooperation with Chinese hospitals. More than 1000 Chinese doctors and staff from other departments have worked and studied in our hospital for months or even years, which really added a lot of color to the German Heart Center. Through the joint efforts of Dr. Weng, as well as my assistants Norbert Franz and Meizhu, China has become our

翁医生编著了许多的心脏外科教学书籍,我们也一起制作过图解,这本《心脏外科名家手术手绘图解》凝聚了翁医生毕生的经验和心血,历经三十年磨砺,终于在翁医生家人和刘中民院长以及他的同事们的努力下全部完成。翁医生不会被忘记,他的学识和教导将永世流传。

让我们难过的是,一场重病侵袭了翁医生,也让他数年来受尽煎熬。好一阵子,他不以介怀,因为他的家人和国内的友人们是他的安慰。他用他的一生在帮助和启迪身边每一个人。

谨向我们伟大的外科医生、朋友和同伴,架起中德两国友谊桥梁的翁渝国医生致敬!

Ronald Hetzer

德国心脏中心(柏林)原院长

2017 年 12 月

greatest friendly country. Sometimes, I went to an operating theatre only to find that the people there were all Chinese, and surgeons, assistants and nurses all communicated in Chinese.

Dr. Weng had written a lot of course books on cardiac surgery, and we had also drawn atlas together. *Hand-drawn Atlas of Master Cardiac Surgery*, having been honed by Dr. Weng for 30 years, is finally completed with the help of Dr. Weng's family, his friend Director Liu Zhongmin and his colleagues. The book, embodying Dr. Weng's lifelong experiences and painstaking effort. Dr. Weng will not be forgotten, and his knowledge and instructions will be handed down from generation to generation.

To our sadness, a serious illness hit Dr. Weng, which made him suffer for years. For a long time, he didn't take his illness to heart, for his family and friends in China were his comfort. Dr. Weng had dedicated his entire life to helping and enlightening everyone around him.

Tribute to our great surgeon, friend and companion, Dr. Weng Yuguo, who built the bridge of friendship between China and Germany.

Ronald Hetzer

Former Director of
the German Heart Center (Berlin)
December, 2017

主编简介
Introduction to editor-in-chief

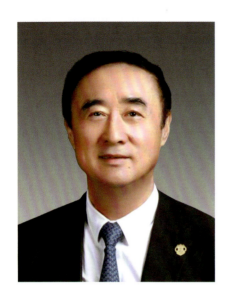

刘中民

主任医师、教授、博士研究生导师,教育部长江学者,俄罗斯工程院外籍院士,法国荣誉军团军官勋章获得者。

刘中民教授从事急危重症和心脏外科工作40余年。2000年初在国内率先开展"柏林人工心脏"和心肺移植治疗终末期心力衰竭的临床研究;同时坚持自主设计研发新型人工心脏,着力推动人工心脏的国产化。

近年来,针对心脏移植供体匮乏、移植后患者生活质量不够理想的现状,他率先进行干细胞治疗心力衰竭的临床研究,以推动心力衰竭治疗从"有创"到"微创",乃至"无创"的细胞治疗,并获得国家多种类、多途径、多项目的临床备案批准,也获得国家食品药品监督管理局细胞新药的转化和审批。

刘中民教授牵头建设心力衰竭专科和心脏外科2个上海市医学重点专科,获批上海市心力衰竭中心和上海人工心脏与心衰医学工程技术研究中心;承担国家高技术研究发展计划(863计划)和国家干细胞重大研发专项、国家自然科学基金等国家项目20余项。作为第一发明人,2项人工心脏发明专利技术获得授权并分别实施转让。作为第一完成人获国家科技进步奖二等奖1项、省部级奖5项、上海医学科技奖二等奖3项和中华医学科技奖二等奖1项,授权发明专利10多项(转移转化5项)。主编《实用心脏外科学》等专著13部,主编国家级规划教材2部,发表SCI论文83篇(影响因子408),他引1283次。被评为上海领军人才和上海市医学领军人才。

现任职务：

同济大学灾难医学工程研究院院长

同济大学附属东方医院终身教授、名誉院长

同济大学学术委员会和校务委员会委员

学术兼职：

中国医师协会心血管外科医师分会第五届会长

中华医学会灾难医学分会主任委员、创始主任委员

中华预防医学会灾难预防医学分会创始主任委员

世界灾难与急救医学会理事

亚太灾难医学协会副主席

中国整形美容协会副会长

中国干细胞产业联盟理事长

国家干细胞转化资源库临床级干细胞资源库负责人

中国整形美容协会干细胞研究与应用分会会长

中国中西医结合学会干细胞与再生医学专业委员会主任委员

中国医药生物技术协会再生医学专业委员会副主任委员

上海市医学会干细胞与再生医学分会创始主任委员

上海干细胞临床转化研究院院长

上海市干细胞临床诊疗工程研究中心主任

上海干细胞转化医学工程技术研究中心专家委员会主任委员

湖南湘江实验室副主任、智慧医疗与计算生物研究院院长

海南省干细胞工程中心主任

海南博鳌乐城先行区干细胞专家顾问委员会主任委员

国家级成果奖励：

国家科技进步奖二等奖

何梁何利基金科学与技术进步奖

光华工程科技奖

主编简介

Introduction to editor-in-chief

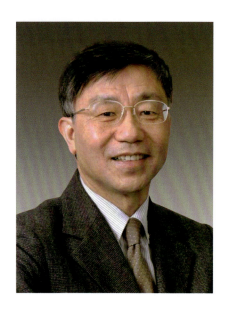

翁渝国

主任医师、教授、博士研究生导师。

翁渝国医生是世界上开展心脏辅助装置植入手术最多的心脏外科医生之一,也是世界上首先使用小儿心脏辅助装置的医生,给四百余位心力衰竭临终患者安装不同的心脏辅助装置,成功率达 80% 以上;在上海开展了亚洲第一例人工心脏手术;为一万余例患者做心内直视手术包括肺移植、心脏移植、心肺联合移植。曾应邀去剑桥大学附属医院,斯坦福大学附属医院,中国香港、澳门、台湾等地区医院进行疑难心脏病手术。

作为炎黄子孙翁渝国医生身居德国,心系祖国故土,关注中国心脏外科的学术进展;他经常回国参加学术会议,做学术报告,手术演示;和中国北京、上海、厦门、昆明、福州、青岛、镇江、台北等地的医院建立各种形式的合作关系,定期为国内数十家医院讲学示范手术义诊;为国内近千名心脏外科医生提供到柏林心脏中心进修学习的机会,现在这些医生都已成为当地医院的心胸外科主干力量。

学术兼职:

德国心胸血管外科协会会员,欧洲心胸血管外科协会会员;

Journal of Thoracic and Cardiovascular Surgery 审稿人,《中国心血管病研究》名誉主编;

先后聘为上海第二医科大学(现上海交通大学医学院)、同济大学附属东方医院、北京医科大学北京医院、广东省心血管研究所、福建医科大学、江苏理工大学、镇江医学院、宁波大学医学院、中山医科大学、第三军医大学、第四军医大学、兰州医学院、青岛医学院、暨南大学名誉教授；沈阳军区总院北方医院心脏外科顾问；中德心脏中心（北京）教授。

工作经历：

1964—1970　北京协和医学院医疗系求学；

1970—1978　陕西省人民医院普通外科、外科轮转住院医生及心胸血管外科主治医师；

1979—1981　考入中国医学科学院心血管研究所、中国协和医科大学研究生院，北京阜外医院心胸外科主治医师；

1982—1985　德国心脏中心（慕尼黑）心胸血管外科主治医生并攻读博士学位；

1985—1987　德国奥格斯堡中心医院心胸科副主任医生；

1987—2008　德国心脏中心（柏林）副院长，德国洪堡大学教授；

2008　洪堡大学终身教授，退休。

学术业绩：

1984 年起开展新生儿大动脉转位的根治手术（Switch），完成 400 余例；

1986 年起临床开展同种主动脉移植物手术，完成 600 余例；

1987 年起开展心脏移植，完成 1 300 余例；

1988 年成功开展主动脉弓部及胸腹主动脉瘤手术；

1989 年起开展肺移植及心肺联合移植，完成 300 余例；

1989 年起临床使用心脏辅助装置或人工心脏，柏林人工心脏，体外型；

1990 年开展背阔肌动力性心肌成形手术；

1991 年改良 Norwood 手术治疗新生儿左心发育不全综合征；

1992 年开展体内植入型心脏辅助装置（Novacor）技术，4 位患者已经带泵存活 4 年；

1993 年开展激光在冠心病外科上的使用；开展体内植入型心脏辅助装置（TCI）技术；为 1 位患者一次替换四个心脏瓣膜成功；

1994 年世界首次采用心脏辅助装置降低左心负荷治疗终末期扩张型心肌病成功；

1995 年为体重仅 1 600 克的早产儿成功进行完全肺静脉畸形引流心下型根治手术；

1997 年为患者做体外携带人工心脏手术，创造存活长达 4 年的世界纪录；

1998 年完成世界首例体内植入型轴流心脏辅助装置（De Bakey-VAD）；

1999 年开展机器人在心外科手术中的应用；

1999 年完成体内全植入型人工心脏，患者存活 3.5 年；

2001 年领导开发新型微型轴流泵 Incor I 的动物实验和临床试验成功，并获得欧洲共同体 CE 证书；

2002 年开始在临床上使用 Incor I，患者最长健康生活已经超过 2 年；

2003 年开始第三代心脏辅助装置 Dura Heart 的临床试验；

2004 年临床应用全人工心脏（CardioWest）；开始干细胞临床使用治疗终末期心力衰竭。

主编简介

Introduction to editor-in-chief

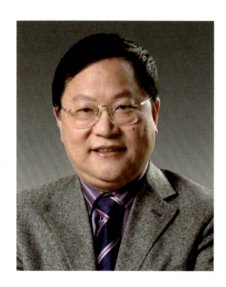

刘锦纷

小儿心胸外科专家、教授、主任医师、博士生导师,1993 起享受国务院政府特殊津贴。

从事小儿先天性心脏病、小儿胸外科疾病的一线临床工作 50 年,主刀各种先天性心脏病、胸外科手术超过 6 000 余例,其中复杂手术超过 80%;为新生儿复杂先天性心脏病外科、功能性单心室、三尖瓣下移畸形锥形重建、先天性肺发育畸形、儿童纵膈肿瘤及漏斗胸治疗领域权威。

职务:

曾任新华医院副院长、上海儿童医学中心院长,现任上海市小儿先天性心脏病研究所名誉所长,国家心血管病专家委员会先天性心脏病专业委员会顾问。

学术兼职:

中华医学会小儿外科学分会第六、第七届心胸外科学组组长,卫生部新型农村合作医疗先天性心脏病项目专家组成员。

2008 年成为美国胸外科协会会员、2010 年起任世界小儿心脏外科协会管理委员会委员和 *World Journal for Pediatric and Congenital Heart Surgery* 杂志副主编。主译《小儿心脏外科学》《先天性心脏病外科综合治疗学》《先天性心脏病临床治疗:从婴儿期到成年期》等专著。以通讯作者和第一作者发表 SCI 收录文章 40 余篇,负责和完成国家自然科学基金面上项目、973 计划项目子课题等国家重要基金 6 项。

获奖：

曾获得"宋庆龄儿科医学奖"、"宋庆龄樟树奖"、国家科技进步奖二等奖、教育部科技进步奖二等奖、中华医学科技奖三等奖、上海市先进工作者、上海医学发展"特殊贡献奖"、上海市科技进步奖一等奖和上海医学科技进步奖三等奖等奖项。

序
Preface

我国婴幼儿心血管外科起步相对较晚，直到 20 世纪 70 年代，我们通过自主研发小儿人工心肺机等儿童专用器械设备，开始了婴幼儿先天性心脏病的手术治疗。但近二十年，随着我们对外交流增加，走出去，请进来，这一领域发生了翻天覆地的变化。无论数量、质量，还是疑难复杂程度，心脏外科手术都有了很大的进步，手术死亡率明显下降。更可喜的是年轻一代技术骨干力量正在快速成长。

据中华医学会胸心血管外科学分会统计，我国能开展先天性心脏病外科手术的单位多达七百余家，但水平参差不齐，治疗效果差别很大。提供一本高质量的婴幼儿心脏外科手术图解，给临床一线工作的专业人员参考学习，显得十分必要。先天性心脏病种类繁多，解剖结构复杂，特别是一些疑难复杂病例手术难度较高。有时仅靠文字描述很难表达清楚，而一本好的手术图解却能收到事半功倍的效果！

China's cardiovascular surgery for infants and young children started relatively late. It was not until the 1970s that pediatric congenital heart surgeries were performed using China's self-developed artificial heart-lung machines and other specialized equipment for children. However, in the last two decades, with the increase of international exchanges and the implementation of the "Bring In and Go Out" policy, there were witnessed dramatic changes in the field. Great progress has been made in cardiac surgery, not only in difficulty and complexity but also in quantity and quality, with surgical mortality rates decreasing significantly. Even more gratifying is the rapid growth among the young generation of technical backbones.

Statistics from the Chinese Society for Thoracic and Cardiovascular Surgery show that over 700 hospitals or centers can provide congenital heart surgery in our country. However, the treatment effects may vary considerably due to the uneven operational levels. Therefore, those front-line medical professionals are in great need of a high-quality atlas of pediatric cardiac surgery for study and consultation. With so many kinds of congenital heart disease and the complex anatomical structure of heart, especially some very difficult and complex surgeries, words alone are not always able to express the idea clearly, but a good surgical atlas can achieve twice the result with half the effort !

本图解编写者都是长期从事先天性心脏病外科工作的临床医生，具有较丰富的临床手术经验。他们以先天性心脏病解剖特征为切入点，详细描述手术步骤、操作要点及注意事项。本书以手绘图片为主，配有文字说明，力求做到图文并茂、简明易学。此外，本书还配有英文翻译，提供给年轻医生学习参考，特别是便于对英文参考书的学习理解。同时为我们打开国门，走向世界，向共建"一带一路"国家推广学习。

本图解基本涵盖先天性心脏病的所有手术。每章先介绍疾病的解剖类型，再详细描述多种手术方法。我相信本书对临床一线的心血管专业人员会有很大的学习参考价值。期待中国的小儿心血管外科事业百尺竿头，更进一步。特作此序，以飨读者！

2024 年 2 月

All of the authors of this atlas are congenital cardiac surgeons with extensive clinical operations experience. By starting with the anatomical characteristics of congenital heart disease, the atlas describes the specific steps, key points, and precautions of the operation in detail. Characterized by plentiful illustrations supplemented with text descriptions, the hand-drawn pictures strives to be concise and easy to study. In addition, by being equipped with the English version, the atlas can serve as a reference book for young doctors to help them learn and understand professional English books. At the same time, the bilingual atlas will open the door for global access, sharing the experiences of pediatric cardiac surgery with Belt and Road Initiative(BRI) countries.

This atlas basically covers all the surgical problems of congenital heart disease. Each chapter begins with an introduction to the anatomy of the disease, followed by a detailed description of various surgical approaches. I believe that the atlas is of great value for all cardiovascular professionals on the clinical frontline. I hope Chinese pediatric cardiovascular surgery may continue to make further progress. This preface is specially written for readers !

Ding Wenxiang

February, 2024

前言
Foreword

翁渝国医生是享誉世界的华人心脏外科医生。20 世纪 80 年代，时任汉诺威心脏中心院长的 Ronald Hetzer 教授盛邀他一同创立德国心脏中心（柏林），从此开辟了德国乃至欧洲心脏大血管外科的一个崭新时代。他是世界上少有的个人手术过万例的医生，被德国媒体誉为"拥有一双金手的医生"；也是被德国政府规定不能同时离开德国的三个医生之一；他有很多个"世界第一"，看过他手术的人无不为他的精湛技艺所折服，所谓"化繁为简""出神入化""化腐朽为神奇"，在他的手里体现得淋漓尽致！除了高超的医术，他为人极其谦和、热情，为中国培养了一千余名心脏外科医生和心肺转流术灌注师、护理人员等。很多医生如今已经成为中国心脏外科领域的大家，他为中国心血管事业的发展作出了不可磨灭的贡献。

Dr. Weng Yuguo, a world-renowned Chinese cardiologist, co-founded the German Heart Institute in Berlin at the invitation of Professor Roland Hatzer, the then Director at Hanover Heart Center, in the 1980s, ushering in a new era for cardiac vascular surgery in Germany, and even the whole of Europe. He was acclaimed by the German media as "Der Arzt mit den goldenen Händens" (the doctor with golden hands), for he was one of the few doctors worldwide to have personally performed more than 10 000 surgeries. He was also one of three doctors who were prohibited by the German government from leaving Germany simultaneously. He developed many of the world's firsts, and those who observed his operations were deeply impressed by his superb surgical skills. These skills are worthy of the praise they have received, which is the so-called "simplifying the complex" "reaching the acme of perfection" and "turning the bad into good". Despite his achievements, he was very modest and enthusiastic to help others. He trained more than 1 000 cardiac surgeons, cardiopulmonary bypass perfusionists, and nurses for his country. Most of these trainees have become masters in the field in China. He has truly made indelible contributions to the development of Chinese cardiovascular research and practice！

我与翁医生的相识是在 20 世纪 90 年代初期,当时我还在仁济医院任心胸外科副主任,翁医生指导我完成了心脏外科生涯的第一例搭桥手术。从那之后,我们可谓亦师亦友。1998 年春节刚过,我第一次前往柏林进修学习,翁医生夫妇亲自开车到泰格尔机场接机。那年冬天也是少有的寒冷,到处冰天雪地,虽然我从上海出发时做了充足的准备,仍然无法抵挡柏林的严寒。翁医生看在眼里,第二天就让他的夫人陈家大姐送来了又厚又暖的皮夹克,这种他乡雪中送炭的温暖至今还铭刻在我的心里。

在柏林学习期间,翁医生在生活上无微不至地关心我和每一个到柏林学习的中国医护人员。考虑到很多人初到柏林,人生地不熟,他常常利用手术的间隙亲自驾车去机场接机。在手术技巧上,他不厌其烦、细心讲解、耐心带教,总是能把复杂的手术变得很简单,把危重的患者处理得很安全,德国的医生和护士都喜欢跟他上台。也正是由于翁医生的言传身教,使我(还包括很多先后去柏林的中国医生)在很短时间里,就学习和掌握了当时在国内看不到的病例和没有的技术,例如极低体重(不到 500g)早产儿先天性心脏病的手术、多种品牌人工心脏的植入和心肺联合移植等,当然还有现代化医院的建设和管理。为了把德国心脏中心(柏林)的信息系统复制回来,我专门买了一台笔记本

It was in the early 1990s that I became acquainted with Dr. Weng. At that time, I was the deputy director of cardiothoracic surgery at Renji Hospital. Under Dr. Weng's instruction, I completed my first bypass surgery as a cardiac surgeon. Since then, he has become my teacher and friend. Just after the Lunar New Year in 1998, I went to Berlin for the first time for further study, and Dr. Weng and his wife drove to Tegel Airport to pick me up. It was, indeed, an extremely cold winter, with everything covered in heavy snow, and I could not still almost cope with the bitter cold here in Berlin, albeit full preparations before my departure from Shanghai. His wife brought a warm leather jacket on the second day. That is still in my mind today.

During my study in Berlin, Dr. Weng took meticulous care of me, as well as every Chinese medical staff member at the Center. Considering that many of us were new to Berlin and had no friends, he would often take advantage of any spare moment, even a break between surgeries, to pick us up at the airport. When conveying instructions, he would go to great lengths to explain every surgical technique and patiently demonstrate them. He could always simplify complicated operations and handle critically ill patients safely. Therefore, doctors and nurses in Germany all enjoyed working with him in the surgical theater. Dr. Weng's clear explanations and operation demonstrations enabled me (as well as many Chinese doctors who went to the Center) to quickly understand the cases unseen and master the techniques unavailable in China at that time, such as surgery for premature congenital heart disease infants weighing less

电脑，翁医生帮我和分管院长打招呼，破例让我全部下载，使上海市东方医院的信息系统在国内较早地与国际接轨。由于有翁医生的穿针引线和积极推动，上海市东方医院成为国内第一个中德合作医院，时任德国心脏中心(柏林)院长 Hetzer 教授 2000 年 5 月第一次到上海，看到浦东的发展深有感触地说："我们来得太晚了！"自此之后的 20 年间，由于翁医生的辛勤耕耘和精心呵护，上海市东方医院和德国心脏中心(柏林)的合作都被双方政府称为中德合作的典范。我也送了很多年轻医生、护士和学生前往柏林学习，他们在翁医生的指导下如今也都成为了业务骨干。

早在柏林学习期间，我和翁医生就在探讨如何把翁医生自己的手术经验通过图解的形式出版，让更多热爱心脏外科专业的医生学习。开始先是采用线条图的方式，但是很难体现翁医生的手术精髓。后来又采用先进的计算机绘图技术，翁医生仍然不满意，因为计算机操作人员难以理解翁医生手术的原

than 500 g, the implantation of various brands of artificial hearts, combined heart-lung transplantations, and the construction and management of modern hospitals. I specially bought a laptop to copy the information system used by the German Heart Center. Dr. Weng communicated with the director in charge, who finally made an exception for me to download the system so that the information system at Shanghai East Hospital, where I worked, could be in line with international standards early on. Thanks to Dr. Weng's communication and promotion, Shanghai East Hospital became the first Sino-German cooperative hospital in China. Later, when Professor Hetzer, the then director of the German Heart Center (Berlin), visited Shanghai for the first time in May 2000, he was deeply impressed by the development of Pudong and sighed that they came too late. In the two decades since then, through Dr. Weng's efforts, the cooperation between Shanghai East Hospital and the German Heart Center (Berlin) has been regarded as a model of Sino-German cooperation by both governments. I also sent many young doctors, nurses, and students to study in Berlin. Thanks to Dr. Weng's guidance, they are now the backbones of this field.

As early as when I was studying in Berlin, Dr. Weng and I had discussed sharing his personal surgical experiences in the form of a medical atlas to allow more cardiac surgeons to learn from him. Unfortunately, the line drawings used previously could not reflect the essence of Dr. Weng's surgery. Although advanced computer graphics technology was later adopted, Dr. Weng was still unsatisfied because the computer operators could not understand the

创性，不能把翁医生的手术理念和操作要点原汁原味地传授给年轻医生。最后，我在国内专门请了一位人体解剖绘图专家朱女士并送到德国，全程陪同翁医生，按照翁医生画的每一个手术步骤的草图，一边理解一边画图，这一待就是六年。2008年翁医生患病，我前往柏林看望，那个时候他已经决定放下手术刀，全身心投入书稿的撰写和绘图当中，书中的每一幅图稿从翁医生手绘起稿、画师修稿，到最后定稿、上色都要经过一遍遍打磨，直到能完全反映翁医生的手术技巧和思路。我们俩也经常就图稿细节讨论到深夜。可以说每一幅图解都是翁医生一生学术的总结和经验的凝练，都反映了他对心血管外科的热爱和对患者的负责。

2015年翁医生的身体状况变差了，我把他从德国接回来，住在上海市东方医院里，一是方便照顾他的健康，二是方便我们讨论书稿，住院期间他仍然绘图到深夜，不过我们的讨论倒是方便了很多，不用再通过邮件或者越洋电话了。那时，我有一个想法，就是把这套图谱命名为《翁渝国心脏外科手术图谱》，但他婉言拒绝，理由是这里面除了他本人的经验和创新，还有德国同事的配合，以及前人的经验教训，所以还是通俗一点，就定位在"心脏外科手术图解"。全书初稿共有

originality of the surgeries, and the graphics could not accurately impart his surgical concepts and operations. Finally, Ms. Zhu, a Chinese specialist in human anatomy illustration, was invited to come over here with these drawings and cooperated with Dr. Weng in Germany. She studied and made sense of all the sketches of the surgical operation procedures by Dr. Weng throughout the following six years. In 2008, when Dr. Weng became ill, I went to Berlin to visit him. At that time, he decided to stop performing any more surgery and devote himself to the writing and drawing of the atlas. Each illustration in the book was hand-painted by Dr. Weng, revised by Ms. Zhu, and finally finalized and colored. Each illustration has been polished over and over until it fully reflects the essence of Dr. Weng's surgery. Dr. Weng and I often discussed the details of the atlas late into the night. It can be said that each illustration is a summary of Dr. Weng's lifelong academic experience, reflecting his passion for cardiovascular surgery and his responsibility to patients.

In 2015, Dr. Weng's health deteriorated. I invited him to return from Germany and hospitalized him at Shanghai East Hospital, which made it convenient for me to care for him and discuss the atlas simultaneously. During his hospitalization, he continued to draw illustrations late into the night, but we were finally able to communicate face-to-face rather than through emails or overseas phone calls. I had suggested the book be titled *Weng Yuguo Cardiac Surgery Atlas*, but he politely refused my proposal. He explained that in addition to his own experiences and innovations, there were also contributions from German colleagues and pre-

手绘彩图 2 000 余幅,均为原创,汇聚了翁医生毕生的心血。2017 年 5 月,翁医生弥留之际,拉着我的手做了最后的嘱托,希望这本图解能够早日出版,供更多的心脏外科医生、医学生、公众学习、参考、科普。2017 年 6 月 26 日 13 时 48 分,我的良师挚友翁渝国医生仙逝,我和翁医生的家人一起陪伴他走完了最后一程。追悼会上,翁医生的同学、同事、学生 500 多人前来送行,斯人虽逝,往事如烟,历历在目,潸然泪下。为了完成翁医生的遗愿,在他走后的几年里,我又邀请刘锦纷教授、李颖则教授共同完善本图解的撰写,并按翁医生的要求将图解分为小儿和成人两册,分别恭请丁文祥教授和胡盛寿院士作序。出于对翁医生的了解和尊敬,两位心脏外科大家欣然命笔,为本书出版增添了浓墨重彩,在此表示衷心感谢!经人民卫生出版社慎重批准,将本书分为《成人心脏外科名家手术手绘图解》和《小儿心脏外科名家手术手绘图解》两册,按中英文对照形式出版,以此告慰翁医生在天之灵。也希望更多的年轻医生从中感悟到心脏外科的深奥和技巧,收获更多前人的经验和爱心。

decessors, so *Atlas of Cardiac Surgery* was a more appropriate title. The book boasts more than 2 000 original hand-drawn color illustrations, all of which embody Dr. Weng's lifelong efforts. In May 2017, shortly before Dr. Weng passed away, he took my hand and made a final request. He hoped that this atlas could be published quickly for cardiac surgeons, medical students, and public learning and reference. At 13: 48 on 26th, June, 2017, Dr. Weng Yuguo, my close teacher and friend, passed away. Dr. Weng's family and I accompanied him on his last journey. At the memorial service, more than 500 of Dr. Weng's classmates, colleagues, and students came to see him off. Although Dr. Weng passed away, my memories of him are still vivid and make me shed tears unconsciously. To realize Dr. Weng's unfinished wish, I worked hard over the following years with Professor Liu Jinfen and Professor Li Yingze on improving the collection of drawings, which, at the request of Dr. Weng, is classified into two volumes: Children and Adults. I have invited Professor Ding Wenxiang and the Chinese Academy of Engineering (CAE) Academician Hu Shengshou to write prefaces for these two volumes. Out of understanding and respect for Dr. Weng, these two masters of cardiac surgery agreed without hesitation to write the prefaces, adding luster to the publication of this book. I would like to express my heartfelt thanks to them here. After careful consideration, the People's Medical Publishing House has approved the publication of this book in both Chinese and English, and it is divided into two volumes: *Hand-drawn Atlas of Master Cardiac Surgery in Adults* and *Hand-drawn Atlas of Master Cardiac Surgery in Children*. It is hoped that the publication of the book will comfort Dr. Weng in heaven and that more young doctors will realize the profoundness of cardiac surgery skills and gain more experience and compassion from their predecessors.

刘中民

中国医师协会心血管外科
医师分会会长
俄罗斯工程院外籍院士
上海市东方医院 / 同济大学
附属东方医院名誉院长
2024 年 2 月

Dr. Liu Zhongmin

President of Cardiovascular Surgeon Branch, Chinese Medical Doctor Association

Foreign Academician of Russian Academy of Engineering

Honorary President of Shanghai East Hospital/ East Hospital Affiliated to Tongji University

February, 2024

Contents

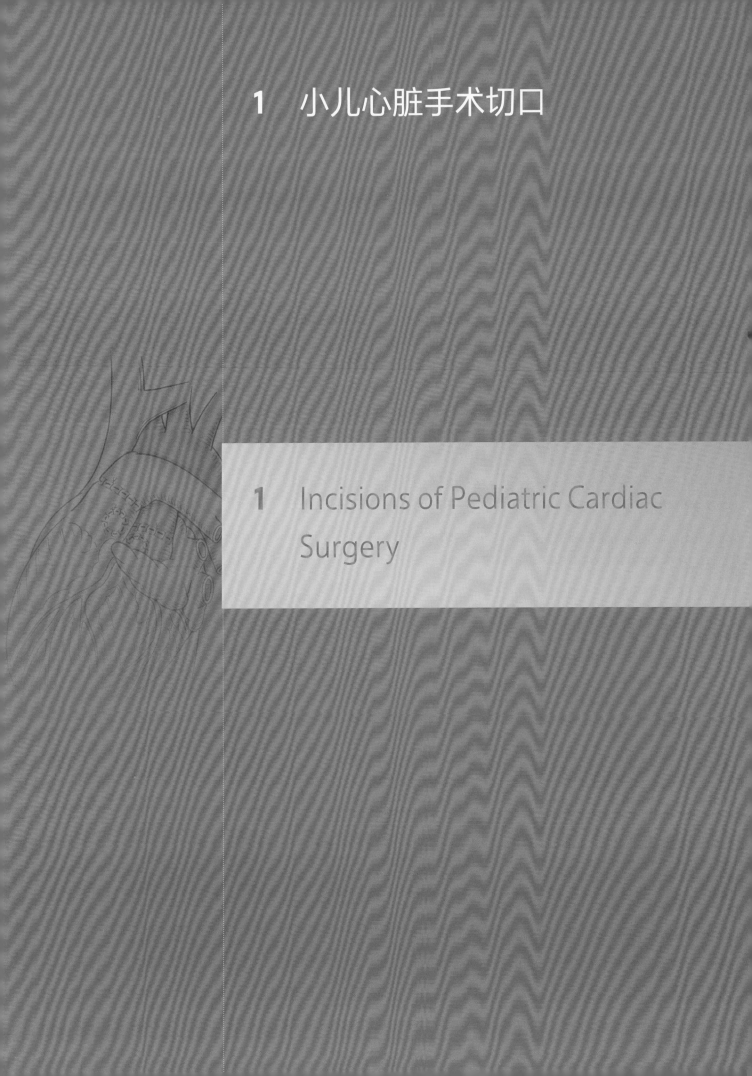

1 小儿心脏手术切口

1 Incisions of Pediatric Cardiac Surgery

一、胸骨正中切口　I. Median Sternotomy

这是儿童先天性心脏病最常选用的手术切口,其优点是解剖暴露清晰,操作容易,尤其对新生儿和小婴儿(图 1-1)。

This is the most common surgical incision for congenital heart disease in children, which has the advantage of clear anatomical exposure and easy manipulation, especially in newborns and infants (Figure 1-1).

图 1-1　胸骨正中切口
A. 患儿平卧,胸骨正中切口,切除部分剑突,分离胸骨后。
B、C. 电锯锯开胸骨。

Figure 1-1　Median sternotomy
A. With the child lying supine, part of the xiphoid process is resected, and the sternum is separated via a median sternal incision.
B, C. Cut through the sternum with a sternal saw.

Continued

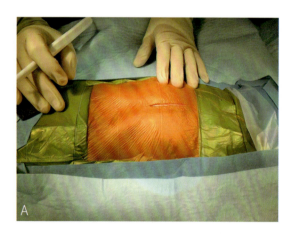

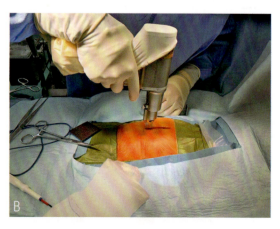

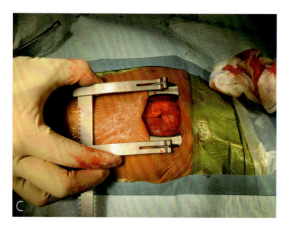

图 1-1（续）

D. 必要时去除部分胸腺组织,特别是做大动脉手术,如主动脉弓中断、大动脉错位等。

E、F. 剪开心包,取下部分心包组织用0.6% 浓度的戊二醛固定备用,将心包悬吊固定。

Figure 1-1 cont'd

D. If necessary, remove some thymic tissue, especially in surgeries of great arteries such as for interruption of aortic arch, malposition of great arteries.

E, F. Cut the pericardium open, remove part of the pericardial tissue and fix it with 0. 6% glutaraldehyde for later use. Suspend the pericardium and fix it.

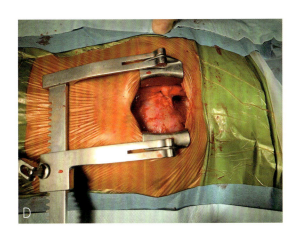

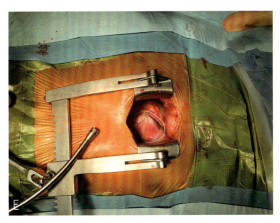

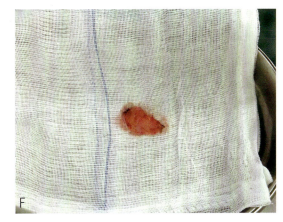

二、右侧腋下切口

II. Right Vertical Infra-axillary Thoracotomy

这是目前开展侧切口微创手术常选用的切口。这类切口手术仅适用于相对简单的体外循环手术患者，如房间隔缺损（atrial septal defect, ASD）、室间隔缺损（ventricular septal defect, VSD）等（图 1-2）。

The incision is commonly used for lateral mini-incision surgery. This type of incision is only used in patients undergoing relatively simple extracorporeal circulation procedures, such as those for atrial septal defect (ASD), ventricular septal defect (VSD)(Figure 1-2).

图 1-2　右侧腋中线切口
A. 患儿左侧卧位，右腋中线切口。
B. 一个胸骨撑开器撑开，经第 4 肋间进胸。
C. 切开心包，并将之悬吊固定。

Figure 1-2　Right vertical infra-axillary thoracotomy
A. With the child in the left lateral decubitus position, a right vertical infra-axillary incision is made.
B. A rib spreader is used to open the chest, and the heart is accessed through the fourth intercostal space.
C. Cut the pericardium open, and then suspend and fix it.

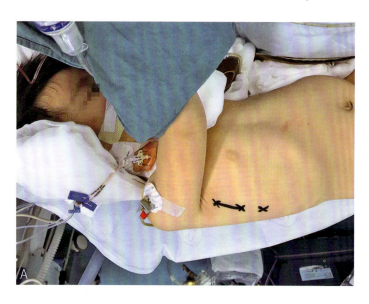

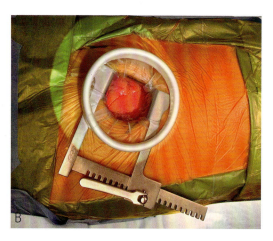
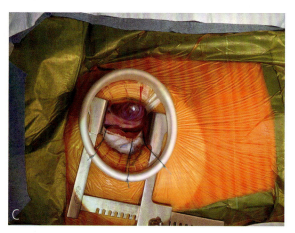

三、左后外侧切口

III. Left Posterolateral Thoracotomy

这类切口主要适用于动脉导管未闭（patent ductus arteriosus，PDA）、单纯型主动脉缩窄、双主动脉弓、血管环等血管畸形（图1-3）。

This type of incision is mainly used in surgeries for vascular malformations such as patent ductus arteriosus (PDA), simple coarctation of the aorta, double aortic arch, vascular ring (Figure 1-3).

图1-3 左后外侧切口
A. 患儿右侧卧位，与乳头平行做弧形切口，在肩胛骨下方向脊柱中间向上延伸。

Figure 1-3 Left posterolateral thoracotomy
A. With the child in the right lateral decubitus position, an arcuate incision is made parallel to the nipple and extended upward from below the scapula toward the middle of the vertebral column.

Continued

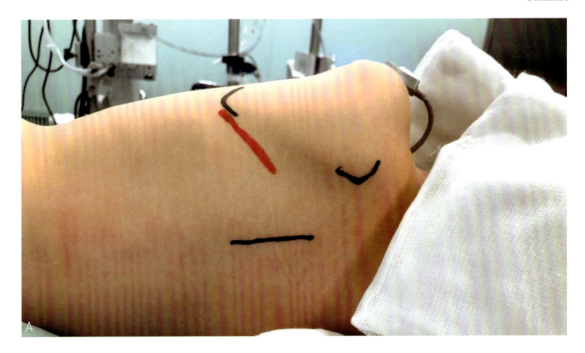

图 1-3（续）

B. 切断部分背阔肌，经第 3 肋间进胸，大多在心包外操作。

Figure 1-3 cont'd

B. The heart is accessed through the third intercostal space after part of the latissimus dorsi muscle is severed. The operation is mostly done outside the pericardium.

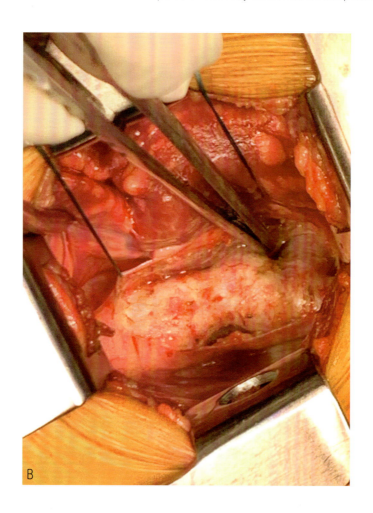

四、二期胸骨开胸手术

IV. Secondary Sternal Thoracotomy

随着手术复杂程度的提高,二期开胸手术患者十分普遍,关键技术是谨慎分离胸骨后粘连,防止出血(图 1-4)。

With the increased complexity of the surgery, the patients undergoing second-stage thoracotomy are common. The key technique is to separate the retrosternal adhesions carefully to prevent bleeding (Figure 1-4).

图 1-4 **二期胸骨开胸手术**
A. 胸骨正中原切口进胸。

Figure 1-4 Secondary sternal thoracotomy
A. Access the heart through the original median sternal incision.

Continued

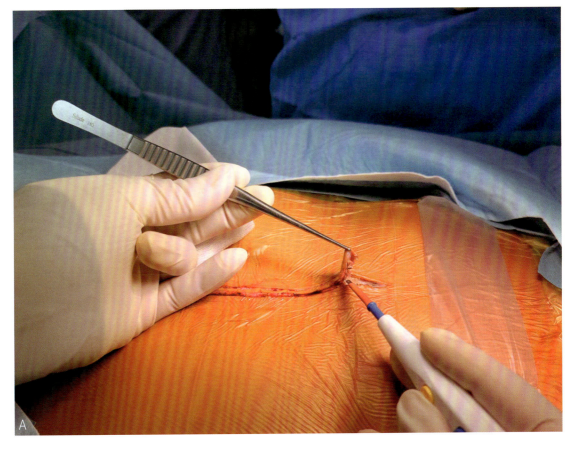

图 1-4（续）

B. 从胸骨下端用两把带齿拉钩上提，逐
步分离胸骨后粘连组织，再用摆锯逐步
锯开胸骨。对胸骨后粘连严重的患者，
则可采用股动、静脉插管，先建立体外
循环。

Figure 1-4 cont'd

B. The retrosternal adhesive tissue was gradually separated from the sternum by lifting up from the lower end of the sternum with two toothed pulling hooks. The sternum is then gradually opened with a pendulum saw. For patients with severe retrosternal adhesions, femoral artery and vein cannulation can be used to establish extracorporeal circulation first.

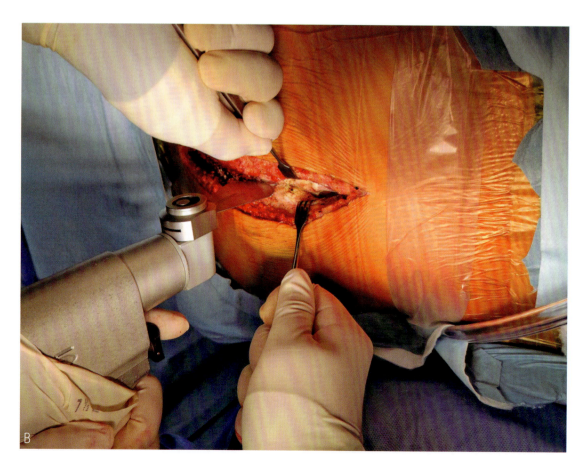

五、胸腔切口或胸骨切口关胸

V. Chest Closure for Thoracotomy or Sternotomy

仔细检查无出血点,患儿生命体征平稳,则常规关胸(图 1-5)。

After careful examination, if there is no bleeding and the patient's vital signs are stable, the chest is closed routinely (Figure 1-5).

图 1-5　胸腔切口或胸骨切口关胸
A. 儿童胸腔切口可用 2-0 可吸收线,经肋骨上缘直接缝合 2~3 针,拉拢即可。

Figure 1-5　The chest closure for thoracotomy or sternotomy
A. A thoracic incision in children can be pulled together after 2-3 stitches through the upper rib edge with 2-0 absorbable sutures.

Continued

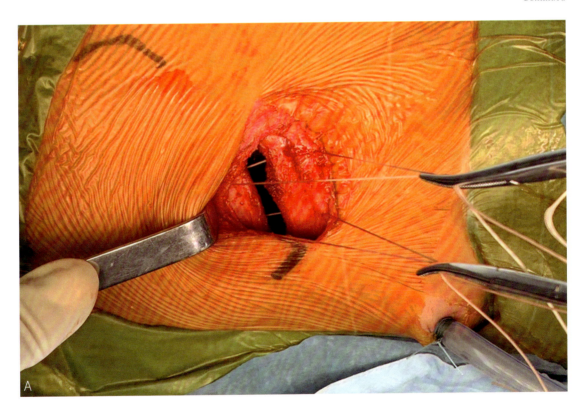

图 1-5（续）

Figure 1-5 cont'd

B. 胸骨正中切口采用 2-0 可吸收线连续缝合,最后打结,将线结埋在胸骨深部,避免凸起影响伤口愈合。

C. 取 3-0、4-0 薇乔缝线,缝合胸骨上肌肉及皮下组织。

B. A median sternal incision can be continuously sutured with 2-0 absorbable sutures and finally tied with a knot. The knot should be buried deeply in the sternum to avoid protuberance affecting wound healing.

C. 3-0 and 4-0 Vicryl sutures are used to suture the suprasternal muscles and subcutaneous tissues of the sternum.

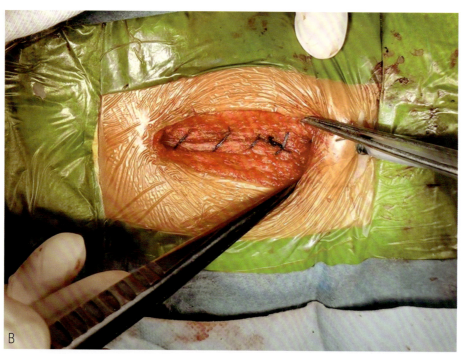

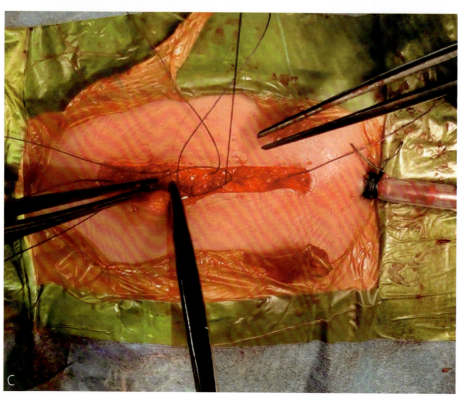

图 1-5（续）

D. 可吸收线皮内缝合皮肤。

Figure 1-5 cont'd

D. Intradermal suturing of the skin with absorbable sutures.

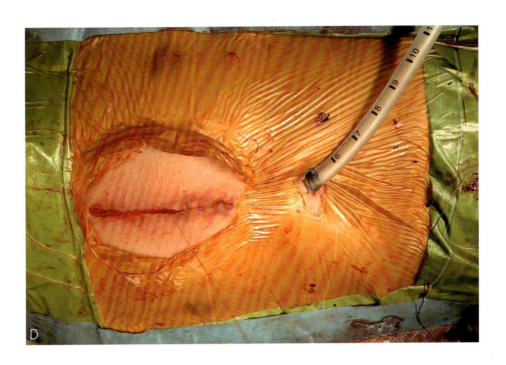

六、延迟关胸

VI. Delayed Chest Closure

新生儿及小婴儿复杂心内畸形矫治后,特别是行体外膜肺氧合(extracorporeal membrane oxygenation,ECMO)的患者常需延迟关胸(图1-6)。

Delayed chest closure is often required after treatment of complex intracardiac malformations in neonates and infants, especially in patients with extracorporeal membrane oxygenation (ECMO) circuit (Figure 1-6).

图1-6 延迟关胸

A. 手术结束后,取一段塑料管道或5ml注射器管,剪成一临时的胸骨撑开装置,将胸骨撑开。

Figure 1-6 Delayed chest closure

A. After the operation, take a piece of plastic tubing or 5ml syringe tube and cut it into a temporary sternal support device to hold the sternum open.

Continued

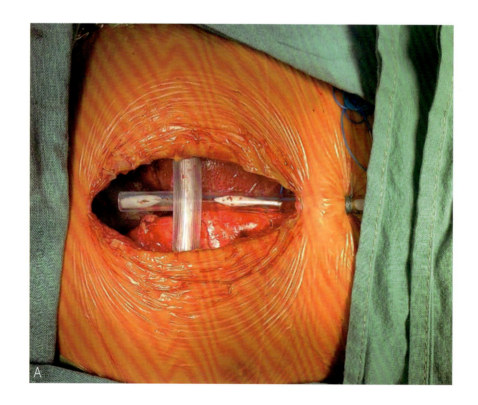

图 1-6（续）

B. 取人工薄膜（通常选用外科手套）剪成相应大小，将皮肤关闭。2~3 天患者状态平稳后，将支撑材料取出。胸骨按常规关闭。

图 1-6 cont'd

B. Cut a piece of artificial membrane (usually surgical gloves) to the appropriate size to close the skin. Remove the support device after 2-3 days when the patient's status is stable. The sternum is closed with the routine procedure.

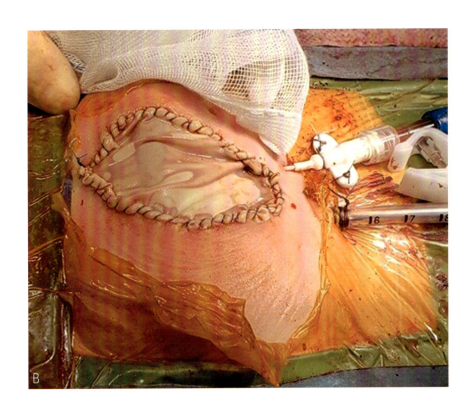

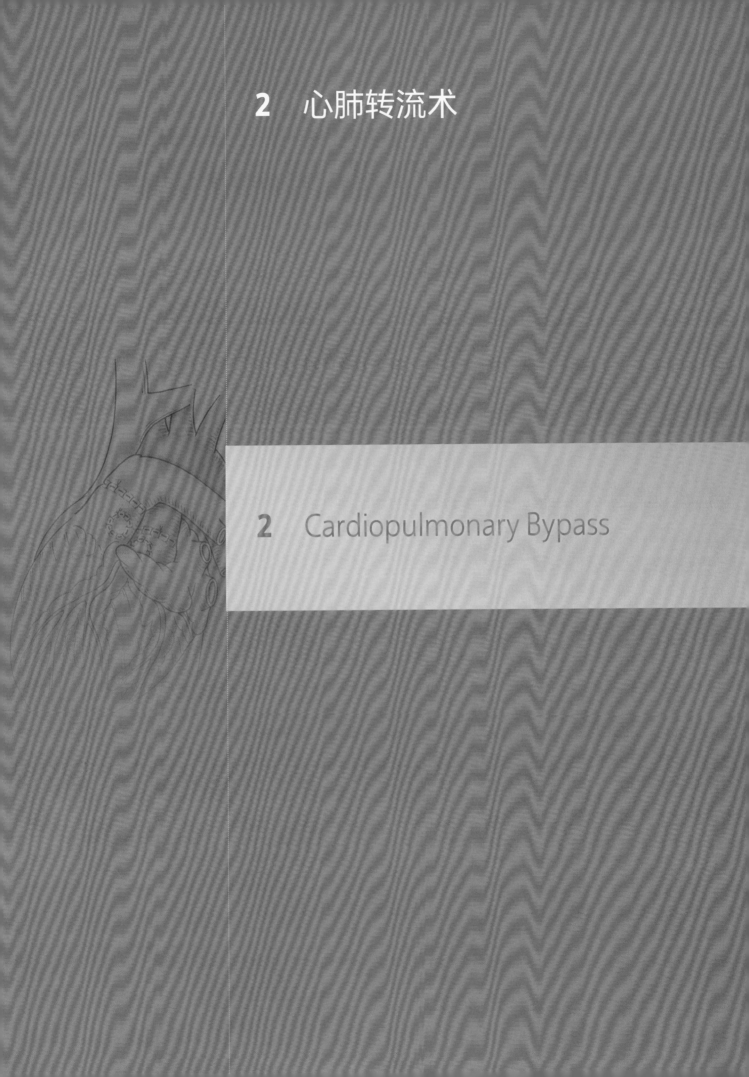

2 心肺转流术

2 Cardiopulmonary Bypass

心肺转流术（cardiopulmonary bypass，CPB）是儿童心脏手术中重要一环。婴幼儿人工心肺机与成人不同，要求管道细，预充容量要小，对血液有形成分破坏更轻。正确的技术方法和合理选择各种氧合器及插管对提高手术成功率、减少并发症十分重要。

Cardiopulmonary bypass (CPB) is an important step in pediatric cardiac surgery. Different from those for adults, the heart-lung machine for infants and young children requires thinner tubing and lower priming volume; hence, it can bring less damage to the formed element of the blood. Therefore, appropriate application of the technique and proper selection of the oxygenators and cannulae can improve the success rate of surgery and reduce its complications.

一、氧合器选择

I. Selection of Oxygenator

儿童心脏手术大多选用膜式氧合器。儿童常用氧合器规格见下表。根据体重选择不同种类氧合器（表2-1）。

In pediatric cardiac surgery, membrane oxygenators are the most common choice. The general specifications of oxygenators for children are shown in the table below. The oxygenators are selected based on the body weight (Table 2-1).

表 2-1　患儿体重与相应氧合器型号
Table 2-1　Patient weight and corresponding oxygenator types

体重 /kg Weight/kg	氧合器型号 Oxygenator types
<5	Terumo Fx05，Dideco Kids 100 等 Terumo Fx05，Dideco Kids100，etc.
5~20	Terumo Fx05，Medtronic Affinity Pixie 等 Terumo Fx05，Medtronic Affinity Pixie，etc.
20~25	Dideco Kids101 等 Dideco Kids 101 etc.
25~60	Terumo Fx15 Terumo Fx15
>60	Terumo Fx25 Terumo Fx25

二、动脉插管　　II. Arterial Cannulae

儿童选择动脉插管一般原则（表 2-2，图 2-1）。

General principles of selecting arterial cannulae for children (Table 2-2, Figure 2-1).

表 2-2　儿童选择动脉插管一般原则

Table 2-2　General principles of selecting arterial cannulae for children

体重 /kg Weight/kg	插管尺寸 /Fr Cannula size/Fr
<5	8
5~10	10
10~15	12
15~30	14
>30	16~18

图 2-1　动脉插管
A. 进口动脉插管。

Figure 2-1　Arterial cannulae
A. Imported arterial cannulae.

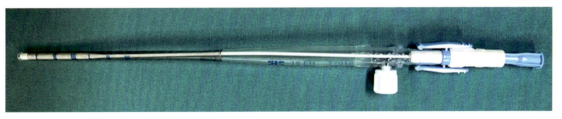
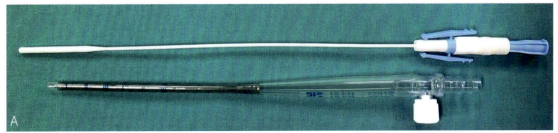

Continued

图 2-1（续）

Figure 2-1 cont'd

B. 不同规格国产动脉插管。

B. Domestic arterial cannulae in different sizes.

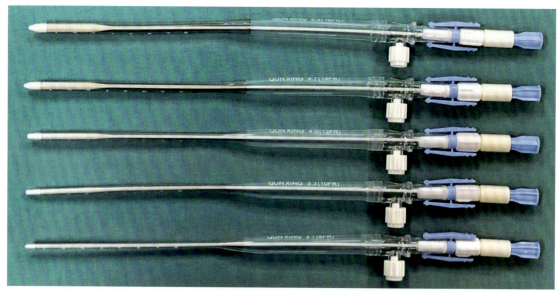

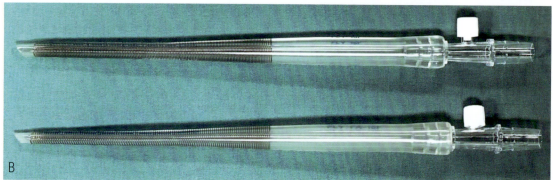

三、静脉插管

Ⅲ. Venous Cannulae

儿童选择静脉插管一般原则（表 2-3，图 2-2）。

General principles of selecting venous cannulae for children (Table 2-3, Figure 2-2).

表 2-3　儿童选择静脉插管一般原则

Table 2-3　General principles of selecting venous cannulae for children

| 体重 /kg | 插管尺寸 /Fr | |
| | Cannula size/Fr | |
Weight/kg	上腔静脉 Superior vena cava	下腔静脉 Inferior vena cava
<3	12	14
<5	14	16
5~10	16	18
10~15	18	20
15~20	20	22
20~30	22	24
>30	26	28

图 2-2　静脉插管

A. 普通静脉插管。

B. 静脉直角插管。

Figure 2-2　Venous cannulae

A. Common venous cannulae.

B. Right angle venous cannulae.

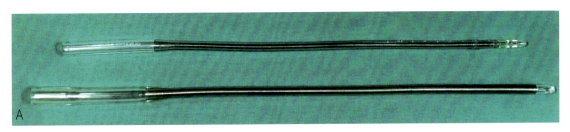

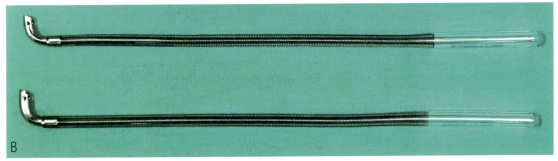

四、左心引流管

术中为避免左心室过胀导致心肌和肺的损伤,通常在主动脉血流阻断后要放置左心引流管。放置位置有两处:①在右上肺静脉和左心房连接处做荷包放置左心引流装置(图 2-3A);②可通过右心房切口,经卵圆孔和房间隔小切口放置(图 2-3B)。常见左心引流管如图(图 2-3C、图 2-3D)。

IV. Left Heart drainage Tube

To avoid myocardial and pulmonary injury by left ventricular overdistension during surgery, a left heart drainage tube is usually placed after aortic occlusion. There are two ways to place it: ① A drainage device is placed at the junction between the right superior pulmonary vein and the left atrium by purse-string suture (Figure 2-3A); ② it can also be placed via a right atrial incision and directed across a foramen ovale and a small incision of the atrial septum (Figure 2-3B). The common left heart drainage tubes are shown in the following figure (Figure 2-3C, Figure 2-3D).

图 2-3　左心引流管

A. 右上肺静脉和左心房连接处做荷包放置左心引流装置。

Figure 2-3　Left heart drainage tube

A. Drainage device was placed at the junction between right superior pulmonary vein and left atrium.

Continued

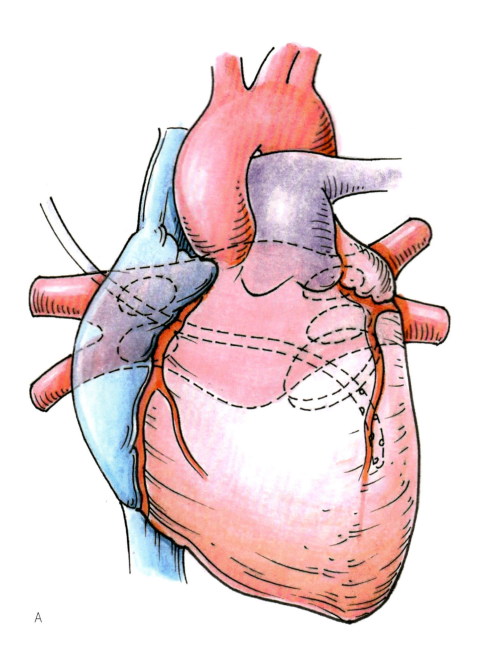

A

图 2-3（续）

B. 经卵圆孔或房间隔小切口放置。

C. 塑料左心引流管。

D. 带弹簧头的左心引流管。

Figure 2-3 cont'd

B. Drainage device placed across a foramen ovale or a small incision of the atrial septum.

C. Plastic left heart drainage tubes.

D. Spring-loaded left heart drainage tube.

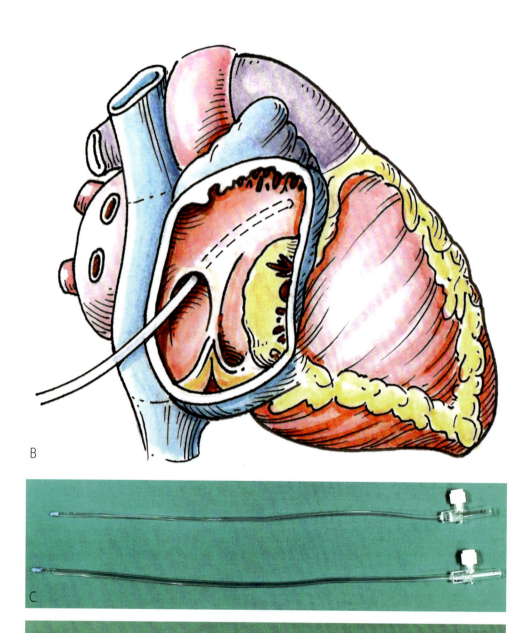

B

C

D

五、股动静脉插管

V. Femoral Arterial and Venous Cannulae

二期手术开胸,有时为确保手术安全,也可采用股动静脉插管心肺转流术(图2-4)。

In second-stage thoracotomy, the cardiopulmonary bypass with femoral arterial and venous cannulation is sometimes adopted to ensure surgical safety (Figure 2-4).

图 2-4　股动静脉插管
A. 股动脉插管。
B. 股静脉插管。

Figure 2-4　Femoral arterial and venous cannulae
A. Femoral artery cannula.
B. Femoral vein cannula.

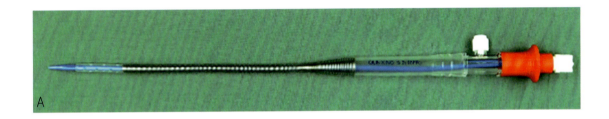

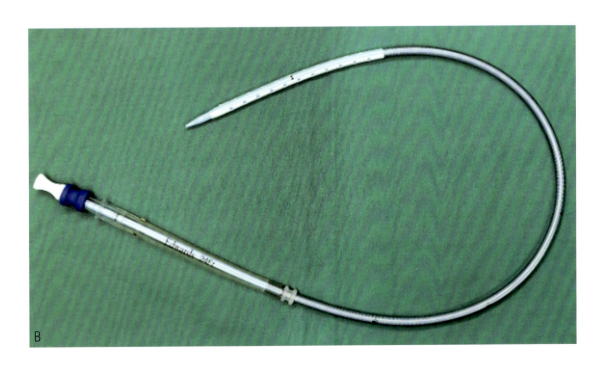

股动静脉插管原则（表 2-4）。

Principles of femoral arterial and venous cannulation (Table 2-4).

表 2-4　股动静脉插管原则

Table 2-4　Principles of femoral arterial and venous cannulation

体重 /kg Weight/kg	插管尺寸 /Fr Cannula size/Fr	
	股动脉插管 Femoral artery cannula	股静脉插管 Femoral vein cannula
15~20	12	15
20~30	15	17
30~40	15	17/19
40~60	15/17	19/21
>60	19	21/23

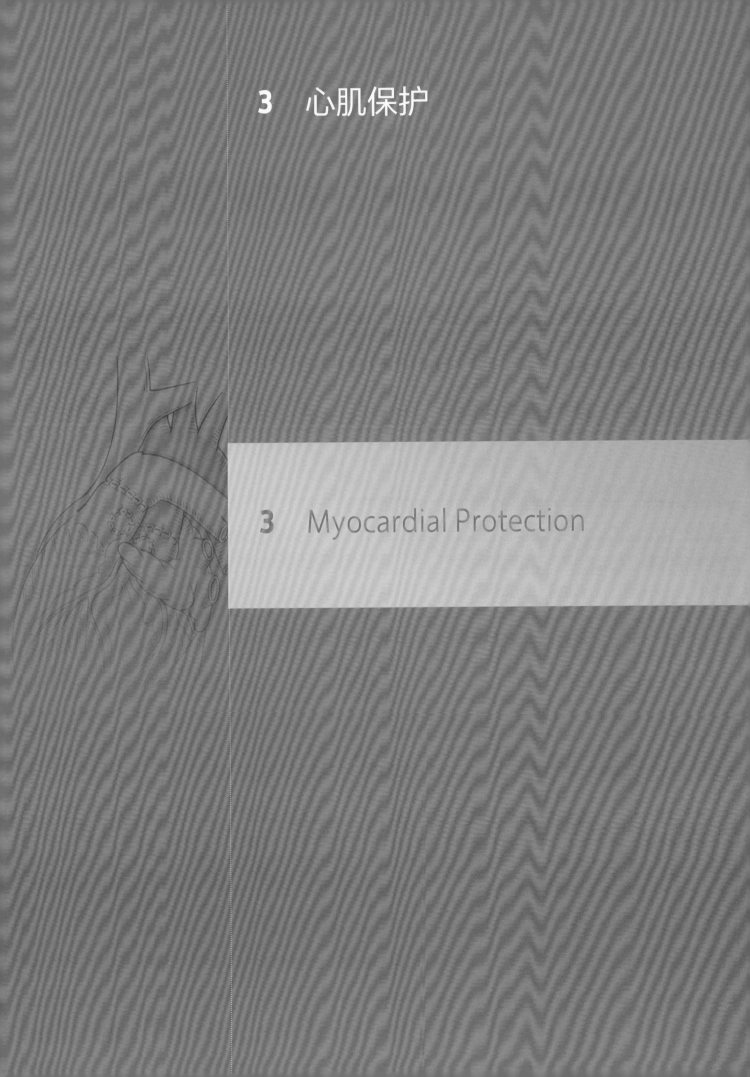

3 心肌保护

3 Myocardial Protection

心肌保护是心脏手术中至关重要的一部分。有许多不同配方的心肌保护液,也有不同的使用方法,但其关键技术是一致的,即通过低温和高钾等暂时停止心脏的收缩活动,为外科手术提供一个安静无血的手术视野。儿童心肌保护液配方主要有两大类:晶体配方溶液和含血心肌保护液。灌注方法也有一次性灌注和间歇多次灌注。

Myocardial protection is an essential part of cardiac surgery. For all the different formulas of myocardial protective fluid and different methods of application, the key techniques are consistent: the heart systole is to be temporarily stopped through hypothermia and a high potassium concentration solution to provide a still, bloodless surgical field. There are two main types of myocardial protective fluid for children: crystalloid cardioplegic solution and blood-based cardioplegic solution. The infusion methods also include single-dose infusion and intermittent multiple-dose infusions.

一、儿童常用的心肌保护液成分

I. Composition of Cardioplegic Solutions Commonly Used for Children

上海儿童医学中心两种不同保护液配方。

Two different types of protective fluid at Shanghai Children's Medical Center.

1. Del Nido 配方 冷血心肌保护液,晶体和血液比例为 4:1(4份晶体、1份血液)。每 500ml 醋酸钠林格注射液中添加 2% 利多卡因3.25ml、20% 甘露醇 6.5ml、10% 硫酸镁 4ml、10% 氯化钾 10ml、5% 碳酸氢钠 10ml。

1. The Del Nido sormula Cold blood cardioplegic solution with crystalloid to blood ratio of 4:1 (4 parts crystalloid, 1 part blood). Add 3. 25 ml lidocaine 2%, 6. 5 ml mannitol 20%, 4 ml magnesium sulfate 10%, 10 ml potassium chloride 10%, 10 ml sodium bicarbonate 5% in per 500 ml sodium acetate ringer's injection.

配制完成后根据患儿体重取适量加入心肌保护液储存袋备用,并预充灌注管道,并循环降温。转流开始后将适量含氧血注入储存袋

After the crystalloid is prepared, a corresponding dose of crystalloid, according to the weight of the patient, is put into the storage bag for later use. Prefill the perfusion tube with the crystal-

完成血液和晶体液的混合, 循环降温维持液体温度 4℃左右。

loid and circulate it to cool down. After the start of the bypass, an appropriate amount of oxygenated blood is injected into the storage bag to mix with the crystalloid and is cooled by circulation to keep the solution's temperature around 4℃.

主动脉血流阻断后用滚轴泵驱动, 在主动脉根部注入, 首次剂量为 20ml/kg, 灌注速度约为 20ml/(kg·min), 最高速度 250ml/min, 灌注时心肌保护液灌注管压力不超过 150mmHg(1mmHg=0.133kPa, 注: 该压力和灌注管道和针头粗细有关)。

After aortic occlusion, the cardioplegia is injected into the aortic root with a roller pump, with a first dose of 20 ml/kg. The perfusion rate is kept approximately at 20 ml/(kg·min) and no more than 250 ml/min, and the perfusion tube pressure should not exceed 150 mmHg (1 mmHg=0. 133 kPa, Note: The pressure is related to the size of the perfusion tube and needle).

预计主动脉血流阻断时间不超过 60~90 分钟者一次灌注, 手术时间较长者可每隔 60 分钟后给予首剂的半量。

Single-dose perfusion is expected when aortic occlusion lasts less than 60-90 min, and for those with longer time, a half dose of the first dose may be given every 60 min.

2. HTK 液 冷晶体心肌保护液, 预充心肌保护液灌注管道后循环降温, 维持液体温度 4℃左右。

2. HTK solution Cold crystalloid cardioplegic solution. Prefilled the perfusion tube with the cardioplegia and circulated it to cool down, making sure the solution's temperature keeps around 4℃. After aortic occlusion, the cardioplegia is injected into the aortic root with a roller pump with a first dosage of 30-50 ml/kg. The initial perfusion rate is kept at about 20 ml/(kg·min), and no more than 200 ml/min. During perfusion, the perfusion tube pressure should not exceed 150 mmHg. After the electrocardiogram shows no electrical activity, decrease the perfusion rate and keep the perfusion for 6-8 min.

主动脉血流阻断后用滚轴泵驱动, 在主动脉根部注入, 首次剂量为 30~50ml/kg, 灌注初期速度约为 20ml/(kg·min), 最高速度 200ml/min, 灌注时心肌保护液灌注管压力不超过 150mmHg。待心电图显示无电活动后, 降低灌注速度, 维持灌注时间 6~8 分钟。

主动脉血流阻断时间 180 分钟以内并且心肌温度较低(低于 25℃), 一次灌注即可, 若超过 180

Single-dose perfusion is expected when aortic occlusion lasts less than 180 min and the myocardial temperature is rather low (less than

分钟并且心肌温度较高酌情添加。

25℃). When the occlusion lasts more than 180 min and the myocardial temperature is rather high, the cardioplegia can be added accordingly.

注意：所灌注的 HTK 液应尽可能用墙式负压吸引排出，不能混入体外循环的转流液，防止低钠血症等情况的发生，以免影响心功能恢复和患儿神经系统预后。

Note: The perfused HTK solution should be aspirated and drained with wall-type vacuum suction as much as possible, and the bypass solution from extracorporeal circulation cannot be mixed to prevent the occurrence of hyponatremia and other conditions, which will affect the recovery of cardiac function and the patient's prognosis.

二、心肌保护方案

II. Methods of Myocardial Protection

低温对心肌的保护十分重要。心肌保护液温度在 4℃。新生儿手术中大多使用 HTK 液 20ml/kg 单剂灌注。婴幼儿手术视手术复杂程度，可使用含血心肌保护液单剂或每隔 60 分钟多次灌注，首次剂量 20ml/kg，之后的复灌剂量为 10ml/kg（图 3-1）。

Hypothermia is important for myocardial protection. During the operation, the temperature of the cardioplegic solution is kept at 4℃. In neonatal surgery, a single-dose infusion of 20 ml/kg of HTK solution was mostly used. Depending on the complexity of the procedure, blood-containing cardioplegic solutions may be used in infants and young children for single-dose infusions or multiple-dose infusions. Multiple perfusions are to be done at intervals of 60 minutes, with an induction dose of 20 ml/kg and reinfusion of 10 ml/kg (Figure 3-1).

图 3-1　心肌保护使用方法
主动脉血流阻断，根部注入保护液。

Figure 3-1　Method of myocardial protection
Aortic occlusion and infusion of cardioplegic solution into the aortic root.

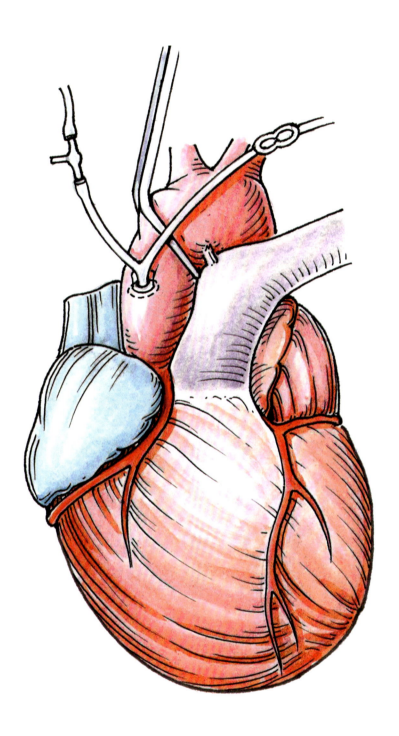

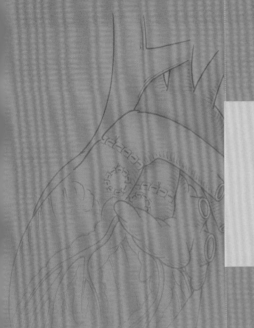

4 姑息性手术

4 Palliative Surgery

姑息性手术，又称减状手术，顾名思义是一种相对简单的手术方法，使患者的症状得到控制或改善。如对严重发绀型患者行体肺分流手术，以增加肺循环血流，改善青紫缺氧。对肺动脉高压患者则可做肺动脉环束术，使肺动脉压力下降，肺血管床得以保护，为今后手术创造条件。

常用手术方式。

Palliative surgery, a type of surgery for symptom relief, is a relatively simple procedure to control and improve patients'symptoms. For example, patients with severe cyanosis can have systemic-pulmonary shunt to increase blood flow in the pulmonary circulation and ameliorate cyanotic hypoxia. In patients with pulmonary arterial hypertension, pulmonary artery banding can be performed to reduce pulmonary artery pressure and protect the pulmonary vascular bed, thus creating appropriate conditions for later operations.

Common Procedures.

一、体循环 - 肺循环分流术

I. Systemic-Pulmonary shunt

1. Blalock-Taussig 分流术 经典 Blalock-Taussig（B-T）分流术通常采用经主动脉弓对侧的胸廓切口完成，第 3 肋间进胸暴露良好。左位主动脉弓使用右侧锁骨下动脉与右肺动脉做端侧吻合。右位主动脉弓则采用左锁骨下动脉与左肺动脉做端侧吻合。

目前临床应用最广泛的方法还是改良 B-T 分流术。通常用 4mm 左右的膨体聚四氟乙烯（expanded poluytetrafluroethylene，ePTFE）人造血管连接体 - 肺血管。其优点是保留患者的自身血管，人工血管可根据患者血管的大小、长度任意选

1. Blalock-Taussig shunt The classic Blalock-Taussig (B-T) shunt is usually accomplished through a thoracotomy on the opposite side of the aortic arch, which provides enough exposure via 3rd intercostal spaces. The right subclavian artery is end-to-side anastomosed to the right pulmonary artery for patients with the left aortic arch. The left subclavian artery is end-to-side anastomosed to the left pulmonary artery for patients with the right aortic arch.

Currently, the most widely used method is the modified B-T shunt. Typically, expanded poluytetrafluroethylene (ePTFE) artificial blood vessels of approximately 4mm are utilized to connect systemic vessels to the pulmonary vessel. Modified B-T shunt not only can keep the patient's own blood vessel but also has two

择;二期手术容易摘除。手术径路目前多采用经胸骨正中切口。其优点是暴露清晰,若术中病情危急,则可采用心肺转流术来实施分流。吻合口大多采用 7-0 或 6-0 Prolene 缝线(图 4-1)。

advantages: the sizes and length of the artificial blood vessel can be customized to meet the different patients'needs, and the artificial blood vessels can also be easily removed at a second-stage operation. The surgery is currently carried out via a median sternotomy, with the advantage of enough exposure and the feasibility of performing cardiopulmonary bypass in case of emergency. Most anastomoses are done with 7-0 or 6-0 Prolene sutures (Figure 4-1).

图 4-1　B-T 分流术
A. 非 CPB 切口位置及患儿体位。

Figure 4-1　Blalock-Taussig shunt
A. The location of incision and the patient's position in non-CPB surgery.

Continued

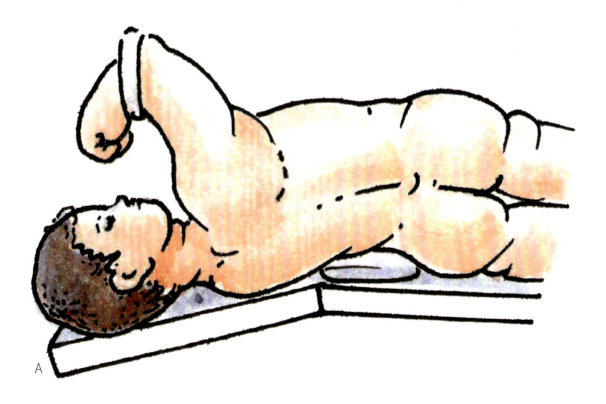

图 4-1（续）

Figure 4-1 cont'd

B. 非 CPB 手术视野。

B. View of surgical field in non-CPB B-T shunt.

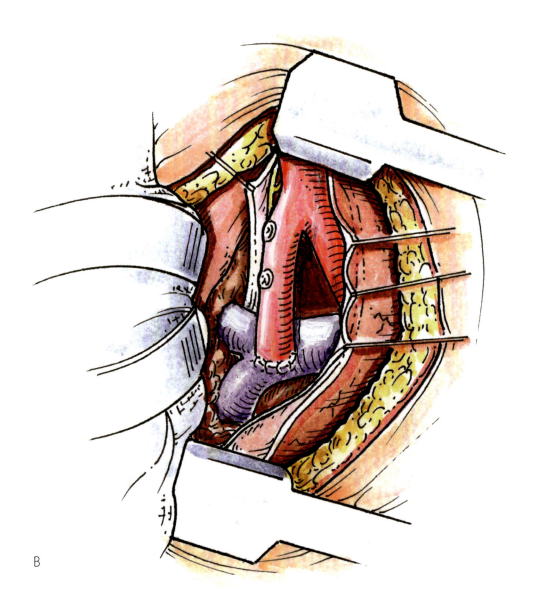

B

图 4-1（续）

Figure 4-1 cont'd

C. 锁骨下动脉吻合口。

C. Anastomosis of conduit and subclavian artery.

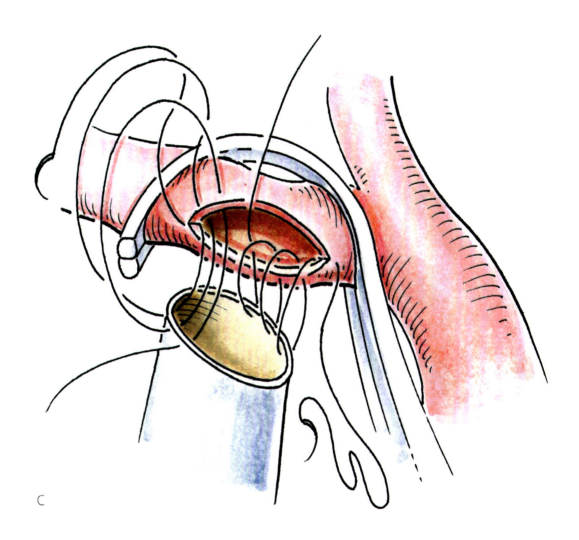

C

2. 中央分流术 对一些肺血管发育极差、年龄小的重症患者可采用中央分流术。用 ePTFE 管道直接在升主动脉和主肺动脉之间做连接。其优点是暴露相对容易。但也有缺点：血流不易控制，二期手术开胸易损伤出血（图 4-2）。中央分流手术大多可在非体外循环心脏不停搏情况下进行，若手术困难，可在体外平行循环下完成。

2. Central shunt The central shunt can be used in some critically ill young children with very poor pulmonary vascular development. An ePTFE conduit is implanted to make a direct connection between the ascending aorta and the main pulmonary artery, with the advantage of relatively easy exposure and the disadvantage of difficult control of the blood flow volume and elevated incidence of injury and bleeding at the second stage of thoracotomy (Figure 4-2). Most central shunt procedures can be performed off-pump beating heart procedure and, if difficult, under extracorporeal circulation.

图 4-2　**中央分流术**
A. 主肺动脉吻合口。

Figure 4-2　Central shunt
A. Anastomosis of conduit and main pulmonary artery.

Continued

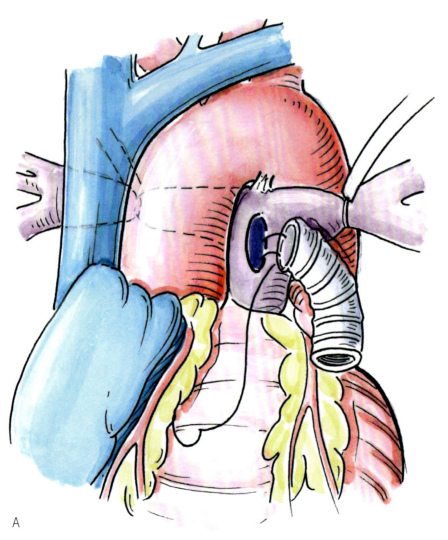

A

图 4-2（续）

B. 升主动脉侧壁吻合。

Figure 4-2 cont'd

B. Anastomosis of conduit and ascending aortic side wall.

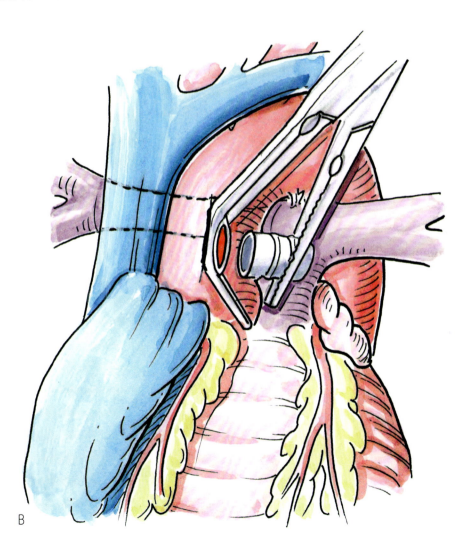

B

图 4-2（续）

Figure 4-2 cont'd

C. 中央分流管道。

C. Conduit of central shunt.

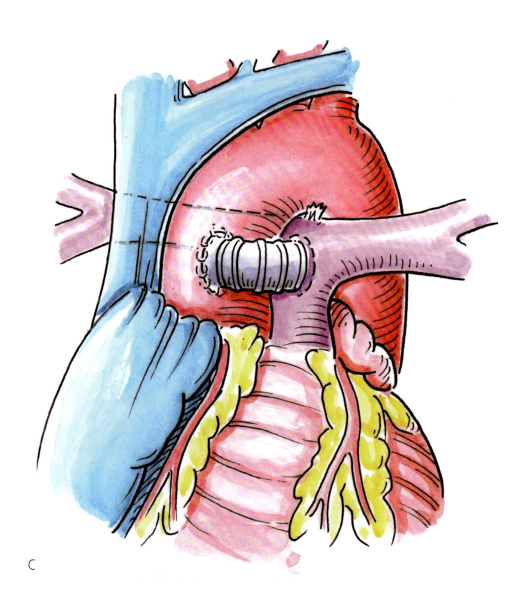

C

3. Waterston 分流术　一种在升主动脉后壁和右肺动脉前壁之间构建吻合的体循环 - 肺循环分流术。手术径路采用右侧胸部切口，将上腔静脉牵开后用一把侧壁钳将右肺动脉和部分升主动脉侧壁钳夹。右肺动脉近、远端分别上两个圈套。切口长度约 3~4mm，用 7-0 Prolene 缝线连续缝合。但其存在

3. Waterston shunt　Waterston shunt is a systemic-pulmonary shunt that connects the posterior wall of the ascending aorta with the anterior wall of the right pulmonary artery. The surgery is carried out via a right thoracotomy. The superior vena cava is retracted, and an anastomosis clamp is used to clamp the right pulmonary artery and partial ascending aortic side wall. Two tourniquets are placed on the proximal and

分流量较难控制,远期右肺动脉扭曲等缺陷,现在极少应用(图 4-3)。

distal ends of the right pulmonary artery, respectively. The incision, which is approximately 3-4 mm long, is closed by a running suture with 7-0 Prolene suture. However, Waterston shunt is rarely used now due to such defect as difficult shunt volume control and the right pulmonary artery distortion in the later period (Figure 4-3).

图 4-3　Waterson 分流术
A. 升主动脉后壁及右肺动脉前壁切口位置。

Figure 4-3　Waterston shunt
A. Position of incisions on the posterior wall of the ascending aorta and the anterior wall of the right pulmonary artery.

Continued

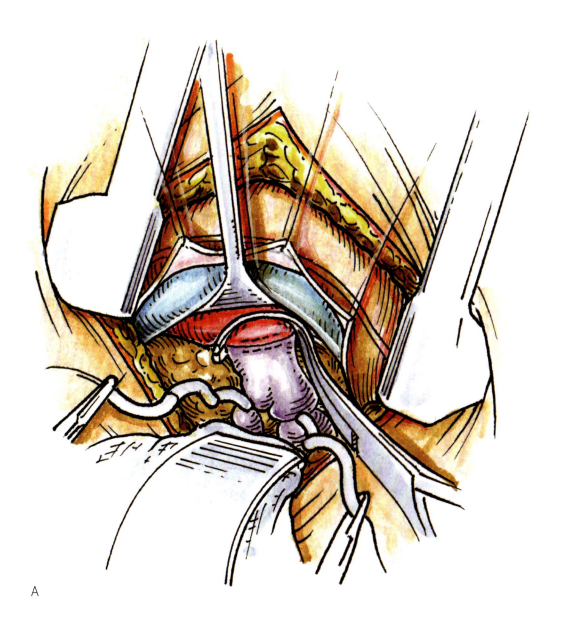

A

图 4-3（续）

B. 侧壁钳钳夹右肺动脉和部分升主动脉侧壁,右肺动脉远端上圈套。

Figure 4-3 cont'd

B. An anastomosis clamp is used to clamp the right pulmonary artery and partial ascending aortic side wall, a tourniquet is placed on the distal end of the right pulmonary artery.

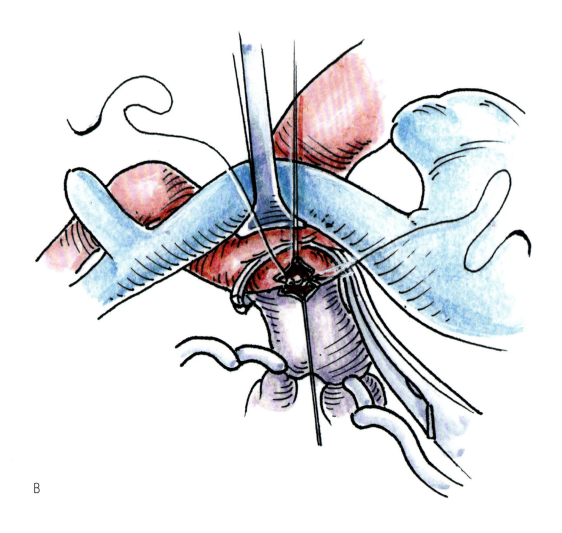

B

4. Potts 分流术　该手术是降主动脉和左肺动脉之间的吻合。可采用左侧胸廓切口径路。用一把特殊的 Potts 阻断钳将降主动脉部分阻断,确保远端血供,左肺动脉近端和远端分别阻断,在主动脉和肺动脉侧壁分别做 3~4mm 切口,然后做侧侧吻合。此方法也因并发症较多,逐渐被淘汰。但近年来有文献

4. Potts shunt　The procedure is an anastomosis between the descending aorta and the left pulmonary artery. Under a left thoracotomy, a special Potts clamp is used to partially occlude the descending aorta, ensuring distal blood supply. Proximal and distal ends of the left pulmonary artery are occluded respectively, and incisions of 3-4 mm on the sidewalls of the aorta and pulmonary artery are made, followed by side-

报道应用 Potts 分流术治疗晚期肺动脉高压患者。通过体肺分流缓解肺动脉高压，并能改善右心功能（图4-4）。

to-side anastomosis. Due to complications, Potts shunt is not routinely performed now. However, the use of Potts shunt in the treatment of patients with advanced pulmonary hypertension has been recently reported in some literature: pulmonary hypertension was relieved, and right heart function was improved (Figure 4-4).

Continued

图 4-4　Potts 分流术
A. 采用左侧胸廓切口径路，主动脉和肺动脉侧壁侧侧吻合。

Figure 4-4　Potts shunt
A. Under a left thoracotomy, the sidewalls of the aorta and pulmonary artery are side-to-side anastomosed.

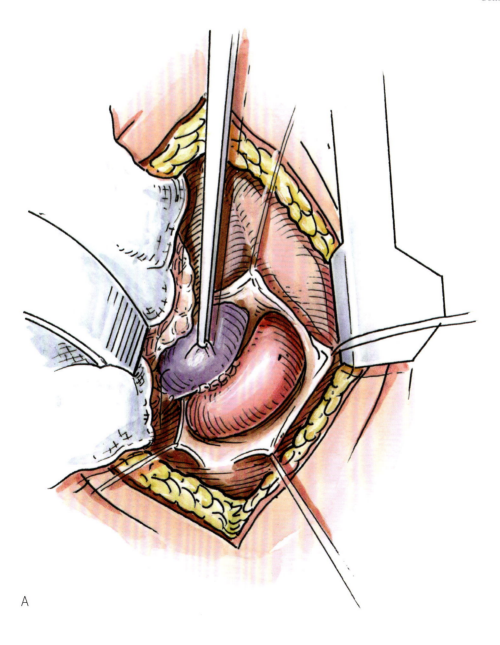

A

图 4-4（续）

Figure 4-4 cont'd

B. Potts 分流吻合口。

B. The anastomotic stoma of Potts shunt.

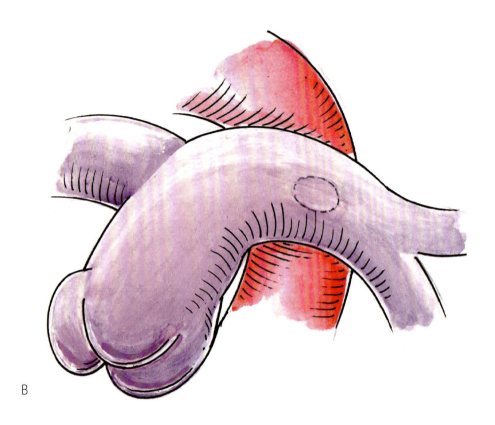

B

5. Melbourne 分流术　该手术主要应用在肺动脉闭锁、自身肺动脉发育极差的患者。将左右肺动脉游离后分别阻断，在升主动脉的右侧壁上一把侧壁钳，做一个 2~3mm 的切口，用 7-0 Prolene 缝线将肺动脉近端直接吻合在主动脉侧壁（图 4-5）。

5. Melbourne shunt　This procedure is mainly used in patients with pulmonary artery atresia and extremely poor development of pulmonary artery. After the left and right pulmonary arteries are dissociated and occluded, an anastomosis clamp is placed on the right-side wall of the ascending aorta to make an incision of 2-3 mm. The proximal pulmonary artery is directly anastomosed to the side wall of the aorta with 7-0 Prolene sutures (Figure 4-5).

图 4-5 Melbourne 分流术

A. 将左右肺动脉游离后分别阻断，在升主动脉的右侧壁上一把侧壁钳，做一个 2~3mm 的切口，用 7-0 Prolene 缝线将肺动脉近端直接吻合在主动脉侧壁。

Figure 4-5 Melbourne shunt

A. After the left and right pulmonary arteries are dissociated and occluded, an anastomosis clamp is placed on the right-side wall of the ascending aorta to make an incision of 2-3mm. The proximal pulmonary artery is directly anastomosed to the side wall of the aorta with 7-0 Prolene sutures.

Continued

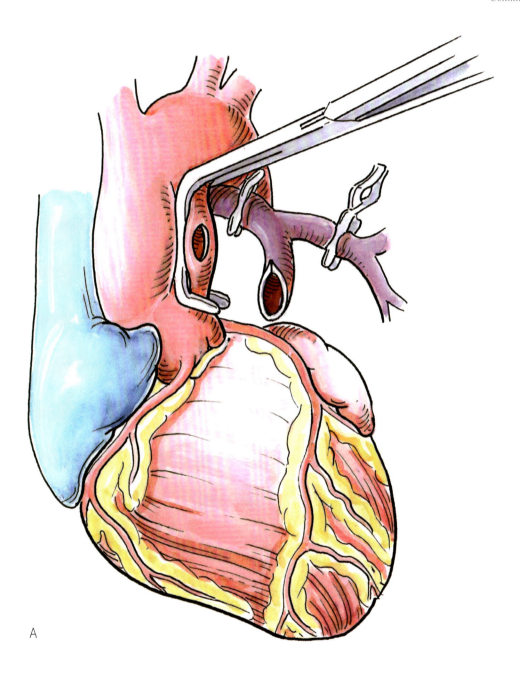

A

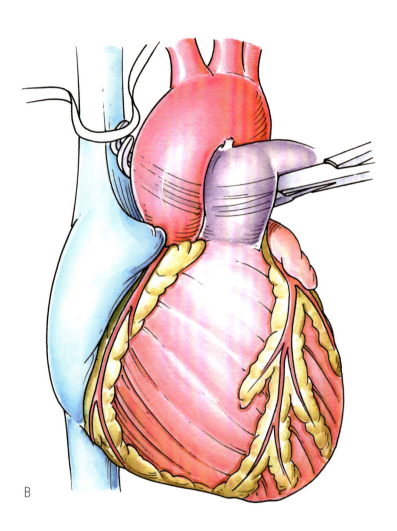

B

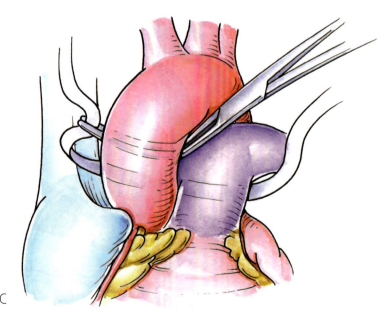

C

图 4-6（续）

D. 在肺动脉环束带两端分别测压，评估肺动脉环束带的松紧程度。通常将肺动脉远端收缩压降至所测得的主动脉收缩压的 50% 以下。环束带需与肺动脉外壁固定 1 针，避免滑动。

Figure 4-6 cont'd

D. Pressure is measured at both sides of the pulmonary artery band to assess the band tightness. The systolic blood pressure of the distal pulmonary artery is usually restricted to less than 50% of the measured aortic systolic pressure. The band needs to be secured to the outer wall of the pulmonary artery via one stitch to prevent band migration.

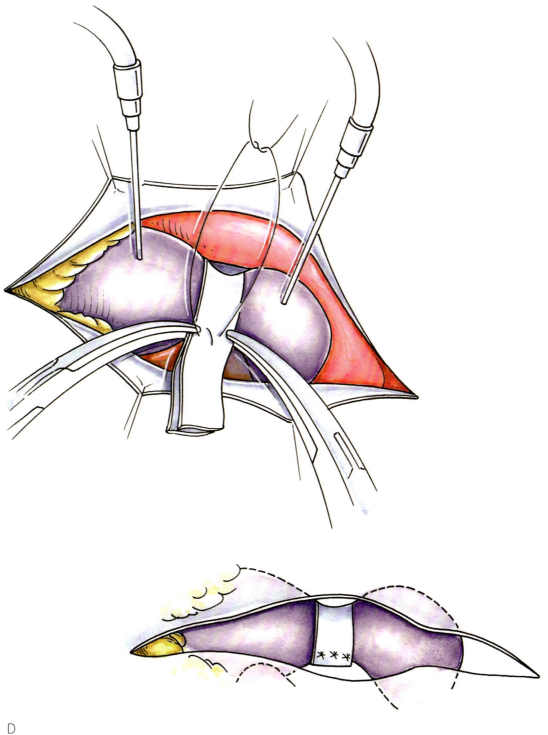

D

三、肺动脉内环束术

III. Intra-pulmonary Artery Banding

对需要心肺转流术同时进行其他心内操作的患者,也可做肺动脉内环束术。在一块 ePTFE 补片中央预先开孔,再将这块补片缝入主肺动脉内。其优点是肺动脉粘连轻,第二次手术分离切除容易(图4-7)。

In patients requiring cardiopulmonary bypass for other intracardiac procedures, intra-pulmonary artery banding may also be indicated. Pre-cut a hole in the center of an ePTFE patch, and then suture this patch into the main pulmonary artery. It has the advantage of little pulmonary artery adhesion and, easy separation and excision at a second operation (Figure 4-7).

图 4-7　肺动脉内环束术

A. ePTFE 补片中央预先开孔。

Figure 4-7　Intra-pulmonary artery banding

A. Pre-cut a hole in the center of an ePTFE patch.

Continued

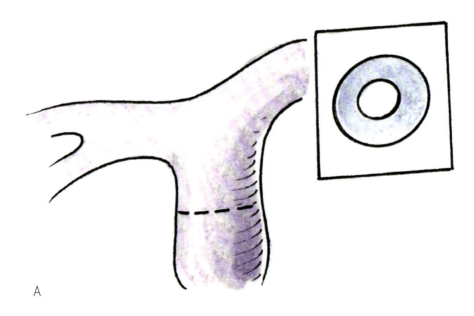

A

图 4-7（续）

B. 将补片缝入主肺动脉内。

C. 肺动脉内环束完成。

Figure 4-7 cont'd

B. Suture this patch into the main pulmonary artery.

C. Intra-pulmonary artery banding completed.

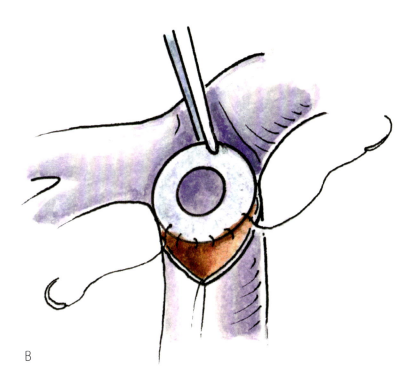

B

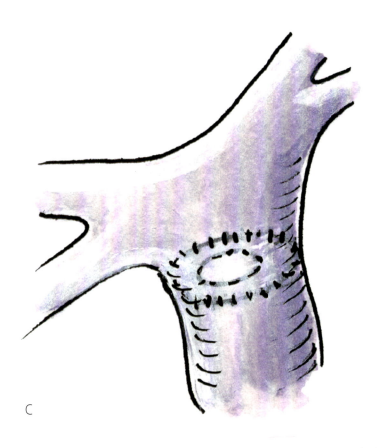

C

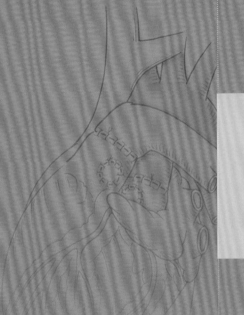

5 动脉导管未闭

5 Patent Ductus Arteriosus

动脉导管未闭（patent ductus arteriosus，PDA）属于心上分流的先天性畸形的一种，胎儿期间动脉导管是连接胎儿主动脉和肺动脉的唯一通道，通常粗约5~15mm，长3~15mm，很少呈较长的管道或者呈瘤样扩张。出生以后数周内导管应自动闭合。如果仍然开放就会造成左向右分流而出现血流动力学的障碍，久而久之引起肺动脉高压变成右向左分流，成为某些心脏手术禁忌证。与其他心内畸形并存时，其作为综合性心脏畸形的一个组成部分而存在，在进行心内畸形手术时须同时处理未闭的动脉导管。

Patent ductus arteriosus (PDA) is one kind of congenital malformation of the supracardiac shunt. As the only channel connecting the aorta and pulmonary artery in fetal life, ductus arteriosus is usually about 5-15 mm in diameter and 3-15 mm long and rarely presents itself as a long duct or an aneurysmal dilatation. Ductus arteriosus usually closes weeks after birth. An open ductus arteriosus causes left-to-right blood shunt and, hence, the hemodynamic disturbances that will result in pulmonary hypertension and, eventually, a right-to-left shunt, as a contraindication to some cardiac surgeries. If other intracardiac malformations are present in addition to a PDA, PDA will be part of a complex cardiac malformation and will be simultaneously treated in intracardiac malformation surgery.

一、解剖分型

I. Anatomical Typing

动脉导管的下端起于左肺动脉根部的后上方，正面看很近于主肺动脉的分叉部，被主肺动脉遮挡而看不清，导管的上端起于主动脉峡部的小弯侧与左锁骨下动脉相对应，但在左锁骨下动脉稍远侧。导管的后方为左主支气管，导管的左前方有左迷走神经经过。喉返神经经导管下缘绕向颈部纵隔胸膜盖在导管侧壁上。

The lower end of ductus arteriosus originates from the posterior part of the root of the left pulmonary artery and is close to the bifurcation of the main pulmonary artery from the front view but is usually shielded by the main pulmonary artery. The upper end of ductus arteriosus originates from the lesser curved side of the aortic isthmus and lies opposite to the left subclavian artery but at the slightly distal side of the left subclavian artery. The left main bronchus is located in the posterior part of the ductus, and the left vagus nerve passes through the front left side of the ductus. Recurrent laryngeal nerve passes through the lateral wall of the ductus from the inferior edge of the ductus towards the cervical mediastinal pleura.

幼儿动脉导管壁比较厚而且弹性好、结实,然而,在成人或肺动脉高压者中,导管的壁会变得薄且脆,而且易钙化,其钙化组织有时可蔓延至主动脉壁。如果合并细菌性心内膜炎则导管壁更加脆弱,在手术切断或结扎时都容易造成撕破出血。

Ductus arteriosus walls are thick, elastic, and strong in young children; however, the walls will get thin and fragile in adults or patients with pulmonary hypertension, and in such cases, the walls are easily calcified, and the calcified tissues sometimes spread to the aortic wall. If complicating with bacterial endocarditis, the ductus walls will get even more fragile, and they are more vulnerable to tearing and rupture during surgical amputation or ligation.

动脉导管未闭分为 5 种类型 (图 5-1)。

PDA is classified into five types (Figure 5-1).

图 5-1　动脉导管未闭分类
A. 管型,外形如管状,最常见。B. 漏斗型,主动脉侧粗,肺动脉侧细,呈漏斗状。C. 窗型,粗而短,类似主 - 肺动脉窗。D. 哑铃型,两端粗,中间细,像哑铃状。E. 动脉瘤型,粗大,呈瘤样膨大。

Figure 5-1　Types of PDA
A. Tubular ductus with tube-like appearance, the most common type. B. Funnel-shaped ductus with a wide aortic orifice and a considerably narrower pulmonary end. C. Window ductus with short and thick duct, like the aorto-pulmonary window. D. Dumbbell-shaped ductus with wide aortic and pulmonary artery ends and a constricted center. E. Ductal aneurysm with aneurysmal dilation.

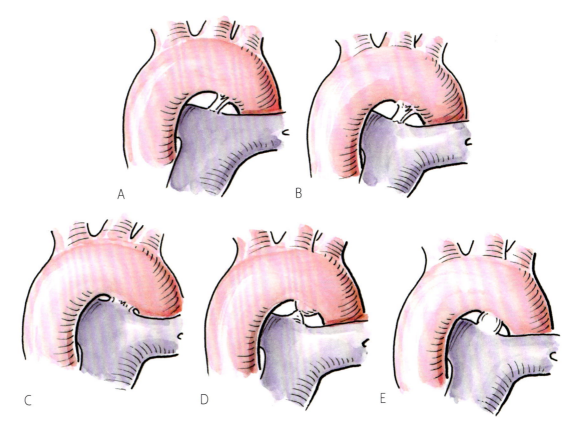

A   B   C   D   E

手术时应注意以下几点。

1. 导管的后方为左主支气管，分离，钳夹，结扎和切断动脉导管注意避免损伤左主支气管。

2. 喉返神经紧绕动脉导管的下缘，呈白色。在游离动脉导管时应尽量避开喉返神经，不要钳夹损伤喉返神经。

3. 单纯动脉导管未闭手术可以通过左侧肋间切口结扎或切断。

对于粗大且伴有肺动脉高压的动脉导管或者合并其他心脏手术，必须进行专门处理：正中进胸心肺转流术辅助下切开主肺动脉显露动脉导管。

Pay attention to the following during the operation。

1. As the left main bronchus lies posterior to the ductus, be careful to avoid injuries during the detachment, clamping, ligation, and transection of the ductus.

2. As the white recurrent laryngeal nerve closely coils around the inferior edge of the ductus arteriosus, be careful to keep away the nerve and not to clamp it in order to avoid any injuries to it when dissociating the ductus arteriosus.

3. Isolated PDA can be ligated or transected from left posterolateral incisions.

Large ductus arteriosus complicated with pulmonary hypertension or other cardiac surgeries shall be treated specifically: a median thoracotomy must be performed with cardiopulmonary bypass, and the main pulmonary artery should be cut through to expose the ductus arteriosus.

二、手术治疗

II. Surgical Treatment

1. 早产儿手术方法 早产儿一般都有动脉导管未闭,出生后即在早产监护室。手术可直接在监护室,保温箱即当手术台(图 5-2)。

1. Surgical methods in preterm infants Preterm infants usually have PDAs and are placed in the neonate intensive care unit (NICU) after birth. The operations can be directly performed in the NICU, with incubators as the operating tables (Figure 5-2).

图 5-2 **早产儿 PDA 手术方法**
A. 早产儿取右侧卧位,左后外侧切口第 4 肋间进胸,切口 2cm 即可。为减少手术出血,切开皮肤后可以使用 100ml 生理盐水加 1~2 滴肾上腺素湿纱布止血。早产儿的所有组织都很脆嫩,一般使用手术刀柄和无创伤镊子即可分离肌纤维。

Figure 5-2 Surgical methods in preterm infants
A. With the infants in the right lateral position, the chest is accessed through the fourth intercostal space with a left posterolateral incision (2 cm is enough). In order to reduce bleeding in surgery, a wet gauze with 1-2 drops of epinephrine in 100 ml physiological saline is used after an incision is cut. As all tissues are very fragile and tender in preterm infants, muscle fibers are usually dissected by scalpel handles and non-invasive forceps.

Continued

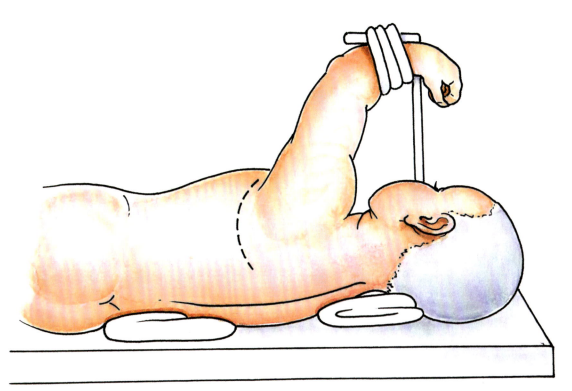

A

图 5-2（续）

B. 切开胸膜前请麻醉师不要膨肺,先切开一个小口,打开胸膜,继续膨肺。用柔软有湿纱布包裹的压舌板轻微把左肺牵开至纵隔方向。有些未闭的动脉导管粗于主动脉弓,在处理动脉导管之前务必确定主动脉弓完整和连续。沿虚线切开胸膜,前侧向肺侧牵开。紧靠胸膜并行于降主动脉旁呈现白色的是迷走神经,其中一个分支正好绕着动脉导管后壁到喉部,称喉返神经。这也是鉴别未闭动脉导管和主动脉弓的标志。

Figure 5-2 cont'd

B. The lung shall not be inflated until a small incision is made and the pleura is cut open. The left lung is slightly retracted towards the mediastinum by a soft tongue depressor wrapped with moist gauze. Some patent ductus are thicker than the aortic arches, so it is essential to make sure that the aortic arches are intact before the treatment of ductus arteriosus. The pleura is incised along the dotted liney and retracted anteriorly to the lung. The white vagus nerve is adjacent to the pleura and parallel to the descending aorta, and one of its branches, called the recurrent laryngeal nerve, twines the posterior wall of the ductus arteriosus all the way to the larynx, which is a marker to distinguish the patent ductus from the aortic arch.

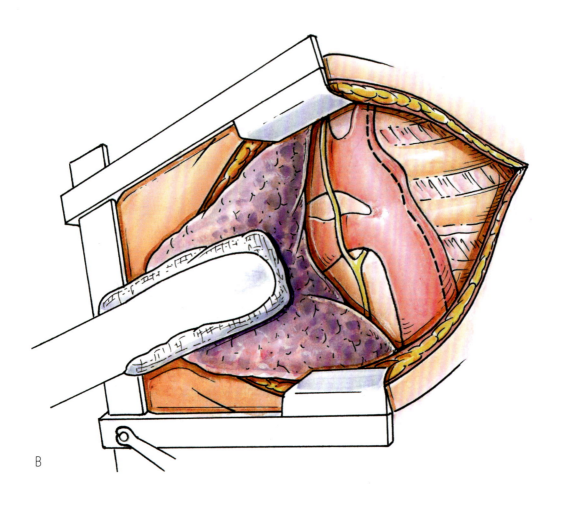

B

图 5-2（续）

C. 早产儿血压不高，导管的压力也不大，为了避免过分的操作可以选择长度合适的银夹或钛夹并行于喉返神经，避开喉返神经在动脉导管的近端和远端各夹一个。

Figure 5-2 cont'd

C. The blood pressure of premature infants is not high, and so is the pressure in the ductus. To avoid excessive movement, choose silver clips or titanium clips of appropriate length, put them parallel to the recurrent laryngeal nerve, and clamp the proximal and distal ends of the ductus arteriosus while keeping off the recurrent laryngeal nerve.

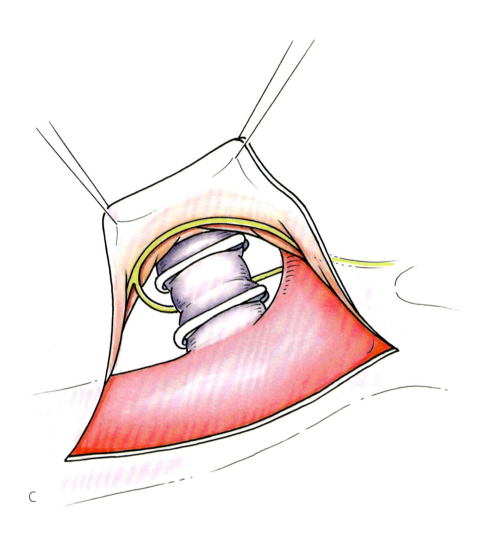

C

图 5-2（续）

D. 也可采取 4 号线或 7 号线在主动脉和肺动脉两端分别结扎。早产儿动脉导管未闭手术，切口小，基本不出血。关胸可以使用 4-0 的 Prolene 缝线 2 针间断贯穿连同肋骨缝合，关胸前膨肺，排气，打结。一般不必放置胸腔引流。

Figure 5-2 cont'd

D. Alternatively, take 4# or 7# sutures to ligate the two ends. Generally, surgeries of PDA in preterm infants with small incisions have minimal bleeding. Chest closure can be performed by two stitches, intermittent sutures through ribs with 4-0 Prolene suture after lung inflation, deflation, and knotting. Chest drainage is generally not necessary.

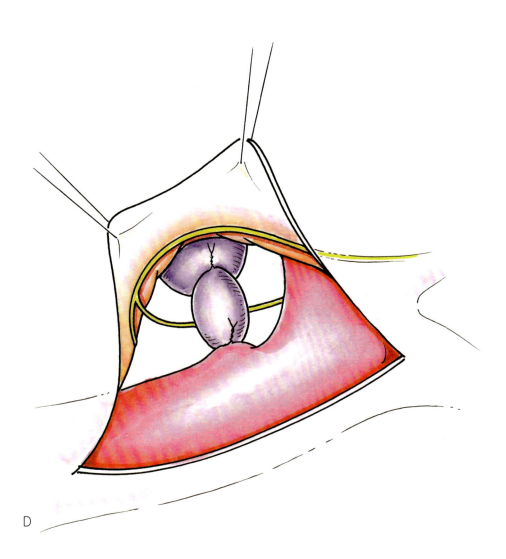

D

2. 婴幼儿的手术方法 单纯的婴幼儿动脉导管未闭，目前都可以通过介入治疗，但是介入治疗失败，或者无法进行介入治疗，外科手术是另一种选择。患儿气管插管，全身麻醉，单肺通气。右侧卧位，后外侧切口，一般长 3~4cm，第 4 肋间进胸。动脉导管显示、鉴别主动脉弓和早产儿一样。手指触摸动脉导管有震颤或者搏动。剪开纵隔胸膜，推开喉返神经，钝性分离未闭动脉导管靠主动脉侧的纵隔胸膜，暴露动脉导管上下两端间隙，用直角钳分离动脉导管后壁。直接取 7 号线或 10 号丝线分别结扎主、肺动脉两侧。对有些比较粗短的未闭动脉导管，为了安全可先分离动脉导管主动脉端上下两侧，用 10 号丝线轻提主动脉，再分离动脉导管后壁，然后再套丝线结扎。结扎时一般采用控制性降压，收缩压通常降至60mmHg。这样结扎更安全，也可避免压力过高、结扎不紧导致动脉导管再通。有些较短未闭动脉导管也可采用切断缝合技术（图 5-3）。

2. Surgical methods in infants and young children Isolated PDA in infants and young children can be treated by interventional therapy now, but if the therapy fails or cannot be performed, surgery is another option. Under general anesthesia with tracheal intubation and one-lung ventilation, the infants are in the right lateral decubitus position, and chests are accessed through the fourth intercostal space with posterolateral incisions (generally 3-4 cm). The identification and differentiation of ductus arteriosus and aortic arches are the same as those in preterm infants. There is a tremor or pulse along the ductus arteriosus when touching with fingers. Cut the mediastinal pleura, push the recurrent laryngeal nerve away, bluntly dissect the mediastinal pleura on the aortic side of patent ductus, expose the spaces between the upper and lower ends of the ductus, and dissociate the posterior wall of ductus by right-angle clamps. Take 7# or 10# sutures to ligate the two ends of aortic and pulmonary arteries. For some relatively large and short patent ductus, firstly separate both upper and lower sides of the aortic end of the ductus for the sake of safety, lift the aorta with 10# suture, separate the posterior wall of the ductus, and then knot it with a suture. Ligation requires controlled hypotension, and the systolic blood pressure usually needs to decrease to 60 mmHg. This makes ligation safer and avoids the reperfusion of ductus arteriosus due to loose ligation and high pressure. Some short patent ductus can also be treated with a technique for cut-off and suture (Figure 5-3).

图 5-3　婴幼儿 PDA 手术方法

A. 游离未闭动脉导管,使用无创镊子或者镊子套上橡皮管轻度短时间夹住连接动脉导管的主动脉近端,用直角钳钝性分离动脉导管下缘和后壁。如果需要时间长,间隙放开夹主动脉的镊子一直到结扎线套过动脉导管。

Figure 5-3　Surgical methods in infants and young children

A. One method of dissociating the patent ductus is to clamp the proximal aorta connecting the ductus arteriosus for a short period of time with atraumatic forceps or rubber-tube-folded forceps and bluntly dissect the inferior edge and posterior wall of ductus arteriosus by using right angle forceps. If it takes a long time, the forceps clamping the aorta are to be released at intervals until the ligature has passed through the ductus.

Continued

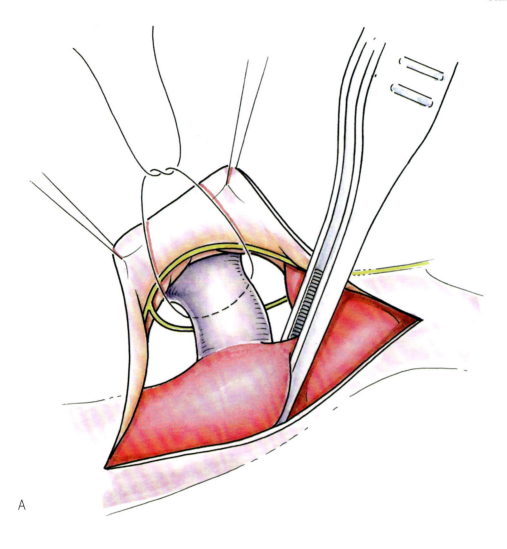

A

图 5-3（续）

B. 使用同样的方法在未闭动脉导管的主动脉侧也穿过结扎线。为避免结扎线滑脱可以使用一头带针的线,无针一头穿过动脉导管后,再使用带针一头缝合穿过动脉导管前壁。

Figure 5-3 cont'd

B. The same approach is taken to cross the ligature over the aortic end of the patent ductus. In order to avoid the slippage of ligature, a needle-attached suture can be used: after the needle-free end of the ligature passes through the ductus, the needle-attached end is used to suture through the anterior wall of the ductus.

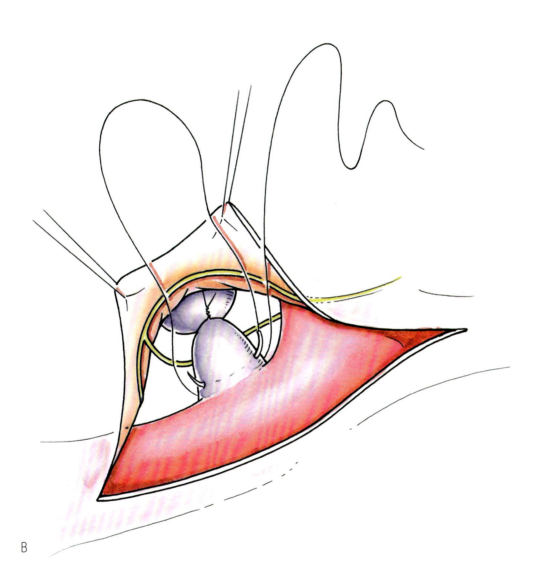

B

图 5-3（续）

C. 动脉导管两端结扎线分别打结。放置结扎线时注意两线之间保持一定距离以便导管切断后有足够残端。

Figure 5-3 cont'd

C. The two ends of ductus arteriosus are sutured separately. When knotting, pay attention to the distance between the two ligations to make sure there are enough stumps at each end after cutting off the ductus.

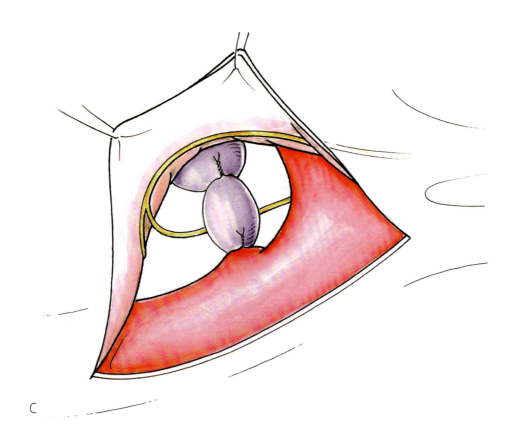

C

图 5-3（续）

D. 切断动脉导管，注意不要切断或者损伤神经。检查两个导管残端是否有出血。

Figure 5-3 cont'd

D. Do not cut off or damage the nerves when cutting ductus. Check whether there is bleeding from both ductus stumps.

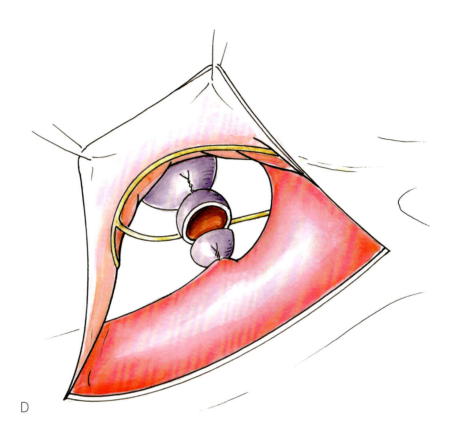

D

图 5-3 (续)

E. 切断的动脉导管一般不会再通。但是主动脉侧的残端导管残余组织很脆弱，手术后有可能因为高血压而撕裂，造成致命性大出血。建议在此残端再做一个加固缝合。缝线多带些健康的主动脉组织。

Figure 5-3 cont'd

E. Generally, a transected ductus arteriosus will not reperfuse. However, the residual tissue of ductus stumps on the aortic side is fragile and may tear after surgery due to high blood pressure, causing fatal massive bleeding. Reinforced stitching is recommended at this stump. The sutures are to be made with more healthy aortic tissues.

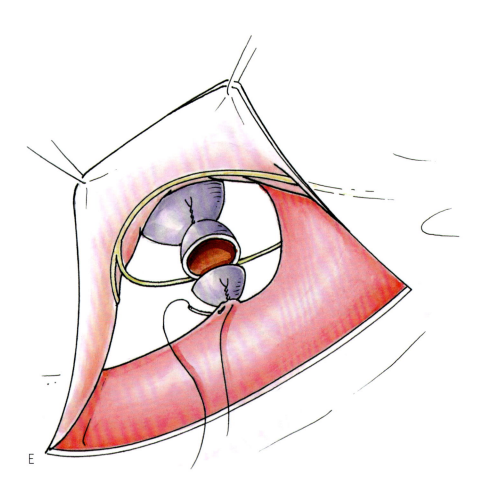

E

图 5-3（续）

F. 动脉导管主动脉侧残端两重缝合。肺动脉残端，因为肺动脉压力低，一般不必处理。

Figure 5-3 cont'd

F. Double suture is needed for the aortic stumps of ductus arteriosus but unnecessary for pulmonary artery stumps since pulmonary artery pressure is low.

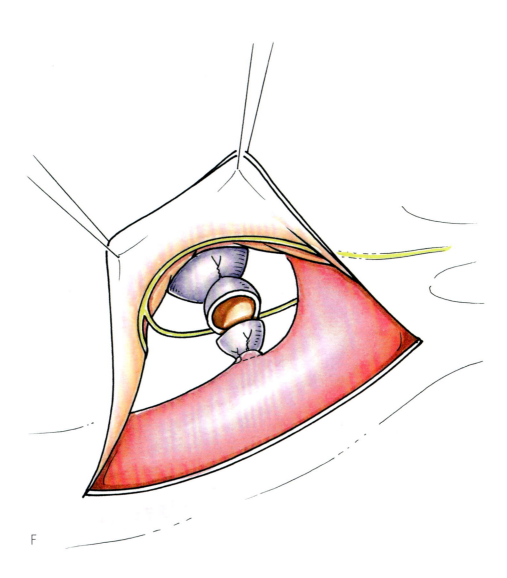

F

3. 复杂动脉导管未闭外科处理 复杂动脉导管未闭的外科处理主要包括肺动脉高压、导管钙化或合并其他心脏手术等。单纯粗大的动脉导管未闭手术，一般不必采用心肺转流术（图 5-4）。

使用左后外侧进胸带垫片直接缝合技术。进胸后显露动脉导管未闭。由于肺动脉高压、导管粗大，甚至钙化，强行分离动脉导管容易损伤周围组织，撕裂导管。复杂动脉导管未闭的显露不同于简单案例，最好不要完全游离未闭动脉导管，仅在导管和主动脉弓窗之间用钝性钳少许分离。

3. Surgical treatment of complex PDA Surgical management of complex PDA is needed when there is pulmonary hypertension, calcification of ductus, or other cardiac procedures in addition to PDA. Simple surgeries of the large patent ductus do not require cardiopulmonary bypass (Figure 5-4).

Direct suture technique with patch after left posterolateral thoracotomy is used. Left posterolateral thoracotomy is performed to expose PDA. Due to the presence of pulmonary hypertension, bulky ductus, and even calcification, forced separation of the ductus arteriosus will risk damaging the surrounding tissue and tearing the ductus. The presentation of complex patent ductus is different from those in simple cases, so it is preferable not to dissociate the patent ductus completely but just slightly separate the ductus arteriosus from the aortic arch window with blunt forceps.

图 5-4 **复杂动脉导管未闭外科处理**

A. 患者取右卧位，左侧向上，后外侧切口，沿肩胛骨后下缘。

Figure 5-4 Surgical treatment of complex PDA

A. The patients are in the right lateral position with the left side upward, and a posterolateral incision is performed along the posterior inferior edge of the scapula.

Continued

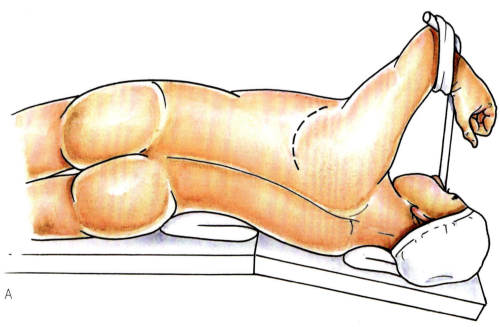

A

图 5-4（续）

B. 准备 4-0 Prolene 无创双头缝线，带垫片。一针缝在导管下缘，另一针在导管上缘，分别穿上垫片，使用无创镊（或带橡皮套镊子）轻轻阻断主动脉，缝线打结。使用同样方法处理另一端。

Figure 5-4 cont'd

B. 4-0 Prolene atraumatic double-needle pledget-supported sutures are prepared at first. One stitch is sewn at the lower edge of the ductus, and the other stitch is sewn at the upper edge, with each stitch attached by a patch. The aorta is gently blocked with atraumatic forceps (or forceps with rubber sleeves) and tied with the suture. The same approach is applied to the other end.

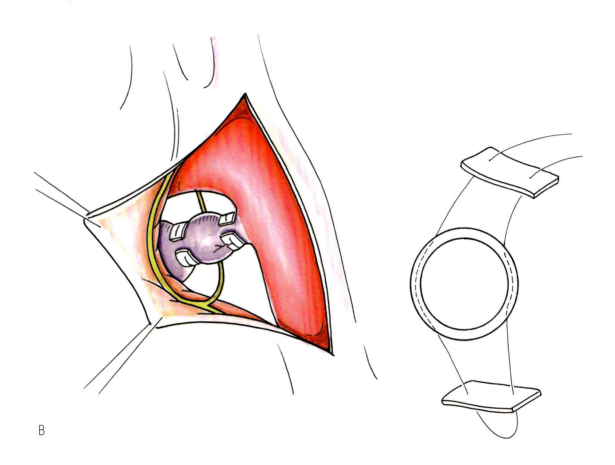

B

图 5-4(续)

C. 对于动脉导管未闭合并严重肺动脉
高压,未闭动脉导管血管瘤样改变、动
脉导管钙化,合并其他复杂心脏病手术
等手术风险高的动脉导管未闭,一般
要采用正中开胸,并在心肺转流术下
手术。

Figure 5-4 cont'd

C. For PDA complicated with severe pulmonary
hypertension, angiomatoid changes, calcification, and other
complex cardiac surgeries, the surgery is to be performed
with a median thoracotomy and a cardiopulmonary bypass.

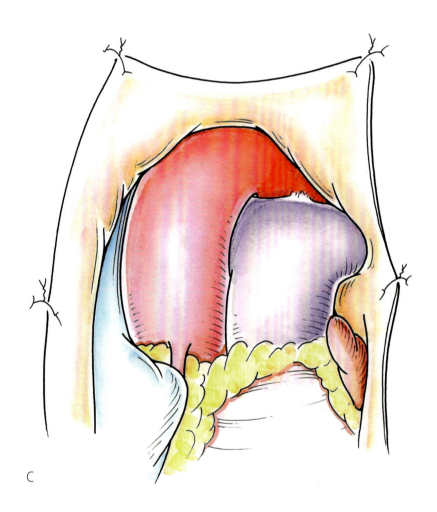

C

图 5-4（续）

D. 在确定必须进行心肺转流术后，全身肝素化，根据需要选择主动脉插管和静脉插管。单纯的动脉导管未闭手术，选择单根右心房插管就可以，在平行循环下处理 PDA。

Figure 5-4 cont'd

D. Once the cardiopulmonary bypass is determined, systemic heparinization is administered, and aortic and intravenous catheters are selected based on the patient's situation. For simple surgery of PDA, only a right atrial catheter is taken to treat PDA in parallel circulation.

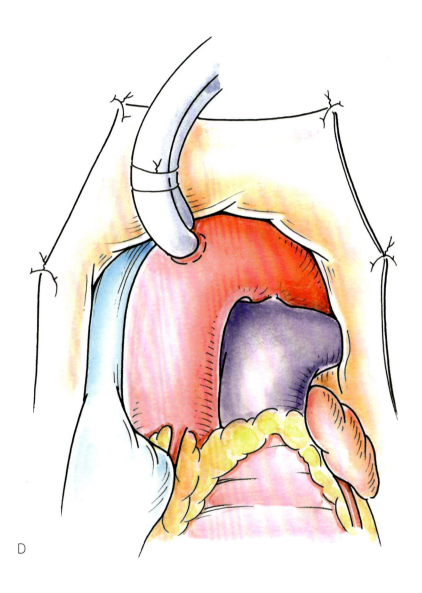

D

图 5-4（续）

E. 游离未闭动脉导管，建议在心肺转流术下进行。心肺转流术稳定后，保持全流量，灌注压维持在 50mmHg 左右。根据动脉导管的不同情况，如压力的大小、导管壁的厚薄、是否钙化或者动脉瘤样改变等，采取不同的方法处理动脉导管未闭。在心肺转流术下，灌注压容易控制，游离导管比较容易，可采用单纯结扎或缝扎。

Figure 5-4 cont'd

E. Dissociation of the patent ductus is recommended to be performed under cardiopulmonary bypass. When cardiopulmonary bypass is stabilized, full flow is secured, and the perfusion pressure is maintained at about 50mmHg. Different approaches are to be used to treat PDA based on the different morphology of ductus arteriosus, such as the indication of pressure, the thickness of the ductus wall, the presence of calcification, or aneurysmal changes. The presence of cardiopulmonary bypass makes it easier to control perfusion pressure and dissociate the ductus, and hence, simple ligation or suture can be used.

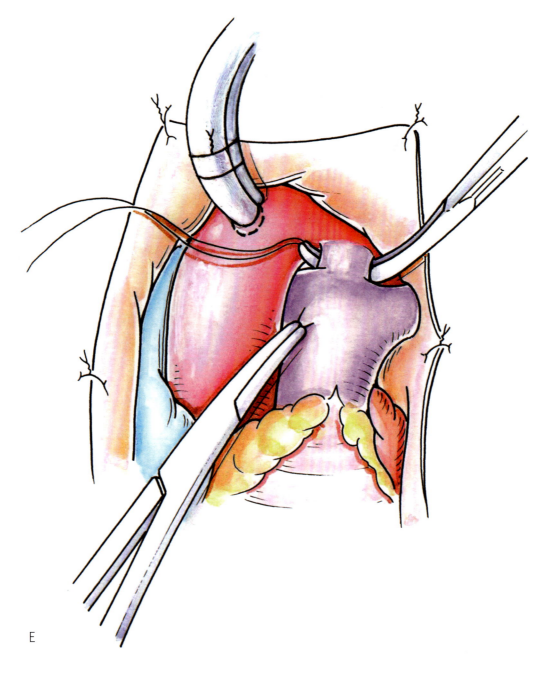

E

图 5-4（续）

F. 对于术后动脉导管再通、粘连、动脉瘤样改变、感染等情况，可以采用深低温、低流量或者短时间停循环，直接切开肺动脉处理开放的动脉导管。必要时用无创血管钳夹住动脉导管。

Figure 5-4 cont'd

F. Certain conditions, such as reperfused ductus arteriosus after surgery or ductus complicated with adhesions, aneurysmal changes, infections, etc., can be treated with deep hypothermic, low-flow, or short-term circulatory arrest, in which ductus arteriosus is treated through direct pulmonary artery incision. If necessary, the ductus arteriosus is clamped with atraumatic clamps.

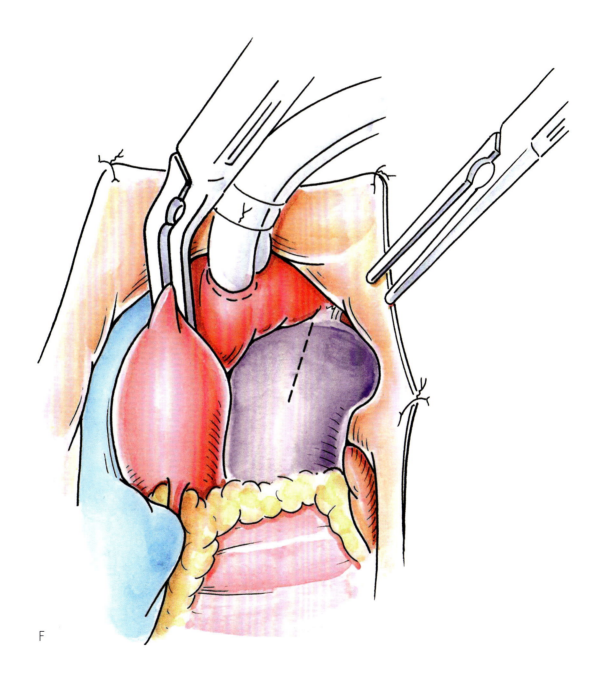

F

图 5-4（续）

G. 短而粗大的动脉导管，如果还有钙化，直接缝合会有再通的可能，一般需要自身心包补片在肺动脉内侧连续缝合闭合动脉导管。

Figure 5-4 cont'd

G. With calcification, a short and large ductus arteriosus may reperfuse after direct suture. Generally, it is necessary to close the ductus with a running suture and pericardial patch implanted to the inner side of the pulmonary artery.

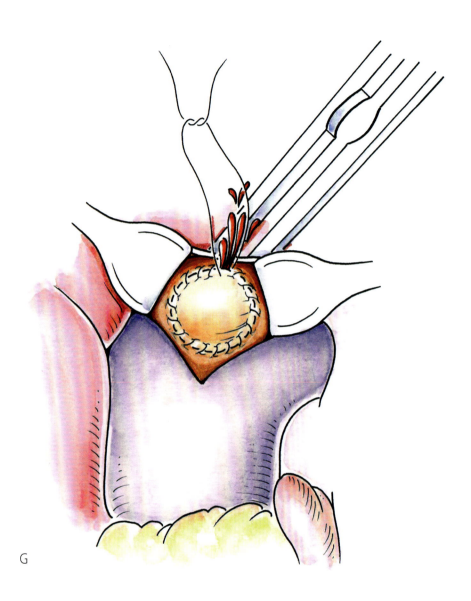

G

图 5-4（续）

H. 补片排气后打结,连续缝合肺动脉切口。

图 5-4 cont'd

H. Tie it after venting the patch. The pulmonary artery incision is to be closed with a running suture.

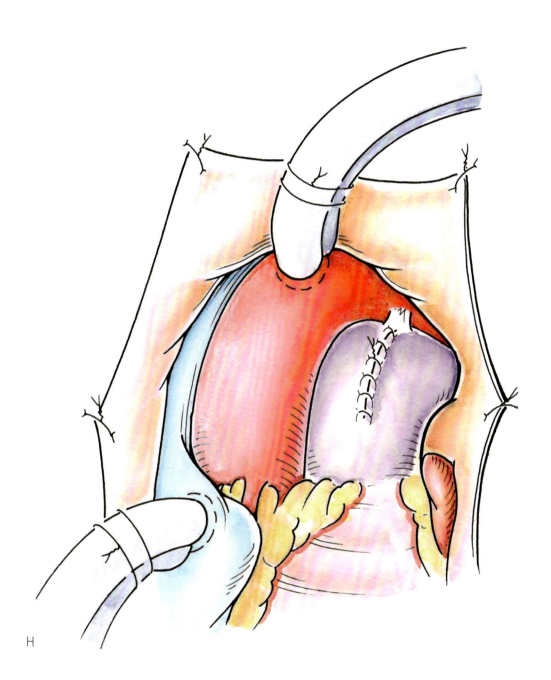

H

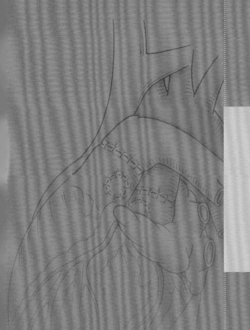

6 主 - 肺动脉窗

6 Aorto-pulmonary Window

主 - 肺动脉窗又称主动脉肺动脉间隔缺损。主动脉瓣和肺动脉瓣发育正常，在升主动脉和主肺动脉的半月瓣的上方有一缺损，造成主动脉和肺动脉的血流互相沟通。其与永存动脉干区别在于前者有两组半月瓣而后者仅一组半月瓣。手术方法可在心肺转流术下直接切开升主动脉（或切开主肺动脉）缝合缺损，如缺损太大必须补片矫正。

The aorto-pulmonary window, also known as the aortopulmonary septal defect (APSD), refers to a defect above the semilunar valve of the ascending aorta and main pulmonary artery while the aortic and pulmonary valves develop normally, resulting in a persistent communication of blood flow between the aorta and the pulmonary artery. It differs from persistent truncus arteriosus in that there are two groups of semilunar valves in the former and only one group of semilunar valves in the latter. Several surgical methods can be used, either to directly incise the ascending aorta (or incise the main pulmonary artery) to suture the defect under cardiopulmonary bypass or to be repaired by pericardial patch if the defect is too large.

一、解剖分型

I. Anatomical Typing

按解剖特点分成三型（图 6-1）。

There are three types according to anatomical characteristics (Figure 6-1).

图 6-1　主 - 肺动脉窗的解剖分型

A. Ⅰ型：主动脉肺动脉间隔近端缺损。相当于紧贴半月瓣上方在主动脉和肺动脉之间形成交通孔，主动脉窦的上缘，此交通孔有时为一很短的管道。

B. Ⅱ型：主动脉肺动脉间隔远端缺损，位于升主动脉后壁，近右肺动脉起源处。

Figure 6-1　Anatomical types of aorto-pulmonary window

A. Type Ⅰ: Proximal defect of the aortopulmonary artery septum. This actually refers to a communicating orifice between the aorta and the pulmonary artery immediately above the semilunar valve at the superior margin of the aortic sinus, which sometimes forms a short conduit.

B. Type Ⅱ: Distal defect of the aortopulmonary artery septum. It is located on the posterior wall of the ascending aorta, usually near the origin of the right pulmonary artery.

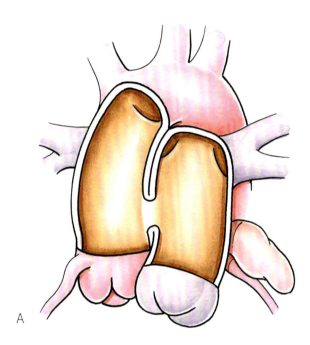

A

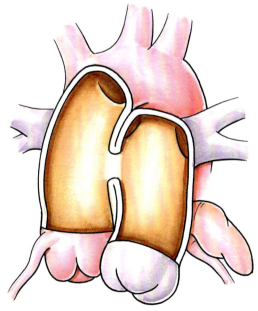

B

图 6-1（续）

Figure 6-1 cont'd

C. Ⅲ型：主动脉肺动脉间隔完全缺损，看起来像是右肺动脉直接起源升主动脉干上。

C. Type Ⅲ: Total defect. It looks as if the right pulmonary artery originated directly from the ascending aortic trunk.

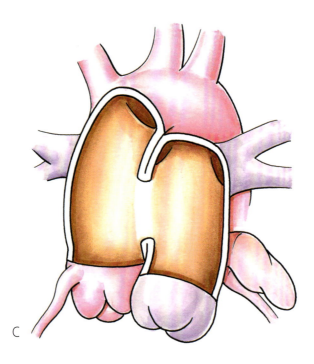

C

二、手术方法

Ⅱ. Surgical Methods

1. 非体外循环或者体外循环心脏不停搏闭合主 - 肺动脉窗　主 - 肺动脉窗诊断明确时应及早手术，避免左向右分流引起肺动脉高压。如果患者合并其他畸形，应同时给予手术修复。可以选择不停搏心肺转流术，在心肺转流术开始时必须阻断左右肺动脉。防止心肺转流术的灌注血通过主 - 肺动脉窗流入肺循环导致灌注肺。主动脉插管靠近主动脉弓，可右心房单根插管，也可上下腔静脉分别插管，还可选择阻断升主动脉，主动脉根部注入心肌保护液，使心脏停搏。主动脉、上下腔静脉插管方法与前文介绍相同，

1. Closure of the aorto-pulmonary window with off-pump or on-pump beating heart procedure　Operation should be considered at the time of diagnosis of the aorto-pulmonary window so as to avoid pulmonary hypertension caused by left-to-right shunt. If other deformities are present, one-stage repair of all defects should be given at the same time. The procedure can be performed under on-pump beating heart cardio-pulmonary bypass. Both left and right pulmonary arteries must be blocked at the beginning of cardio-pulmonary bypass to prevent blood flow from the cardiopulmonary bypass entering the pulmonary circulation through the aorto-pulmonary window that will, in turn, result in perfusion of lungs. Aortic

主 - 肺动脉窗切开后,肺动脉回血不会很多,必要时在主 - 肺动脉窗切开处外加吸引器(图 6-2)。

cannulation is to be close to the aortic arch. It can be single right atrial cannulation or separate superior and inferior vena cava cannulation. Alternatively, after aortic occlusion, cardioplegia can be injected into the aortic root and cardiac arrest is induced. In such cases, the cannulation of the aorta and superior and inferior vena cava is the same as mentioned before, After the window is incised, there is usually limited blood returned to the pulmonary arteries, and if necessary, suction can be applied to the site of the incision (Figure 6-2).

图 6-2 **非体外循环或者体外循环心脏不停搏闭合主 - 肺动脉窗**

A. 少数主 - 肺动脉窗较小,可采用简单的结扎法。

Figure 6-2 Closure of the aorto-pulmonary window with off-pump or on-pump beating heart procedure

A. For a few small aorto-pulmonary windows, ligation can be applied.

Continued

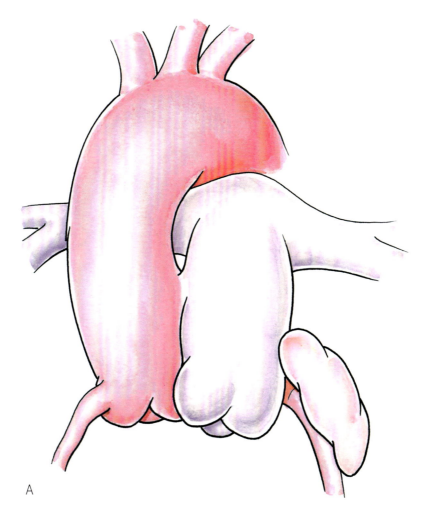

A

图 6-2（续）

B. 术中不慎有可能造成主动脉或者肺动脉出血。所以决定使用结扎方法时要确定主-肺动脉窗不大，主动脉和肺动脉之间有些距离，而且主动脉与肺动脉之间没有太多的粘连。尽管如此，还是建议准备心肺转流术，以防不测。结扎不完全，或者结扎线松脱时主-肺动脉窗有再通的可能。目前临床已经很少应用。

Figure 6-2 cont'd

B. Since there is the risk of bleeding from the aorta or pulmonary artery during the procedure, ligation methods will only be considered if aorto-pulmonary window is small, there is some distance between the aorta and the pulmonary artery, and there is not much adhesion between the aorta and pulmonary arteries. Nonetheless, preparation for cardiopulmonary bypass is still recommended, just in case. Incomplete closure or loose ligatures may cause recanalization of aorto-pulmonary window. At present, it has been rarely used in clinical practice.

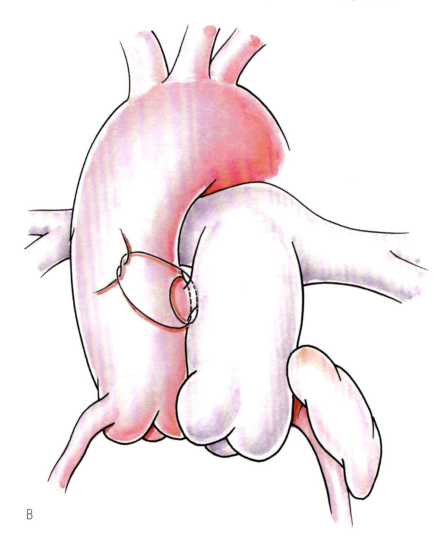

B

图 6-2（续）

C. I 型主 - 肺动脉窗不大, 之间有一定距离而且主肺动脉直径足够大, 可以在心肺转流术下不停搏进行手术。

Figure 6-2 cont'd

C. Type I aorto-pulmonary window is small, the distance between the aorta and the pulmonary artery windows is adequate, and the diameters of main pulmonary arteries are large enough, so that the procedure can be performed under on-pump beating heart cardiopulmonary bypass.

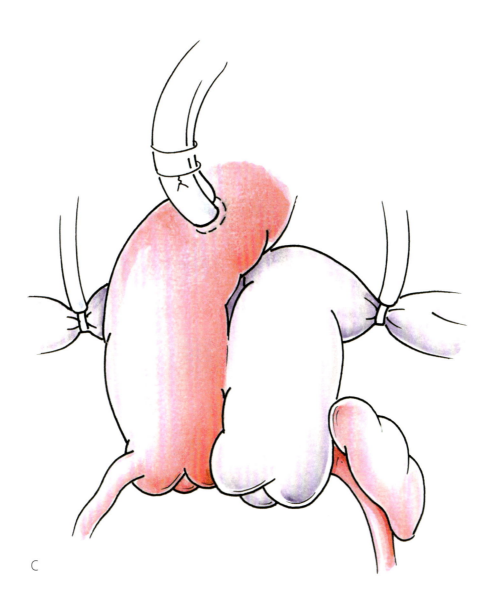

C

图 6-2（续）

Figure 6-2 cont'd

D. 在游离主 - 肺动脉窗后壁后选择升主动脉合适位置，上主动脉侧壁钳。

D. A side-biting vascular clamp is used at the proper position of the ascending aorta after disassociating the posterior wall of the aorto-pulmonary window.

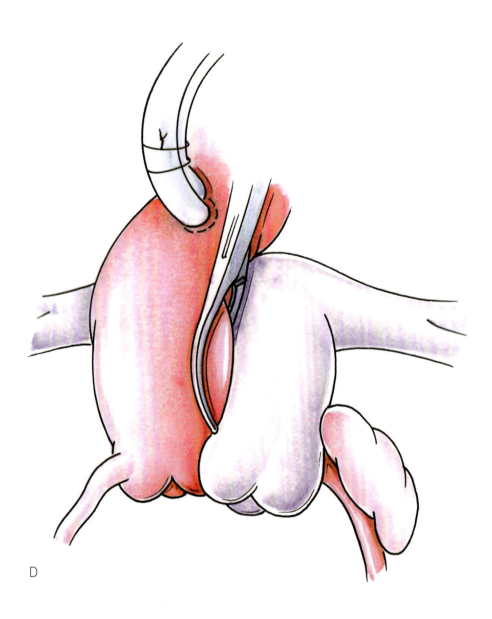

D

图 6-2（续）

E. 尽量保留较多主动脉壁以便升主动
脉缺损处有足够组织直接缝合。

Figure 6-2 cont'd

E. Keep as much aortic wall as possible so that there is
sufficient tissue in direct suturing of the ascending aortic
defect.

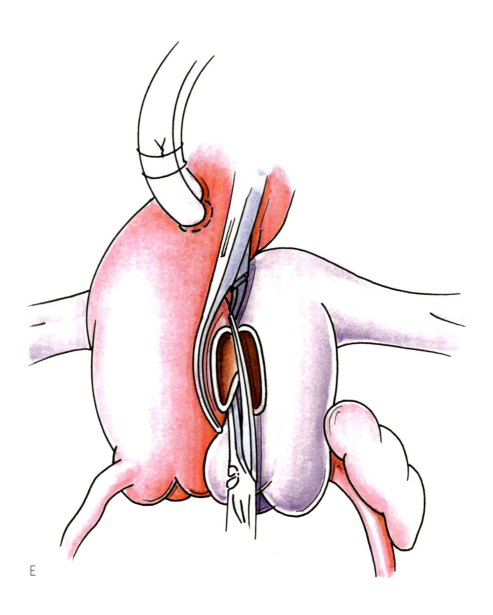

E

图 6-2（续）

F. 主 - 肺动脉窗的组织大部分留给升主动脉直接闭合用。

Figure 6-2 cont'd

F. The tissue of aorto-pulmonary window is mostly reserved for direct closure of the ascending aorta.

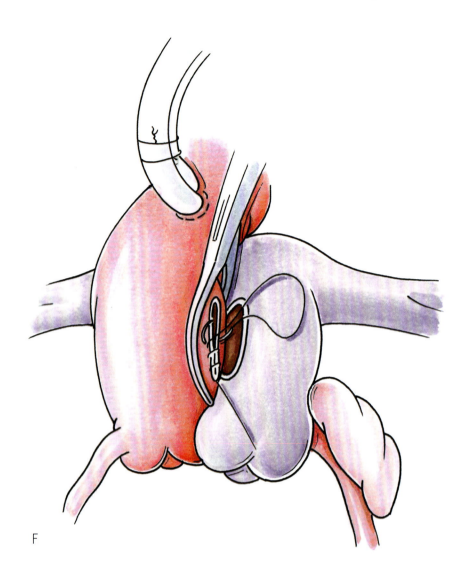

F

图 6-2（续）

G. 肺动脉切口可直接缝合关闭。

Figure 6-2 cont'd

G. Pulmonary artery can be closed directly.

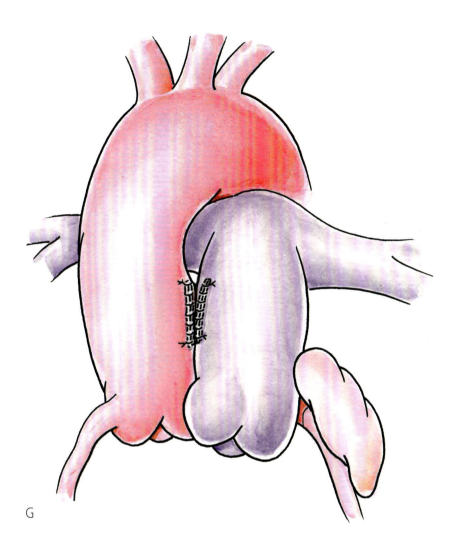

G

图 6-2 (续)

H. 若肺动脉缺损较大, 一般使用补片或者患者自身心包补片修补。

Figure 6-2 cont'd

H. If the pulmonary artery defect is large, a patch or autologous pericardial patch is commonly used for repair.

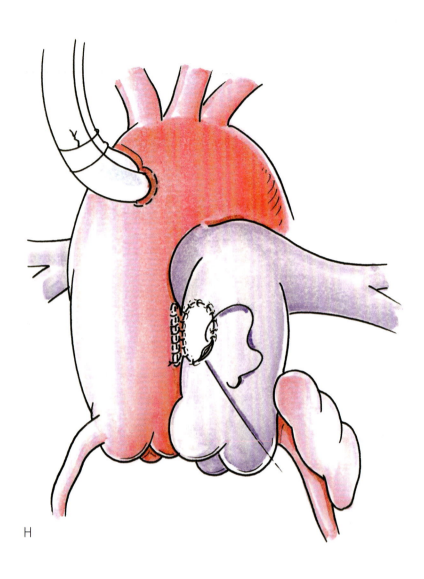

H

2. 补片修补主 - 肺动脉窗

（1）"三明治"修补方法：Ⅱ型和Ⅲ型主 - 肺动脉窗因为缺损大，而且缺损直接在主动脉和肺动脉后壁，可以保留缺损后壁。手术需要心肺转流术，婴幼儿可以直接深低温、停循环（图 6-3）。

2. Patch closure of aorto-pulmonary window

(1) Sandwich patch method: Since the defects of the type Ⅱ and type Ⅲ aorto-pulmonary windows are large and are usually located on the posterior wall of the aorta and pulmonary arteries, their posterior wall can be preserved. The procedure requires cardiopulmonary bypass or, in infants and young children, deep hypothermic circulatory arrest (Figure 6-3).

图 6-3 "三明治"修补方法
A. 开胸后，主动脉、腔静脉插管。游离左右肺动脉，分别圈套肺动脉阻断带。

Figure 6-3　Sandwich patch method
A. After thoracotomy, the aorta and the vena cava are cannulated. The left and right pulmonary arteries are disassociated, and each is blocked with a pulmonary artery controller.

Continued

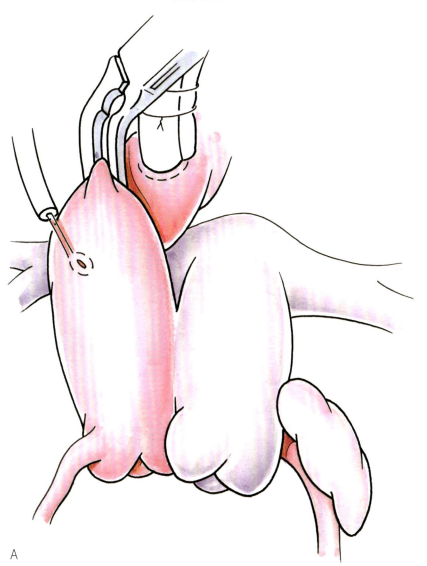

A

图 6-3（续）

B. 阻断主动脉血流、灌注心肌保护液，心脏停搏后可以逐步切开和扩大主 - 肺动脉窗，保留后壁，解除肺动脉阻断带。仔细检查，确认主动脉和肺动脉瓣膜完整，冠状动脉起源无错位，注意避免损伤。

Figure 6-3 cont'd

B. After aortic occlusion and cardioplegic arrest induced by perfusion of cardioplegic solution, the aorto-pulmonary window can be incised and enlarged gradually, the posterior wall should be preserved, and then the pulmonary artery controllers can be relieved. Make sure the aortic valve and the pulmonary valve are intact, and there is no transposition at the origin of the coronary artery to avoid any injuries.

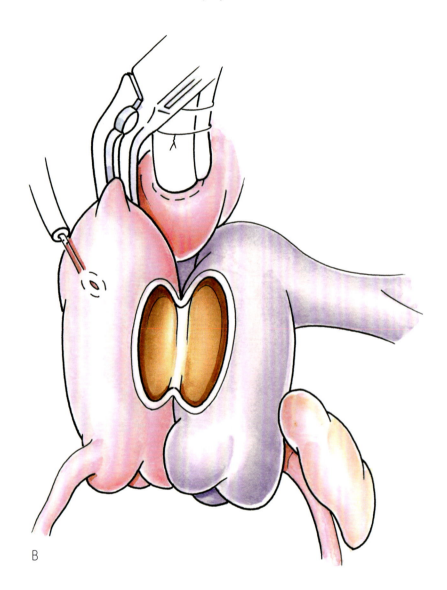

B

图 6-3 (续)

C. 选择大小合适的补片, 嵌入主 - 肺动脉窗。补片材料建议使用 ePTFE 补片, 其柔软、结实, 一般不会钙化。用 5-0 Prolene 缝线。后壁将补片直接和没有切开的主 - 肺动脉窗后缘连续缝合。

Figure 6-3 cont'd

C. A patch of appropriate size is selected for embedding in the aorto-pulmonary window. An ePTFE patch is recommended, for it is soft and strong and generally will not be calcified. 5-0 Prolene suture is usually applied. On the posterior wall, the patch is directly sutured to the intact posterior rim of the aorto-pulmonary window.

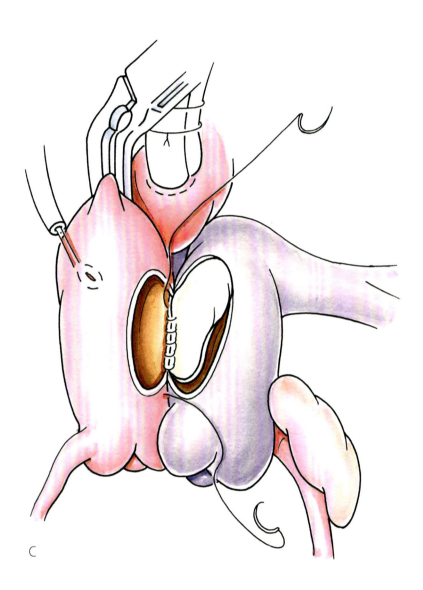

C

图 6-3（续）

图 6-3 cont'd

D. 前壁缝线从缺损上下两端把补片缝在主 - 肺动脉窗之间。

D. On the anterior wall, the patch is sutured between the aorto-pulmonary window from both the superior and inferior ends of the defect.

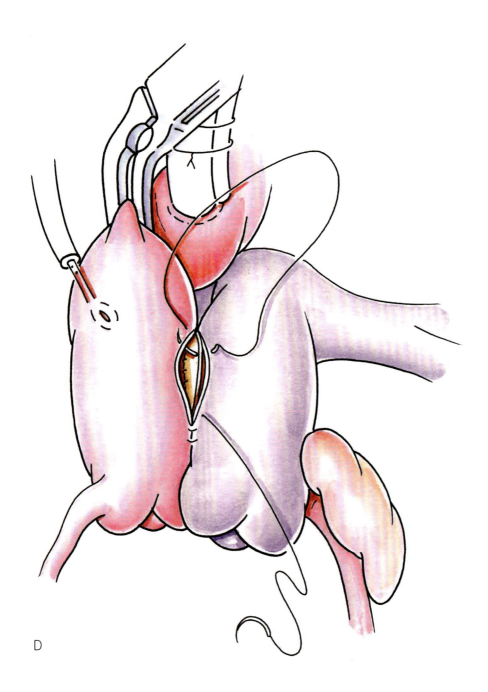

D

（2）经肺动脉切口修补：有主 - 肺动脉窗的患者大多合并肺动脉高压、肺动脉明显增粗。采用经肺动脉切口修补暴露较容易。缺损修补大多应用自身心包补片或牛心包补片，也可应用 ePTFE 补片（图 6-4）。

(2) Transpulmonary incision repair: Most patients with aorto-pulmonary window are complicated with pulmonary hypertension, and their pulmonary arteries are markedly dilated. Therefore, exposure is easier with a transpulmonary artery incision, and most defects are repaired with either a autologous pericardial patch or a bovine pericardial patch. An ePTFE patch is also an alternative (Figure 6-4).

图 6-4　**经肺动脉切口修补**
A. 虚线为肺动脉切口示意图。

Figure 6-4　Transpulmonary incision repair
A. The dotted line presents the schematic diagram of pulmonary artery incision.

Continued

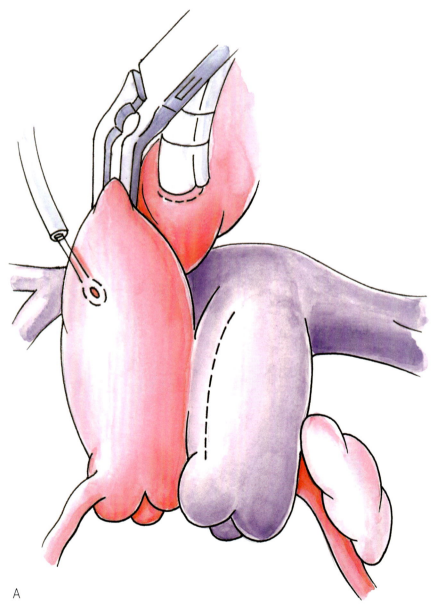

A

图 6-4(续)

Figure 6-4 cont'd

B. 切开主肺动脉,暴露缺损。

B. The main pulmonary artery is incised to expose the defect.

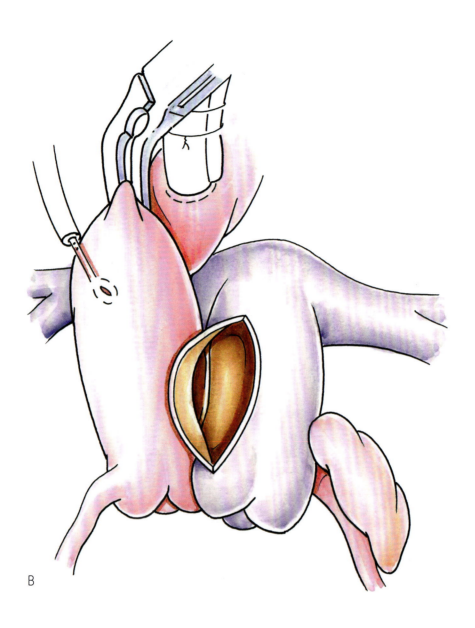

B

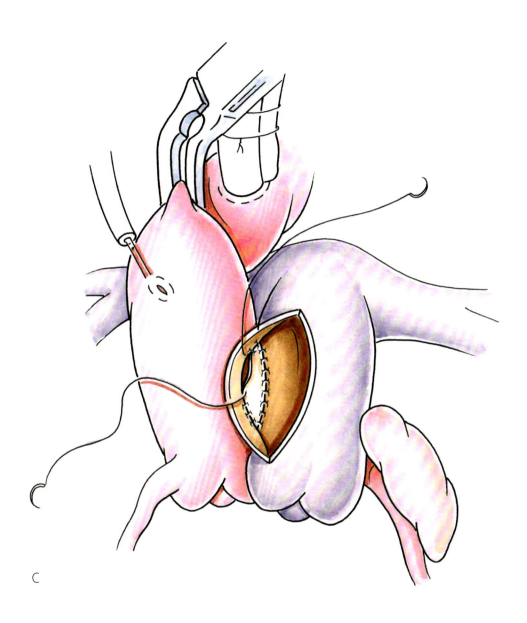

C

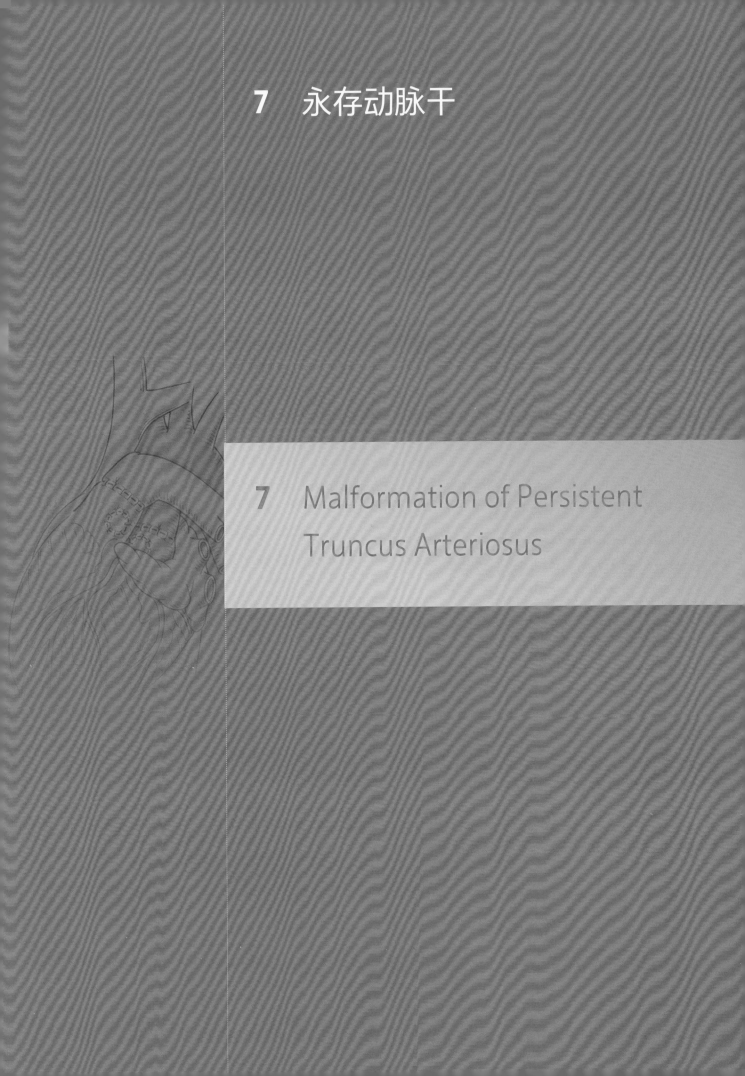

7 永存动脉干

7 Malformation of Persistent Truncus Arteriosus

永存动脉干是指单一的动脉干起源于心脏，骑跨在室间隔上，同时发出体循环和肺循环两组大血管。根据著名病理学家 Van Praagh 分型，共分四大类。

Persistent truncus arteriosus (PTA) is a single arterial trunk that arises from the heart, straddles the ventricular septum, and supplies both the systemic and the pulmonary circulations. There are four categories, according to the famous pathologist Van Praagh.

一、解剖分型

I. Anatomical Typing

永存动脉干分型（图 7-1）。

Anatomic classification of PTA (Figure 7-1).

图 7-1　永存动脉干分型
A. A1 型：较小的主肺动脉起源于动脉干的左侧壁。

Figure 7-1　Anatomic classification of PTA
A. Type A1: A small main pulmonary artery arises from the left wall of the truncus arteriosus.

Continued

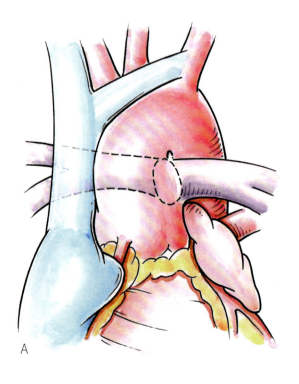
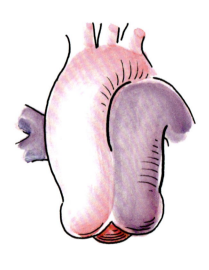

图 7-1（续）

B. A2 型：肺动脉各自起源动脉干侧壁，相互靠近，也可能相距较远。

C. A3 型：单根肺动脉起源于动脉干侧壁，左右相距较远，通过动脉导管或侧支血管向对侧供血。

Figure 7-1 cont'd

B. Type A2: Pulmonary arteries originate from the lateral walls of the truncus arteriosus, which are closely positioned to each other or widely separated from each other.

C. Type A3: A single pulmonary artery which is widely separated from the other one origins from the lateral wall of the truncus arteriosus with either a ductus or collateral vessel supplying the contralateral side.

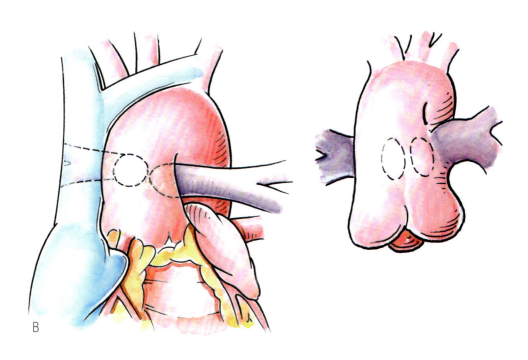

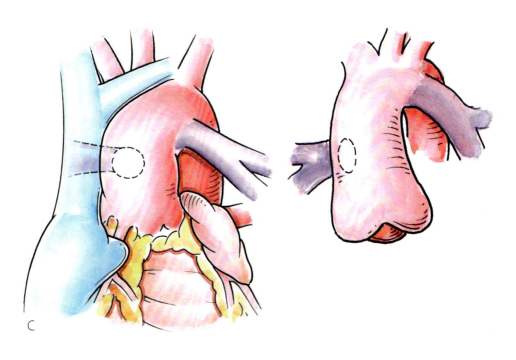

图 7-1（续）

Figure 7-1 cont'd

D. A4 型：永存动脉干主动脉弓离断。

D. Type A4: Truncus arteriosus with an interrupted aortic arch.

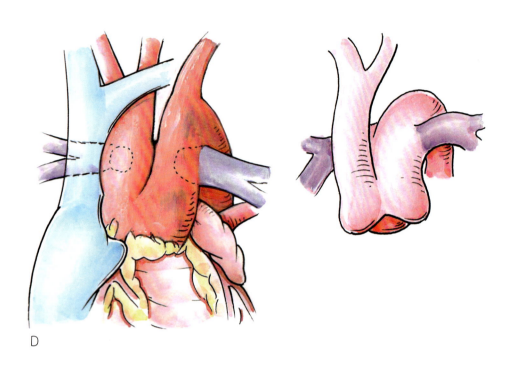

D

二、手术方法

II. Surgical Methods

1. 心肺转流术建立方法 通常采用主动脉高位插管。主动脉阻断钳也要尽量高位，这样有足够空间做肺动脉离断和主动脉重建手术。心肺转流术前必须先将主肺动脉或左右肺动脉圈套收紧，避免灌注肺（图 7-2）。

1. Methods for cardiopulmonary bypass High aortic cannulation is used to establish the cardiopulmonary bypass. The aortic blocking clamps should also be placed as high as possible, allowing adequate space for pulmonary artery detachment and aortic reconstruction. Before cardiopulmonary bypass, the main pulmonary artery or the left and right pulmonary arteries must be tightly constricted to avoid perfusion of the lungs (Figure 7-2).

图 7-2　心肺转流术建立方法　　　　　Figure 7-2　Methods for cardiopulmonary bypass

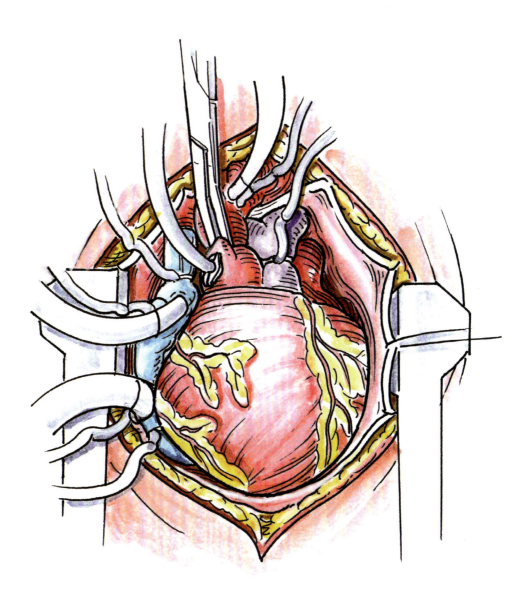

2. 肺动脉直接下拉重建右心室流出道（图 7-3）

2. Reconstruction of right ventricular outflow tract by direct pulling down pulmonary artery (Figure 7-3)

图 7-3　肺动脉直接下拉重建右心室流出道

A. 将肺动脉从升主动脉上离断，用心包补片（自体心包或牛心包补片）将主动脉上缺口关闭。

Figure 7-3　Reconstruction of right ventricular outflow tract by direct pulling down pulmonary artery

A. The pulmonary artery is separated from the ascending aorta, and the supra-aortic defect is closed with a pericardial patch (autologous pericardial or bovine pericardial patch).

Continued

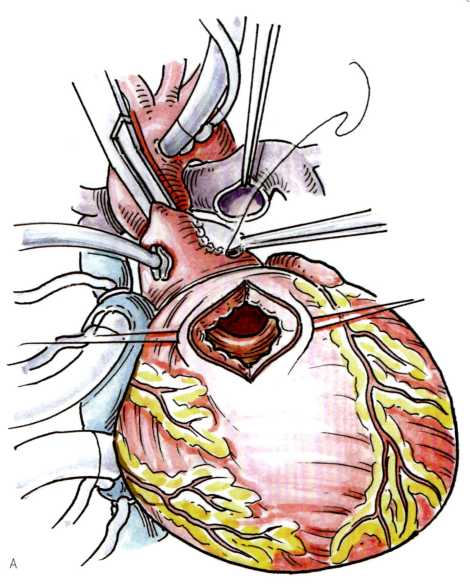

A

图 7-3（续）

B. 经右心室流出道切口用心包补片关闭室间隔缺损。

Figure 7-3 cont'd

B. The ventricular septal defect is closed with a pericardial patch through the right ventricular outflow tract incision.

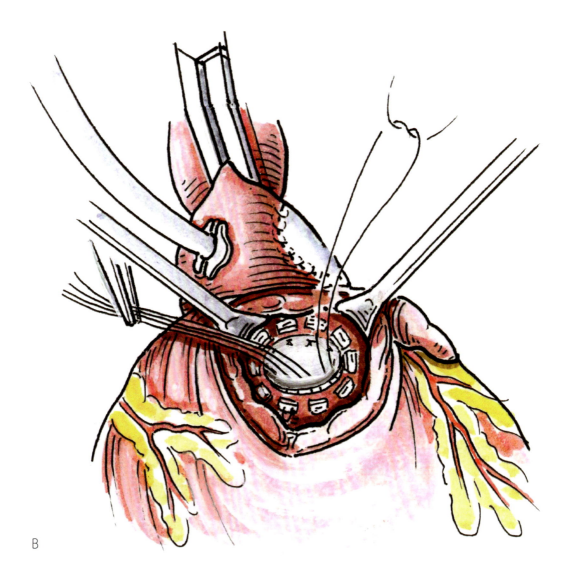

B

图 7-3（续）

Figure 7-3 cont'd

C. 将肺动脉远端充分游离后直接下拉，直接吻合后壁与右心室切口。

C. The distal pulmonary artery is sufficiently freed and directly pulled down, and the posterior wall is directly anastomosed to the right ventricular incision.

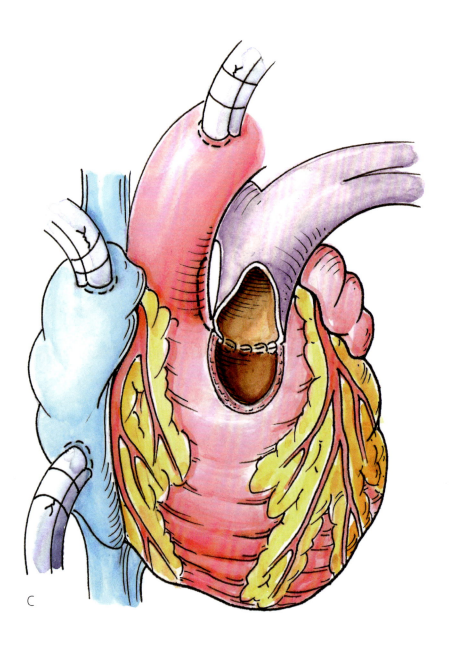

C

图 7-3（续）

D. 用心包补片扩大前壁，补片上可用未固定的自体心包或 ePTFE 薄膜做个单瓣。

Figure 7-3 cont'd

D. The anterior wall is enlarged with a pericardial patch, and a single valve is created with either an unfixed autologous pericardium or a ePTFE membrane.

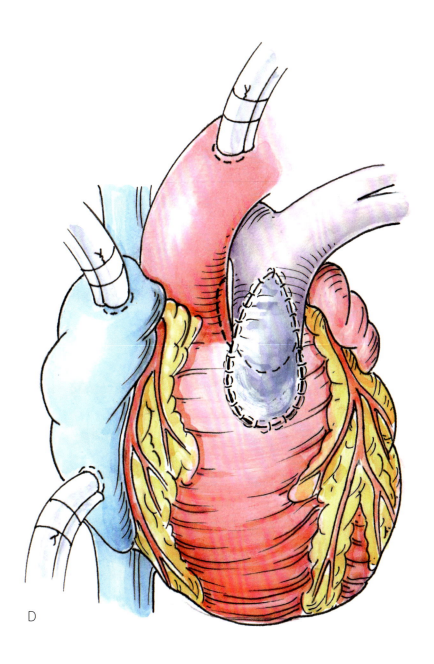

D

3. 用替代材料重建右心室流出道 用同种异体带瓣管道重建肺动脉，采用适当大小的同种异体带瓣管道（图 7-4）。肺动脉材料优于主动脉材料。

3. Reconstruction of the right ventricular outflow tract with alternative materials The valved homograft conduit of appropriate size is adopted to reconstruct the pulmonary artery (Figure 7-4). Pulmonary artery conduit is superior to aortic conduit.

我国因同种异体带瓣管道来源紧缺，目前临床上大多采用异种生物材料，如牛颈静脉管道，或采用 ePTFE 人工血管。管腔内用 ePTFE 薄膜缝制 3 个瓣叶。

Due to the shortage of valved homograft conduit in our country, heterologous biomaterials, such as bovine jugular vein conduit or ePTFE artificial blood vessels, are mostly used in clinical practice at present. Three valve leaflets are sewn with ePTFE membrane in the conduit.

图 7-4　用替代材料重建右心室流出道

A. 将同种异体带瓣管道的远端缝合至左右肺动脉汇合处。近端将瓣环的后 1/3 直接缝合到右心室切口上缘。

Figure 7-4　Reconstruction of the right ventricular outflow tract with alternative materials

A. The distal end of the valved homograft conduit is anastomosed to the right and left pulmonary arteries confluence. On the proximal end, one-third of the annulus is proximally anastomosed to the upper edge of the right ventricular incision.

Continued

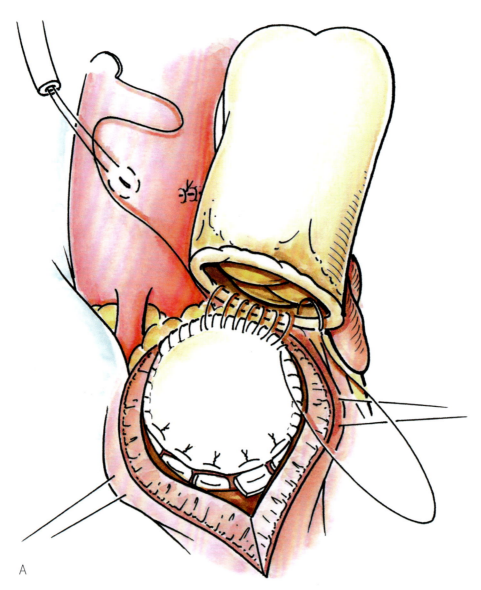

A

图 7-4（续）

B. 前壁取心包补片或 ePTFE 补片剪成"盾牌状"直接将带瓣管道前壁和右心室切口缝合。

Figure 7-4 cont'd

B. Shield-shaped pericardial patch or ePTFE patch is used to connect the anterior wall of the valved homograft conduit and the right ventricular incision.

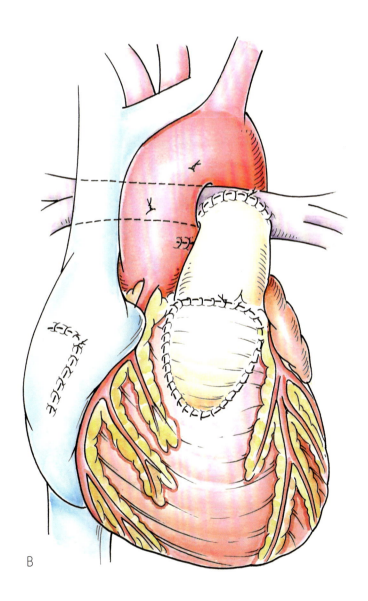

B

4. 永存动脉干合并主动脉弓中断手术方法　这类手术中心肺转流术通常采取深低温、低流量、脑灌注的方法。转流前需将左右肺动脉分别圈套控制（图 7-5）。长段的主动脉中断手术方法将在第九章中介绍。

4. Repair of PTA with interrupted aortic arch　This type of surgery is usually performed under cardiopulmonary bypass with deep hypothermia, low flow, and cerebral perfusion. Before the start of bypass, the bilateral pulmonary arteries must be constricted separately (Figure 7-5). The surgical approach to the long aortic interruption will be described in Chapter 9.

图 7-5　**永存动脉干合并主动脉弓中断手术方法**

A. 体外转流后先充分游离松解主动脉和肺动脉组织。图中虚线表示需做切口的位置。

Figure 7-5　Repair of PTA with interrupted aortic arch

A. After extracorporeal bypass is established, the aorta and pulmonary artery tissues are fully freed. The dotted liney in the figure indicates the location of the incision to be made.

Continued

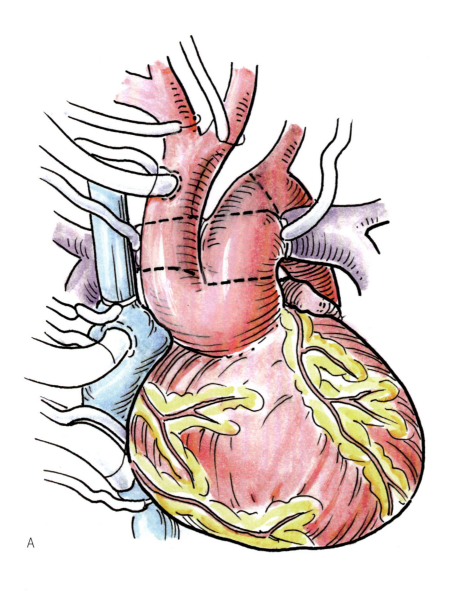

A

图 7-5（续）

B. 将主动脉弓降部直接上拉与升主动脉侧壁做端侧吻合，再将肺动脉做Lecompte 手术换位。用带瓣管道重建肺动脉和右心室连接。

Figure 7-5 cont'd

B. An end-to-side anastomosis is made between the descending part of the interrupted aortic arch and the lateral wall of the ascending aorta. The Lecompte procedure is used for the transposition of the pulmonary artery. The right ventricular to pulmonary artery continuity is reestablished with a valved conduit.

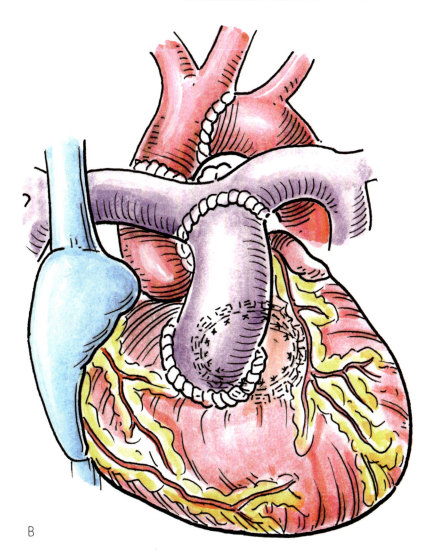

B

5. 主动脉共干瓣膜的修复　永存动脉干的患者常常会合并有不同程度的共干瓣膜反流。对共干瓣膜重度反流的患者必须做瓣叶整形，包括对瓣叶悬吊、切除瓣叶的冗长部分、瓣环交界成形术等（图 7-6）。对大年龄患儿可做主动脉瓣置换。

5. Repair of co-truncated aortic valve　Patients with malformation of PTA often present with varying degrees of truncal valve regurgitation. Valvuloplasty is necessary for patients with severe truncal valve regurgitation. Valve repair consists of cusps suspension, resection of redundant portions of the cusps, annuloplasty of the commissures and so on (Figure 7-6). Aortic valve replacement may be performed in elder children.

图 7-6　**主动脉共干瓣膜的修复**
A. 瓣叶切除和瓣环重建：先将升主动脉横断，显示关闭不全的四叶化动脉干瓣膜，通常会有一个瓣叶明显小。

Figure 7-6　Repair of co-truncated aortic valve
A. Leaflet excision and annular remodeling: After the ascending aorta is transected, the incompetent quadricuspid truncal valve is exposed. One leaflet is usually significantly smaller.

Continued

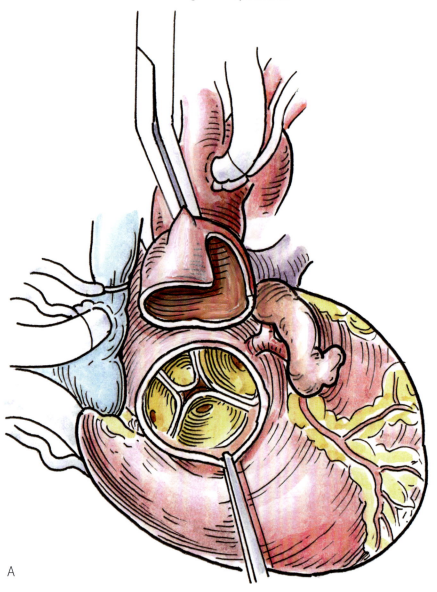

A

图 7-6（续）　　　　　　　　　Figure 7-6 cont'd

B、C. 将该瓣叶切除。　　　　　B, C. This small leaflet is excised.

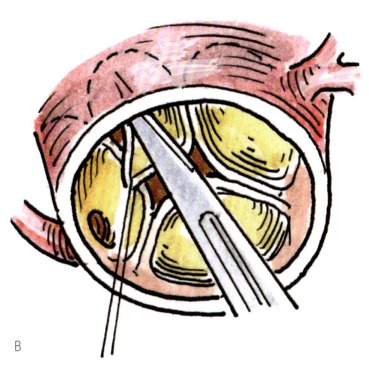

B

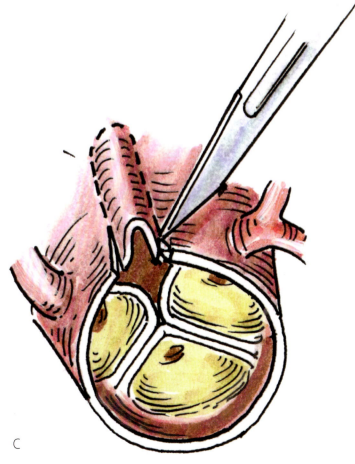

C

图 7-6（续）

D、E. 使用带垫片加强线来收紧瓣环，并将其余瓣膜对合形成一个新的主动脉瓣。

Figure 7-6 cont'd

D, E. The annulus is tightened by using pledget-supported sutures, and the remaining leaflets are aligned and remodeled into a new aortic valve.

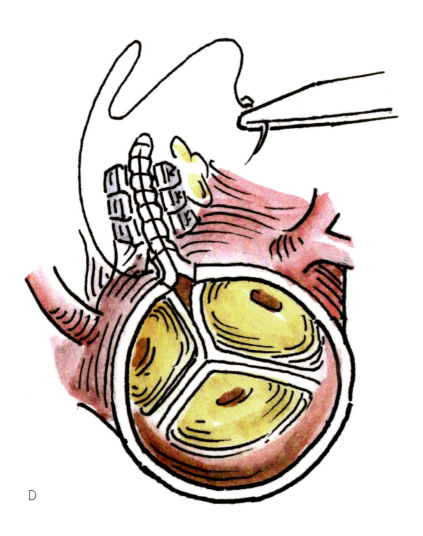

D

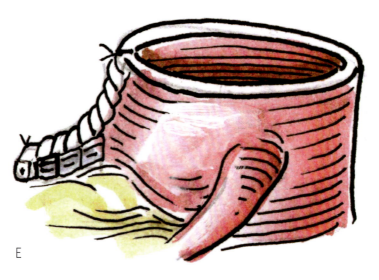

E

图 7-6（续）

Figure 7-6 cont'd

F. 若病变的瓣叶正好靠近冠状动脉开口，则需将冠状动脉开口纽扣状取下，切除病变瓣叶。

F. If the prolapsed leaflet is occasionally located near the coronary sinus, the coronary button should be removed from the affected sinus, and the prolapsed leaflet is excised.

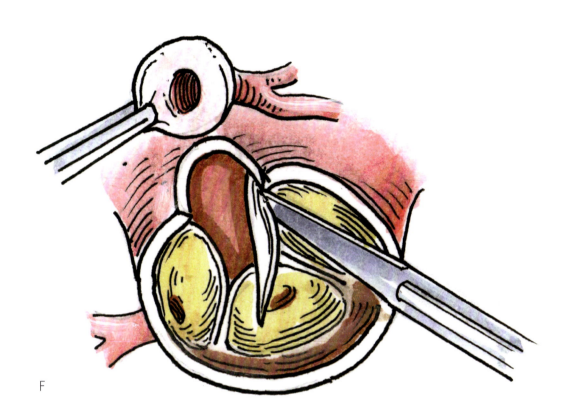

F

图 7-6（续）

G、H. 再将瓣环重新对合，并将冠状动脉开口重新种植。

Figure 7-6 cont'd

G, H. Annulus is then retightened, and the coronary artery button is reimplanted.

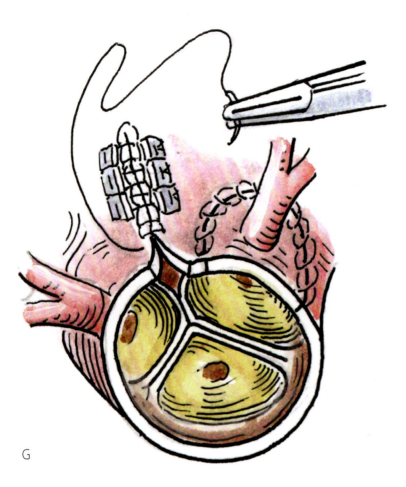

G

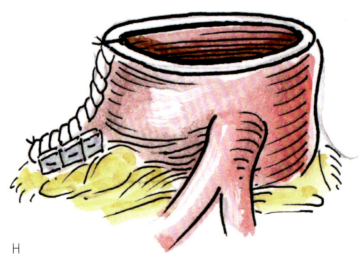

H

8 主动脉缩窄

8 Coarctation of Aorta

主动脉缩窄是一种常见的先天性心脏病,其在所有先天性心脏病中占 5% 至 8%。这类患者通常还合并其他先天性心脏病,最常见的是动脉导管未闭、二叶主动脉瓣、室间隔缺损和二尖瓣畸形。

Coarctation of aorta is a common type of congenital heart disease, accounting for 5% to 8% of all cases of congenital heart defect. It is usually complicated with other congenital heart defeats, among which patent ductus arteriosus (PDA), bicuspid aortic valve, ventricular septal defect, and mitral valve malformations are the most common types.

一、解剖分型

I. Anatomical Typing

婴儿型或"导管前型"主动脉缩窄,其缩窄发生在动脉导管前端,降主动脉的血流主要靠开放的动脉导管来供应。

For the preductal (or infantile) type of coarctation of aorta, there is narrowing at the anterior end of the ductus arteriosus, with the PDA supplying blood flow to the descending aorta.

成人型或"导管后型"主动脉弓缩窄,其缩窄部位实际上位于动脉导管旁,通常较局限,并有一个明显的厚嵴突入管腔,动脉导管关闭或成为韧带(图 8-1)。

For the postductal (or adult) type of coarctation of aorta, the narrowing is near the ductus arteriosus, which usually has a limited size and has a prominent ridge protruding into the lumen of the aorta. In this case, ductus arteriosus will either close or become a ligament (Figure 8-1).

图 8-1　主动脉缩窄的解剖分型
A. 婴儿型或"导管前型"。B. 成人型或
"导管后型"。

Figure 8-1　Anatomical typing of coarctation of aorta
A. Preductal (or infantile) type. B. Postductal (or adult) type.

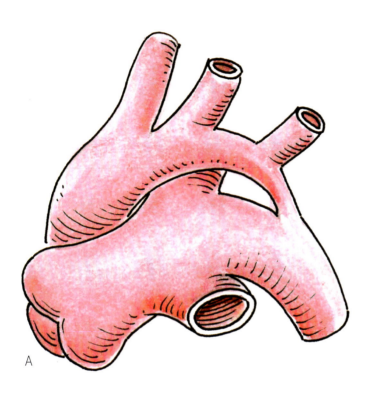

A

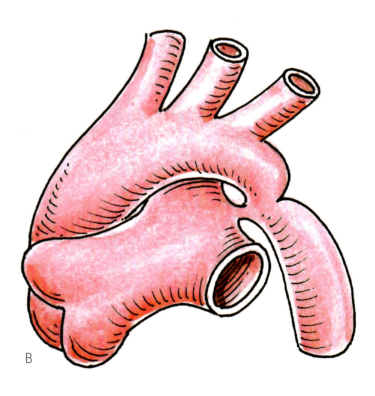

B

二、手术方法

Ⅱ. Surgical Methods

1. 缩窄段切除端端吻合 手术径路：左后外侧第 3 或第 4 肋间进胸。对于合并心脏畸形需要同时治疗心内畸形的患者，则需胸骨正中切口径路（图 8-2）。

1. Resection of the coarctated segment with end-to-end anastomosis Left posterior thoracotomy is usually carried out through the third or fourth intercostal spaces. If patients with coarctation of aorta have other cardiac malformations requiring surgery, a median sternotomy will be indicated (Figure 8-2).

图 8-2 缩窄段切除端端吻合
A. 暴露缩窄段后，充分游离。在缩窄段的两端分别上阻断钳。

Figure 8-2 Resection of the coarctated segment with end-to-end anastomosis

A. After exposure and full dissociation, coarctation forceps are placed on both sides of the coarctated segments.

Continued

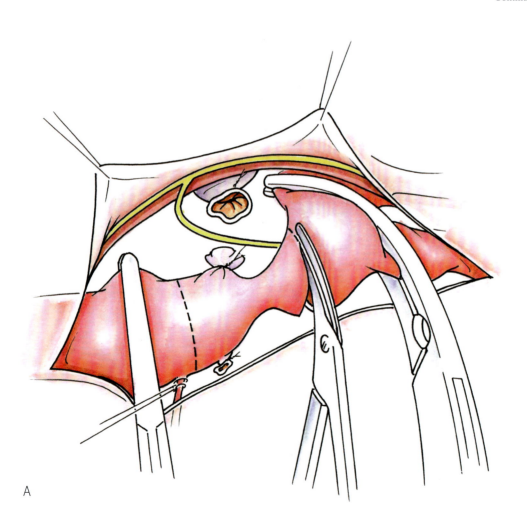

A

图 8-2（续）

B. PDA 结扎切断，将缩窄段切除。

Figure 8-2 cont'd

B. PDA is ligated and divided, and the narrowed segment is excised.

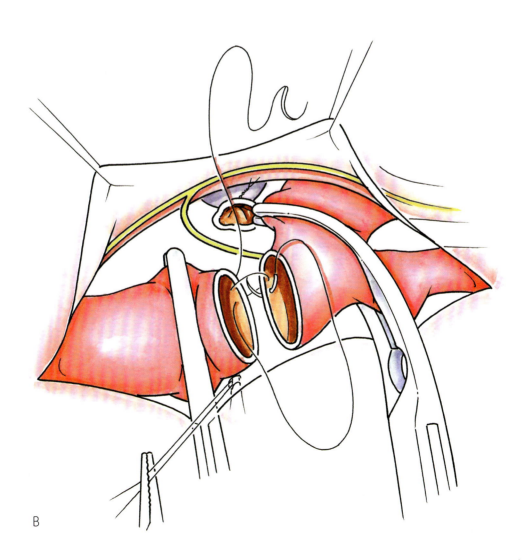

B

图 8-2（续）

C. 取 6-0 或 7-0 Prolene 缝线做连续
缝合。

Figure 8-2 cont'd

C. The anastomosis is constructed with a continuous
suture (6-0 or 7-0 Prolene suture).

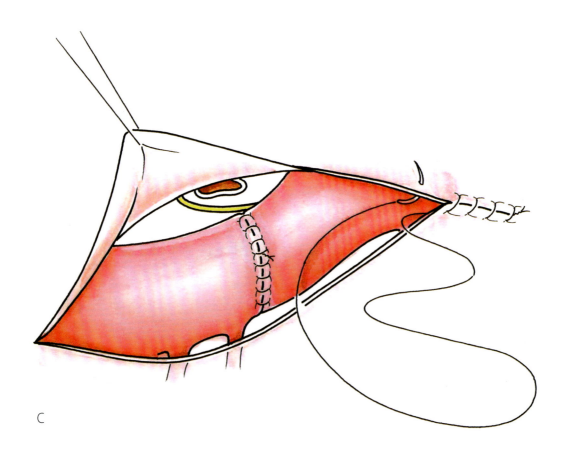

C

图 8-2（续）

D. 对缩窄段相对较长、主动脉弓发育稍差的患儿，也可在主动脉弓下端做一延长切口，虚线显示要切除的区域及延长部位。

Figure 8-2 cont'd

D. For children with a relatively long coarctated segment and hypogenetic aortic arch, an extended incision can also be made at the lower end of the aortic arch. The dotted line shows the area to be resected and extended.

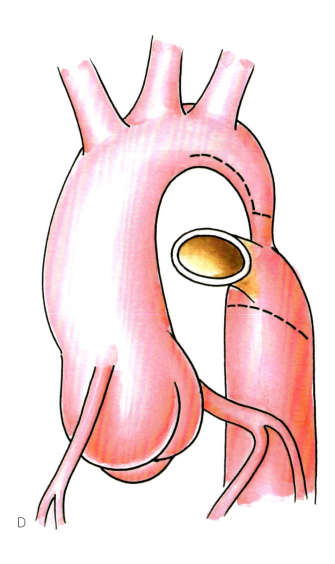

D

图 8-2 (续)

Figure 8-2 cont'd

E~G. 主动脉弓与主动脉远端做端端吻合。

E-G. An end-to-end anastomosis is constructed to connect the distal aorta.

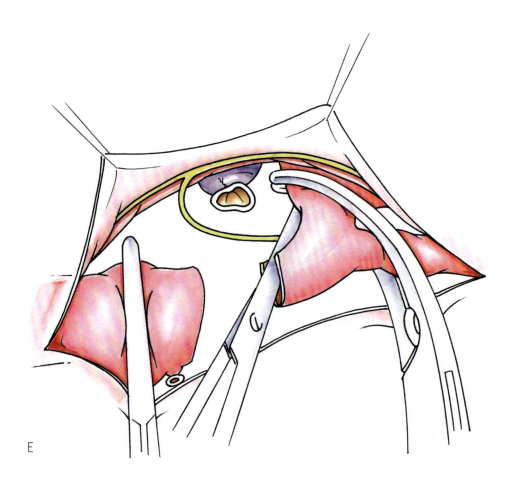

E

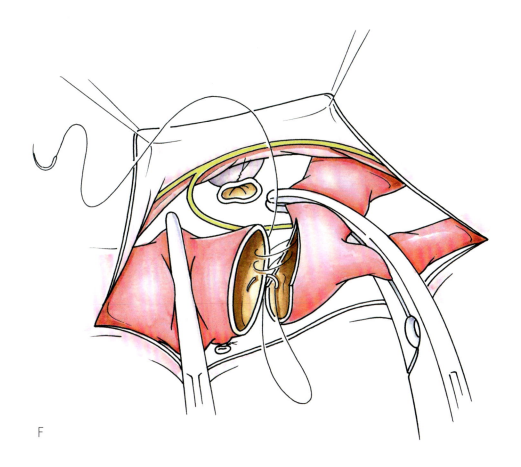

F

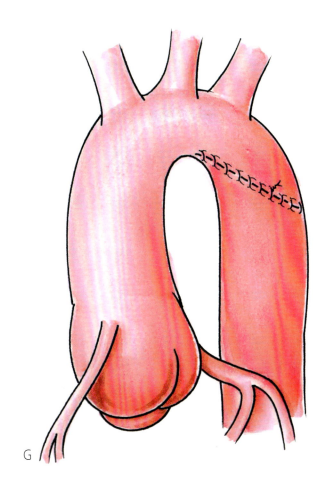

G

2. 补片扩大主动脉成形术　对于较年长、狭窄段较长的患儿可采用补片扩大主动脉方法，手术径路同缩窄段切除端端吻合。根据狭窄段长度取生物补片（同种异体补片、自身心包、牛心包）或人工材料［聚四氟乙烯（PTFE）管道］，剪成相应大小补片做连续缝合修补（图 8-3）。

2. Patch aortoplasty　In elder children with longer coarctated segments, patch aortoplasty may be indicated. With the same entry into the chest as that in the first method, a biological patch (homograft patch, autologous pericardial or bovine pericardial patch) or synthetic patch (polytetrafluoroethylene [PTFE] tube) is selected based on the length of the coarctated segment and cut into the corresponding size for completing running suture of the aorta (Figure 8-3).

图 8-3　补片扩大主动脉成形术
A. 虚线显示需要切开的部位。

Figure 8-3　Patch Aortoplasty
A. The dotted line shows the incision position.

Continued

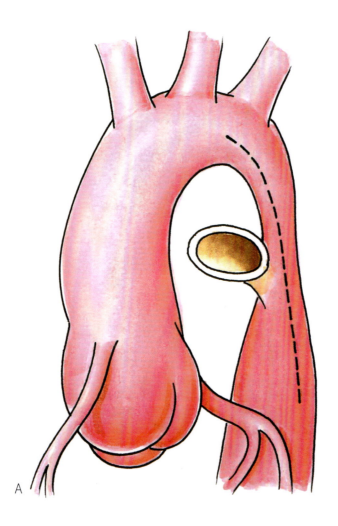

A

图 8-3（续）

B. 根据狭窄段长度剪成相应大小补片。

Figure 8-3 cont'd

B. A patch is cut into the corresponding size based on the length of the coarctated segment.

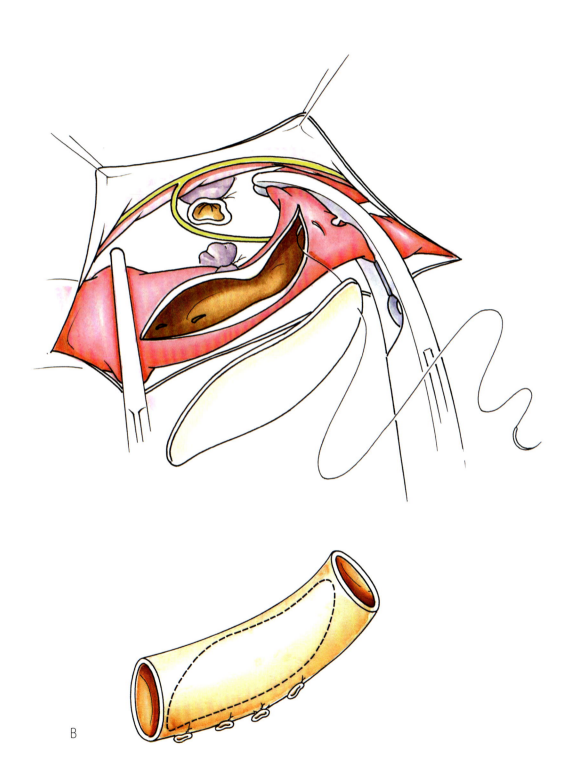

B

图 8-3 (续)

Figure 8-3 cont'd

C. 连续缝合修补。

C. Running suture of the aorta.

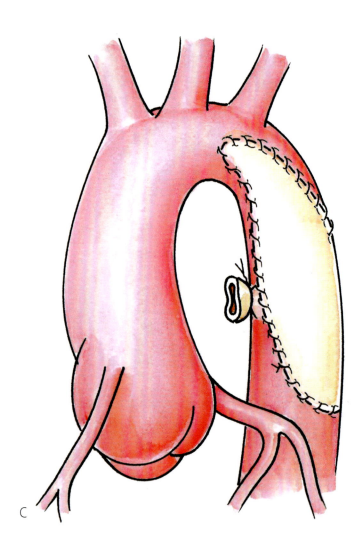

C

3. 左锁骨下动脉切开主动脉成形术 对合并主动脉弓略有狭窄患儿,可采用此方法(图 8-4)。

3. Left subclavian artery incision and aortoplasty Left subclavian artery incision and aortoplasty can be used in children with minor aortic arch stenosis (Figure 8-4).

图 8-4 **左锁骨下动脉切开主动脉成形术**
A. 将左锁骨下动脉先离断,分别将主动脉弓上缘和左锁骨下动脉右侧壁剪开。

Figure 8-4 Subclavian artery incision and aortoplasty
A. Transect the left subclavian artery first and then incise the right wall of the left subclavian artery from the upper edge of the aortic arch.

Continued

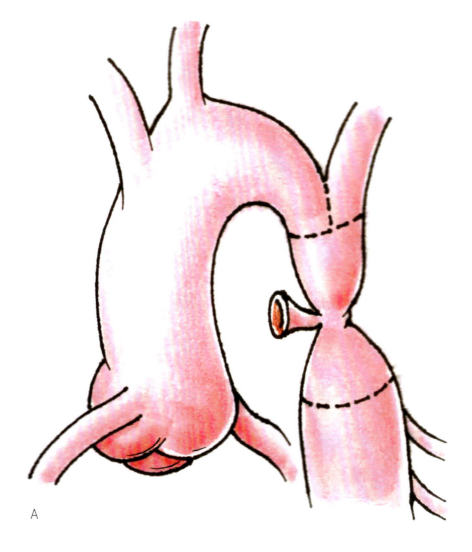

A

图 8-4（续）

Figure 8-4 cont'd

B. 将剪开之血管先做侧侧吻合。

B. Following a side-to-side anastomosis.

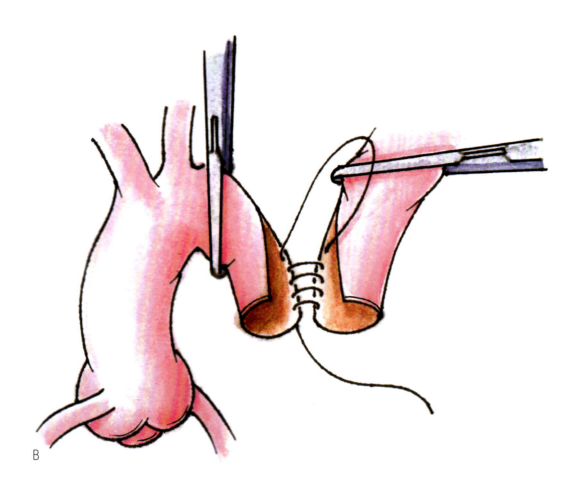

B

图 8-4（续）

C、D. 与降主动脉做端端吻合。

Figure 8-4 cont'd

C, D. The incised vessels are end-to-end anastomosed to the descending aorta.

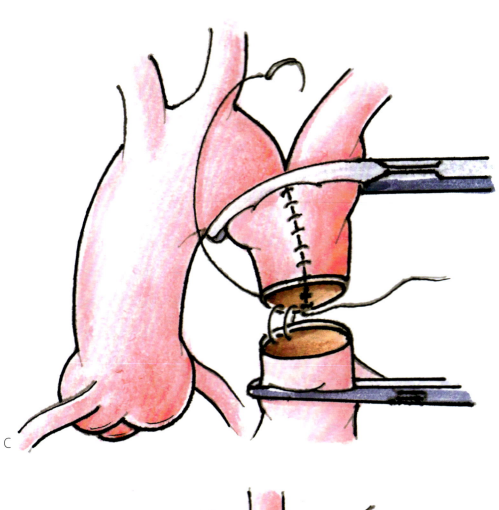

C

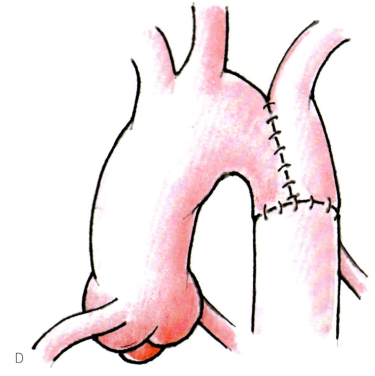

D

4. 左锁骨下动脉下翻主动脉成形术　左锁骨下动脉下翻主动脉成形术的优点包括增加吻合口的生长潜能、避免因使用异体血管材料而导致的术后再狭窄等。但缺点也很明显的，结扎了一条正常的血管，导致左臂血供受影响，现在该方法已很少用了（图 8-5）。

4. Left subclavian flap aortoplasty　Left subclavian flap aortoplasty offers advantages such as increased anastomotic growth ability and the low possibility of restenosis owing to the use of autogenous vascularized materials. However, it fell out of favor now because the ligation of a normal vessel affects the blood supply to the left arm (Figure 8-5).

图 8-5　**左锁骨下动脉下翻主动脉成形术**

A. 结扎左锁骨下动脉，沿虚线所示做切口。

Figure 8-5　Subclavian flap aortoplasty
A. Ligate the left subclavian artery and make an incision along the dotted line.

Continued

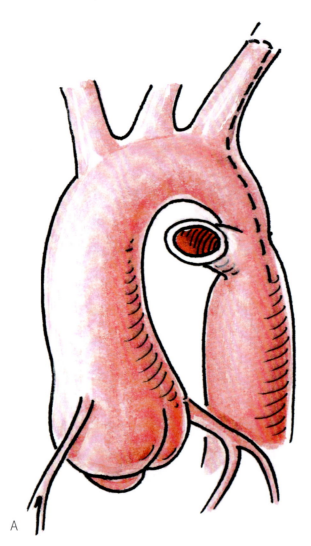

A

图 8-5 (续)
B. 左锁骨下动脉下翻。

Figure 8-5 cont'd
B. The flap of left subclavian artery.

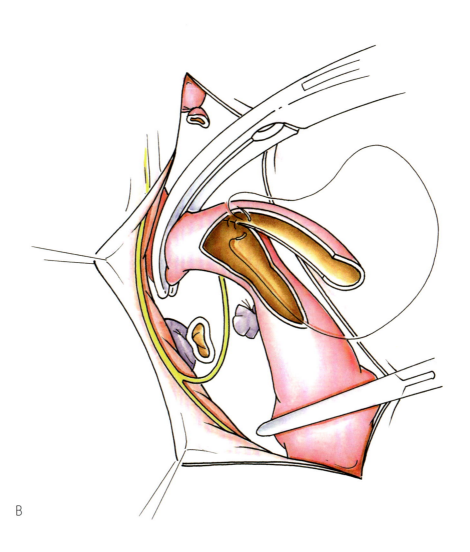

B

图 8-5（续）
C. 连续缝合，主动脉弓成型。

Figure 8-5 cont'd
C. Running suture of the aorta, aortoplasty completed.

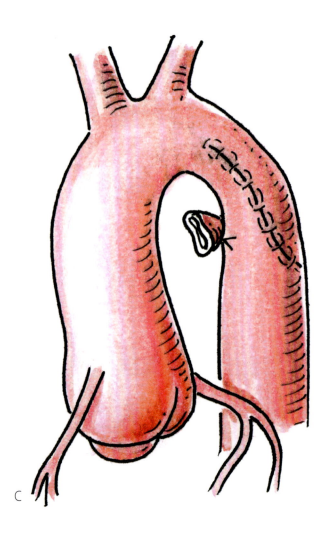

5. 人工血管替换 此方法一般选择年龄在大于十岁、狭窄段超过 3cm 的患儿(图 8-6)。

5. Artificial blood vessel replacement Blood vessel replacement is usually applied to children aged over ten years and with coarctated segments longer than 3 cm (Figure 8-6).

图 8-6 人工血管替换
A. 左侧第 4 肋间隙进胸暴露较清楚。

Figure 8-6 Artificial blood vessel replacement
A. Clear exposure can be achieved by an entry into the chest through the fourth intercostal space.

Continued

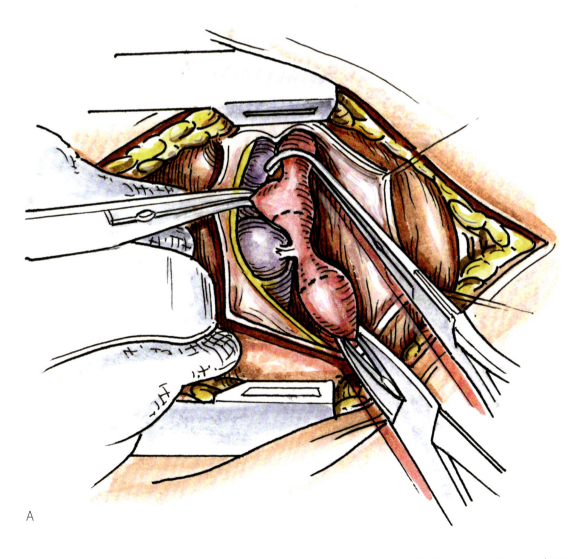

A

图 8-6（续）

Figure 8-6 cont'd

B. 将狭窄的主动脉段切除。

B. The narrowed aortic segment is excised.

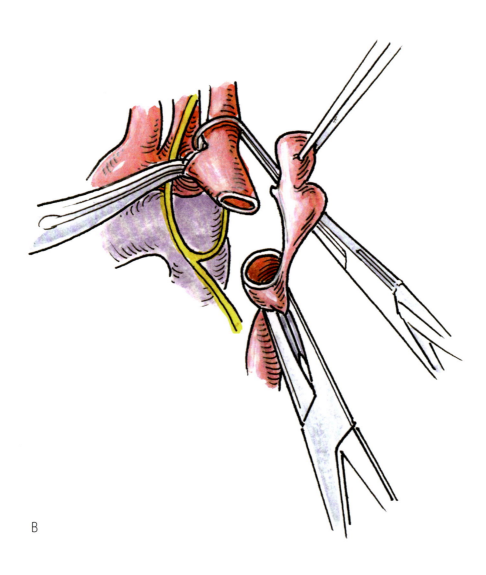

B

图 8-6（续）   Figure 8-6 cont'd

C、D. 取相应大小人工血管（ePTFE 血管），通常直径要大于 16mm，分别做两端的吻合。

C, D. An artificial vessel (ePTFE vessel) of appropriate size, generally greater than 16mm in diameter, is anastomosed to both ends of the aorta.

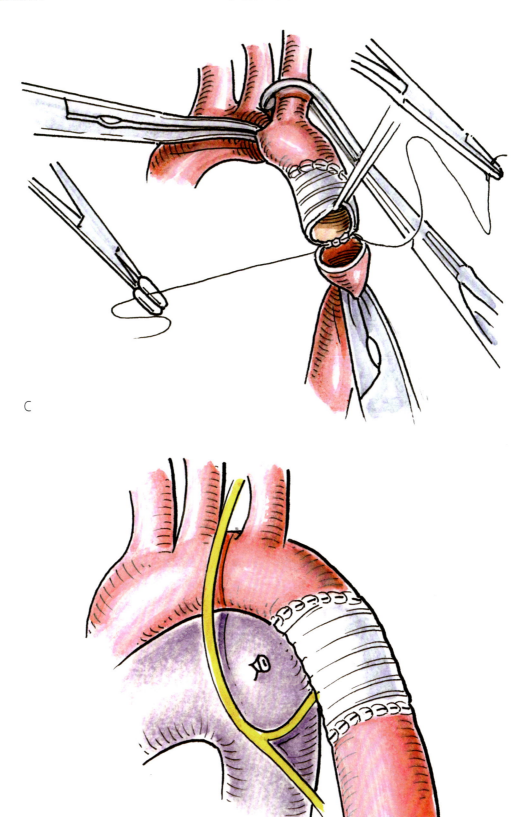

C

D

6. 主动脉弓发育不良　有些主动脉缩窄患者可合并有主动脉弓发育不良。可在处理主动脉缩窄同时扩大主动脉弓部（图 8-7）。

6. Aortic arch hypoplasia　Some patients with coarctation may have aortic arch dysplasia. The aortic arch can be enlarged simultaneously during the repair of coarctation of the aorta (Figure 8-7).

图 8-7　伴主动脉弓发育不良成形术
A. 在深低温脑灌注条件下，将狭窄主动脉剪开并延长至降主动脉。

Figure 8-7　Patch aortoplasty with aortic arch dysplasia
A. The stenotic aorta can be cut open and extended to the descending aorta under deep hypothermic cerebral perfusion.

Continued

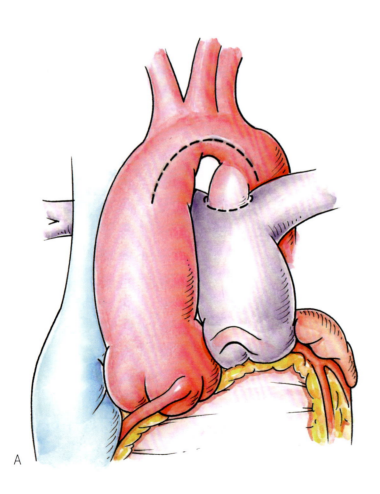

图 8-7（续）

B. 用牛心包补片缝合肺动脉端 PDA
开口。

Figure 8-7 cont'd

B. Bovine pericardial patch is used to close the PDA opening
at the pulmonary artery end.

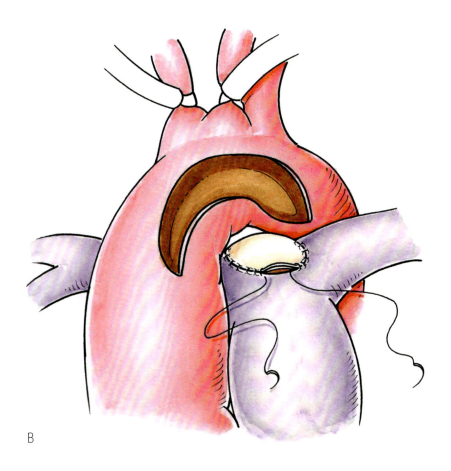

B

图 8-7（续）
C、D. 用牛心包补片缝合扩大主动脉弓部。

Figure 8-7 cont'd
C, D. Bovine pericardial patch is used to enlarge the aortic arch.

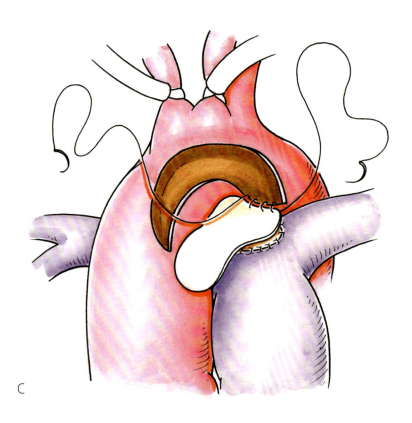

C

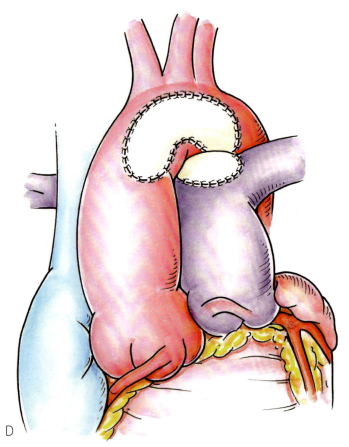

D

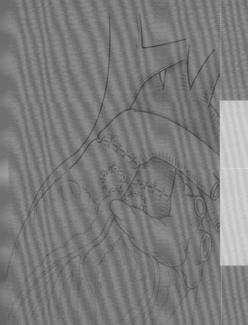

9 主动脉弓中断

9 Interrupted Aortic Arch

主动脉弓中断是一类较罕见畸形，在先天性心脏病畸形中占1.5%。除了必须有动脉导管未闭之外，最常见合并有房间隔缺损、室间隔缺损、左心室流出道的梗阻性病变。

Interrupted aortic arch (IAA) is a rare type of deformity and can only be found in 1.5% of patients with congenital heart diseases. In addition to patent ductus arteriosus (PDA), it is commonly associated with obstructive lesions such as the atrial septal defect (ASD), ventricular septal defect (VSD), and left ventricular outflow tract obstruction (LVOTO).

一、解剖分型

I. Anatomical Typing

根据主动脉中断的位置分为三类（图 9-1）。

There are three categories according to the location of aortic interruption (Figure 9-1).

图 9-1　主动脉弓中断解剖分型
A. A 型：中断在左锁骨下动脉的远端。

Figure 9-1　Anatomical typing of aortic interruption
A. Type A: The interruption occurs distal to the left subclavian arterial origin.

Continued

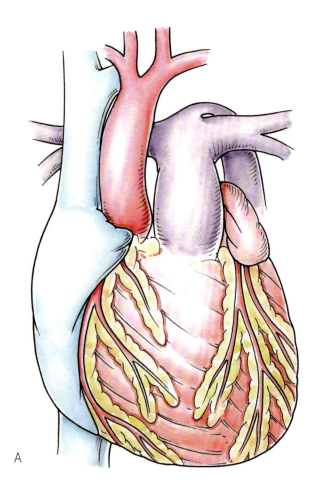

A

图 9-1 (续)

B. B 型 : 中断在左锁骨下动脉和左颈总
动脉之间。

Figure 9-1 cont'd

B. Type B: The interruption occurs between the left common carotid artery and the left subclavian artery.

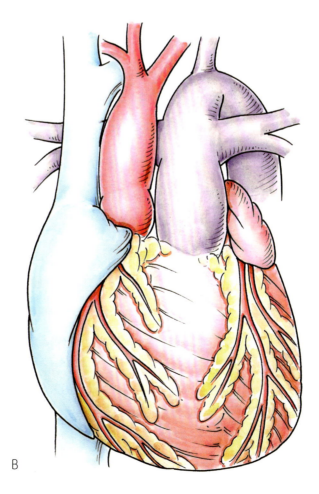

B

图 9-1（续）
C. C 型：中断在左颈总动脉和无名动脉之间，约 10% 的患者会合并有永存动脉干。

Figure 9-1 cont'd
C. Type C: The interruption occurs between the left common carotid and innominate artery, and approximately 10% of the patients will have persistent truncus arteriosus (PTA).

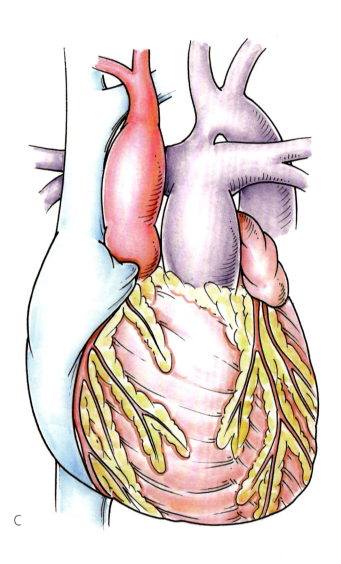

C

二、手术方法

Ⅱ. Surgical Methods

1. 特殊心肺转流术建立方法　主动脉弓中断大多在新生儿期手术，正确的插管是手术的一个重要部分。主动脉灌注管需要两根，用"Y"管连接。一根插在升主动脉偏右侧缘，另一根插在主肺动脉，最好

1. Special cardiopulmonary bypass method　Most cases of the IAA should have surgeries in the neonatal period. The proper cannulation is a crucial part of the procedure. Two aortic cannulae are employed and connected with a "Y" tube, with one inserted into the right edge of the ascending aorta and the

通过 PDA 直接进入降主动脉。在转流开始前将动脉导管近端圈套收紧，或将左右肺动脉圈套控制（图 9-2）。

other into the main pulmonary artery, preferably through the PDA and directly into the descending aorta. Prior to the start of the bypass, either the proximal loop of the ductus arteriosus should be tightened, or the left and right pulmonary artery loop should be controlled (Figure 9-2).

图 9-2　特殊心肺转流术建立方法　　　　Figure 9-2　Special cardiopulmonary bypass method

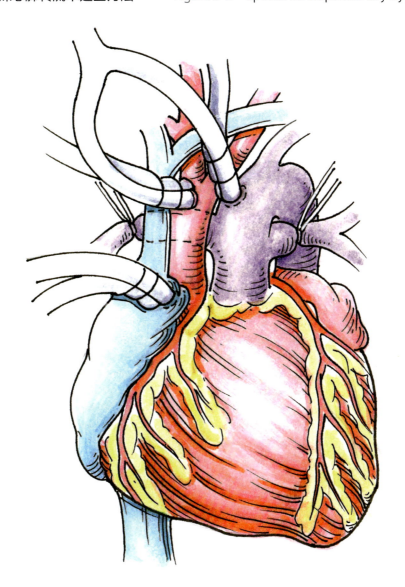

2. 直接端侧吻合　主动脉弓中断位置较近，可充分游离主动脉后做直接端侧吻合（图 9-3）。

2. Direct end-to-side anastomosis　When the two ends of the interrupted aortic arch are close enough, the aortic artery can be dissociated, and direct end-to-side anastomosis can be performed (Figure 9-3).

图 9-3 直接端侧吻合 Figure 9-3 Direct end-to-side anastomosis

图 9-3 直接端侧吻合

A. 连接降主动脉的 PDA 组织必须完全切除。

B. 用自身心包补片将肺动脉切口关闭。

Figure 9-3 Direct end-to-side anastomosis

A. The PDA tissue attached to the descending aorta must be completely excised.

B. The pulmonary artery incision could be closed with an autologous pericardial patch.

Continued

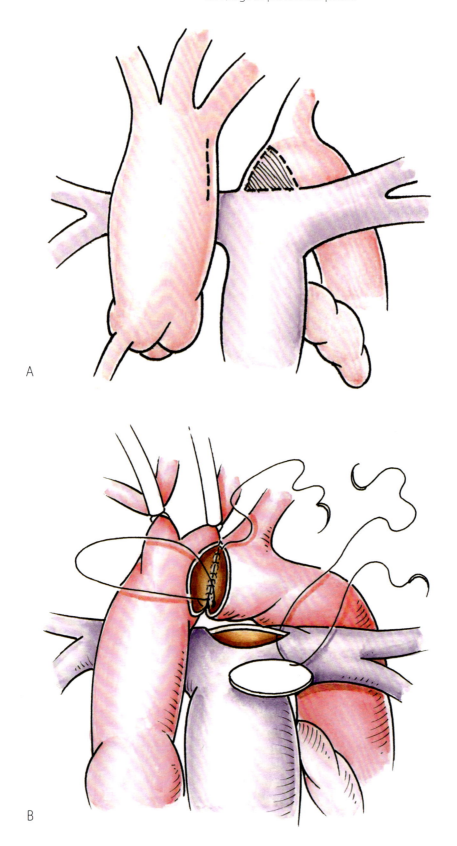

图 9-3（续）

Figure 9-3 cont'd

C. 一般采用 5-0 或 6-0 Prolene 缝线做连续缝合。

D. 若吻合时张力过紧，可将左锁骨下动脉切断松解。

C. 5-0 or 6-0 Prolene sutures may be used for running suture.

D. If the tension is too tight at the time of anastomosis, the left subclavian artery may be dissected free.

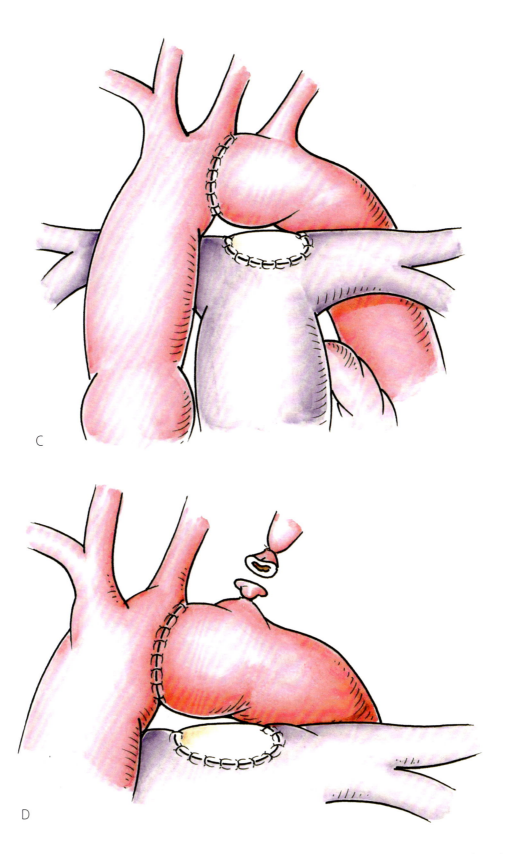

C

D

图 9-3（续）

Figure 9-3 cont'd

E~G. 可在吻合口前壁用心包补片扩大减小吻合口张力。

E-G. A pericardial patch may also be used in the anterior wall of the anastomosis to reduce anastomotic tension.

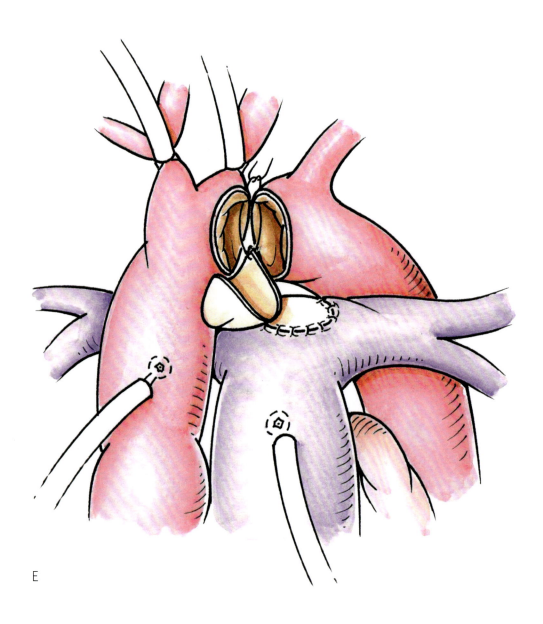

E

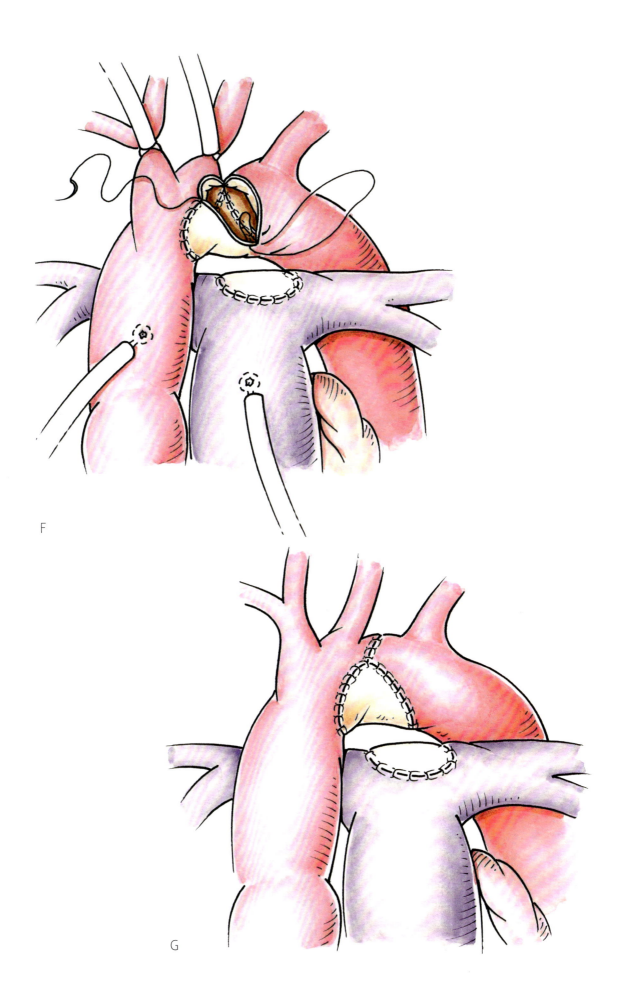

3. 主动脉弓中断合并大动脉转位 这类患者常合并肺动脉高压、主肺动脉严重扩张(图 9-4)。

3. IAA with transposition of great arteries (TGA) Such patients are often complicated with pulmonary hypertension and the severely dilated main pulmonary artery (Figure 9-4).

图 9-4 **主动脉弓中断合并大动脉转位**

A. 手术切口(虚线)。

Figure 9-4　IAA with transposition of great arteries

A. The incision is shown as dotted lines.

Continued

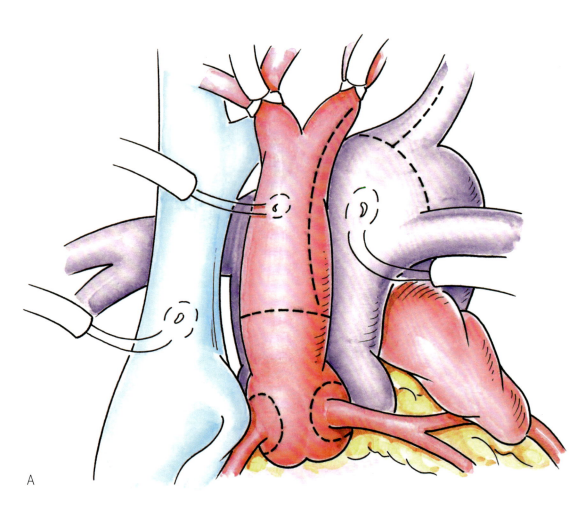

A

图 9-4（续）

B. 大动脉离断，完成冠状动脉移植。

Figure 9-4 cont'd

B. The great arteries are transected, and a coronary artery transplantation is completed.

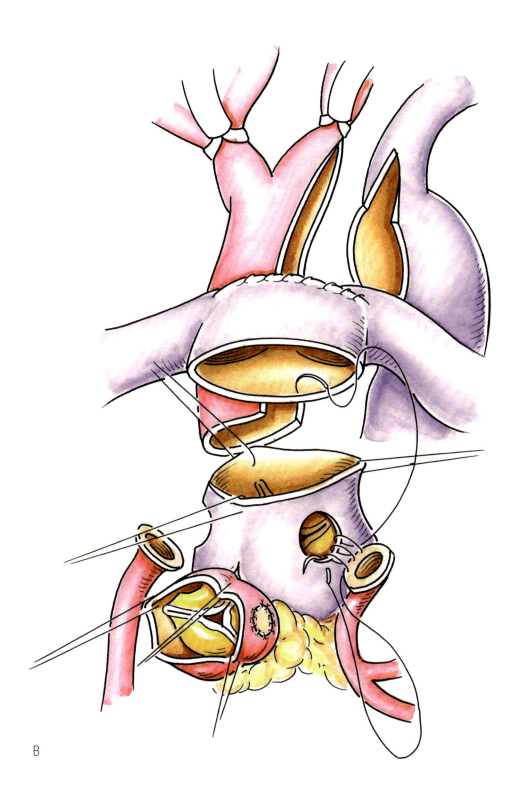

B

图 9-4（续）

C. 远端主动脉弓与升主动脉上端直接吻合，前壁取心包或同种异体补片材料扩大成形，形成新的升主动脉。

Figure 9-4 cont'd

C. The distal aortic arch is anastomosed directly to the upper end of the ascending aorta, and the anterior wall is expanded with pericardial or homograft material to create a new ascending aorta.

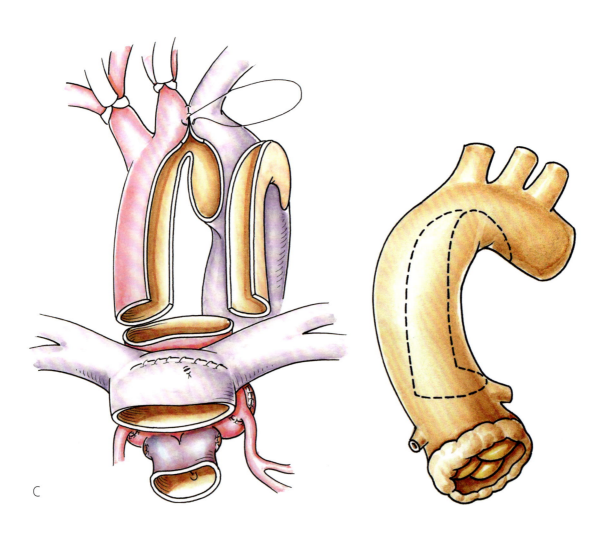

C

图 9-4 (续)

D. 主肺动脉后壁下拉与右室切口上缘直接缝合,前壁取心包补片扩大,必要时可做一个单瓣。

Figure 9-4 cont'd

D. The posterior wall of the main pulmonary artery is pulled down and sutured directly to the upper rim of the right ventricular incision. The pericardial patch in the anterior wall is employed to expand the anterior wall, and a single valve can be made if necessary.

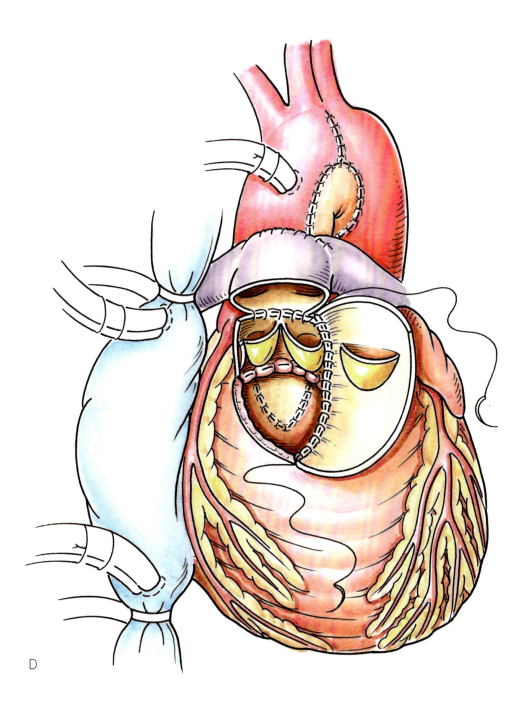

D

4. 主动脉弓中断合并永存动脉干
短段的主动脉弓中断合并永存动脉干手术方法在第七章已有描述。此处重点介绍长段的主动脉弓中断手术方法（图 9-5）。

4. IAA with persistent truncus arteriosus (PTA)
Surgical techniques for short-segment interruption of the aortic arch with PTA have been described in Chapter 7. Here, the focus is on the surgical approach to the long segment interruption of the arch (Figure 9-5).

图 9-5　主动脉弓中断合并永存动脉干
A. 先从升主动脉上将主肺动脉和左右肺动脉离断并充分游离。将 PDA 切断，并切除 PDA 组织直至正常降主动脉组织，如图虚线所示。

Figure 9-5　IAA with PTA
A. The main pulmonary artery and left and right pulmonary arteries are transected from the ascending aorta and fully detached. The PDA is cut, and the PDA tissue is excised until the excision reaches normal descending aorta tissue, as shown in the dotted line.

Continued

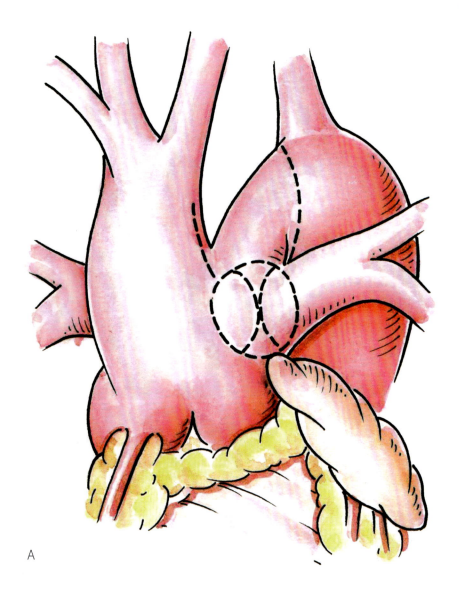

A

图 9-5（续）

B. 这类患者升主动脉与降主动脉之间距离较远,大多须接一段人工血管或生物材料(自体心包或牛心包制成的血管)。

Figure 9-5 cont'd

B. In such patients, since the distance between the ascending aorta and the descending aorta is remote, in most cases, it requires a segment of the artificial vessel or biomaterial (blood vessels made from autologous pericardium or bovine pericardium).

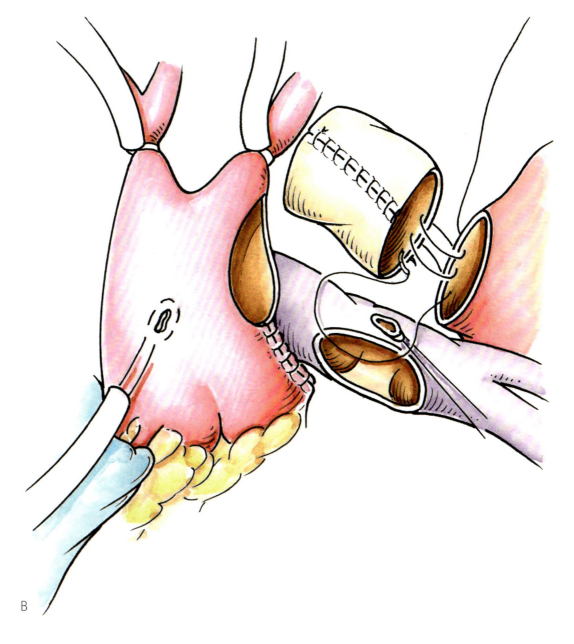

B

图 9-5（续）

Figure 9-5 cont'd

C. 用人工补片关闭室间隔缺损。

C. The VSD is closed with an artificial patch.

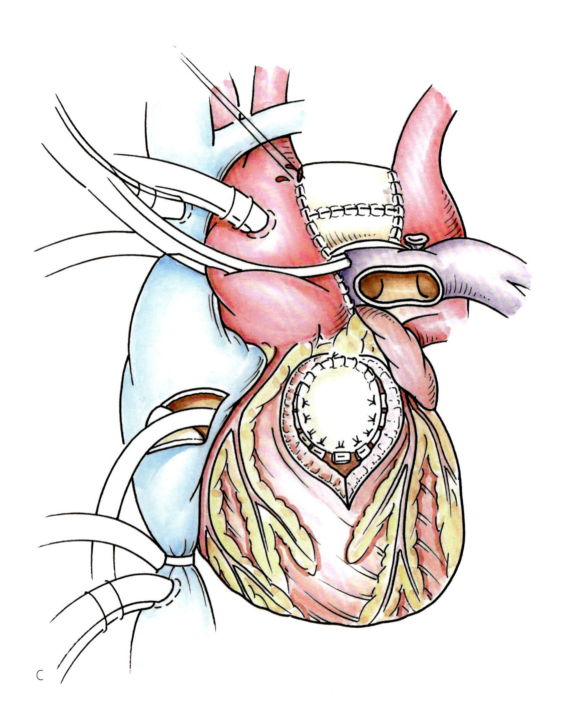

C

图 9-5（续）

D~F. 右心室 - 肺动脉连接大多选用带瓣生物管道和人工管道。

Figure 9-5 cont'd

D-F. The right ventricular-pulmonary artery connections are mostly made with a valved conduit or an artificial conduit.

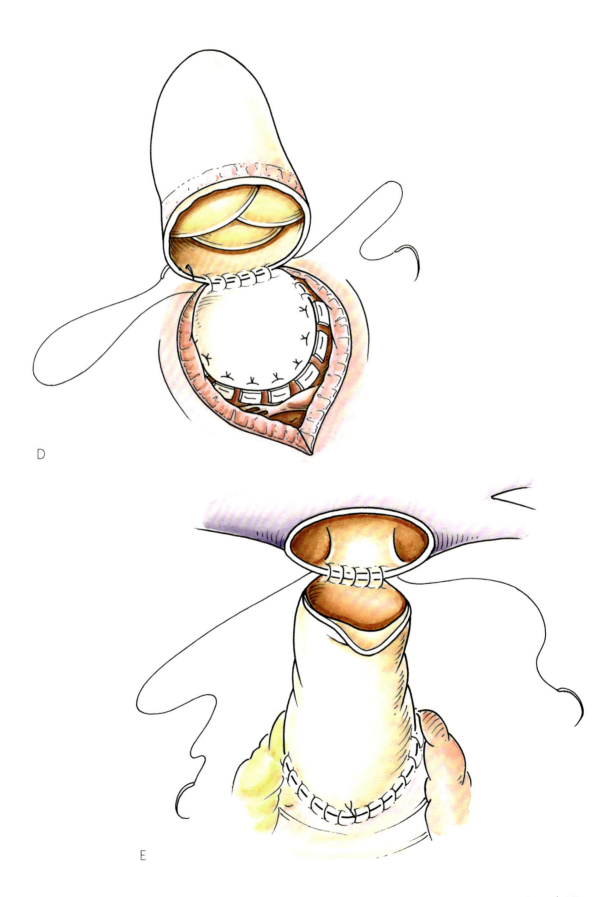

D

E

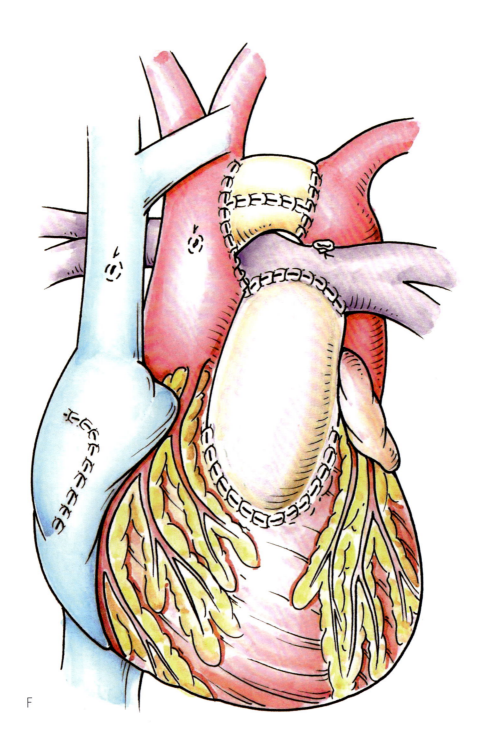

F

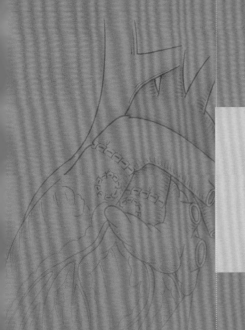

10　血管环和肺动脉吊带

10　Vascular Rings and Pulmonary
Artery Sling

血管环是由于主动脉弓复合体发育异常所致,并可导致气管和/或食管受压。病理分型通常为完全性和部分性血管环两大类。

Vascular ring resulted from abnormal development of the aortic arch complex may cause compression of the trachea or/and esophagus. Based on the pathology, vascular ring are divided into two categories: total and partial vascular rings.

一、解剖分型

I. Anatomical Typing

完全性血管环:①双主动脉弓;②右位主动脉弓合并左位动脉导管韧带。

Total vascular rings: ① Double aortic arch; ② Right-sided aortic arch with left-sided ligamentum arteriosum.

部分性血管环:①无名动脉压迫综合征;②肺动脉吊带;③左主动脉弓伴迷走右锁骨下动脉。

Partial vascular rings: ① Innominate artery compression syndrome; ② Pulmonary artery sling; ③ Left aortic arch with aberrant right subclavian artery.

二、手术方法

II. Surgical Methods

1. 双主动脉弓 包括双弓平衡、右弓优势及左弓优势三类(图10-1)。

1. Double aortic arch Double aortic arch includes three types: balance double arch, dominant right arch, and dominant left arch (Figure 10-1).

图 10-1　双主动脉弓
A. 双弓平衡（A1 横截面，A2 正面）。

Figure 10-1　Double aortic arch
A. Balance double arch (A1 cross-section, A2 front view).

Continued

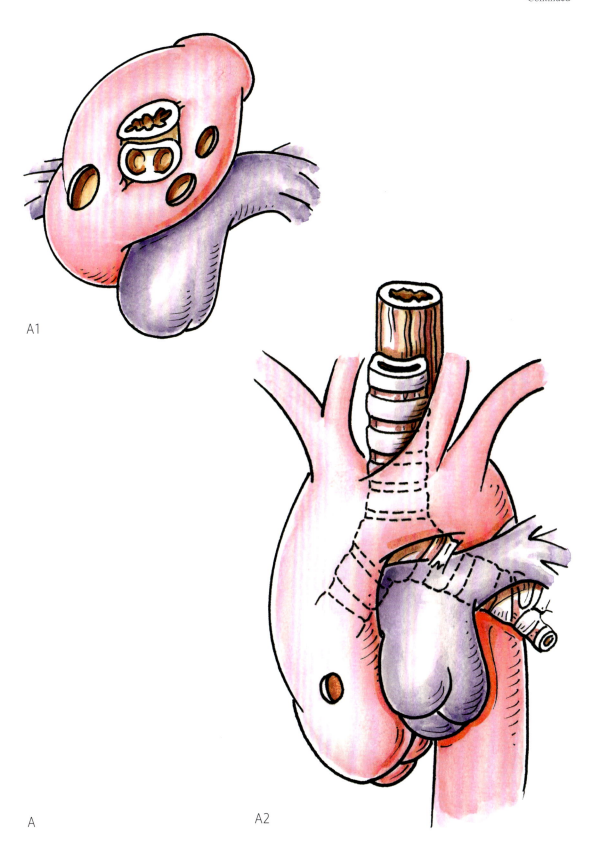

A1

A

A2

图 10-1（续）

Figure 10-1 cont'd

B. 右弓优势（B1 横截面，B2 正面）。

B. Dominant right arch (B1 cross-section, B2 front view).

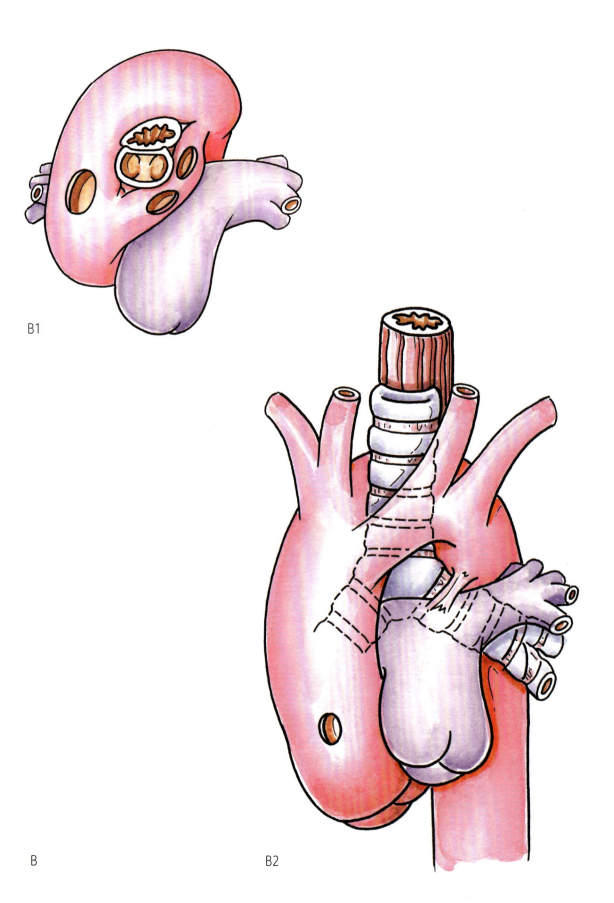

B1

B

B2

图 10-1（续）

C. 左弓优势（C1 横截面，C2 正面）。

Figure 10-1 cont'd

C. Dominant left arch (C1 cross-section, C2 front view).

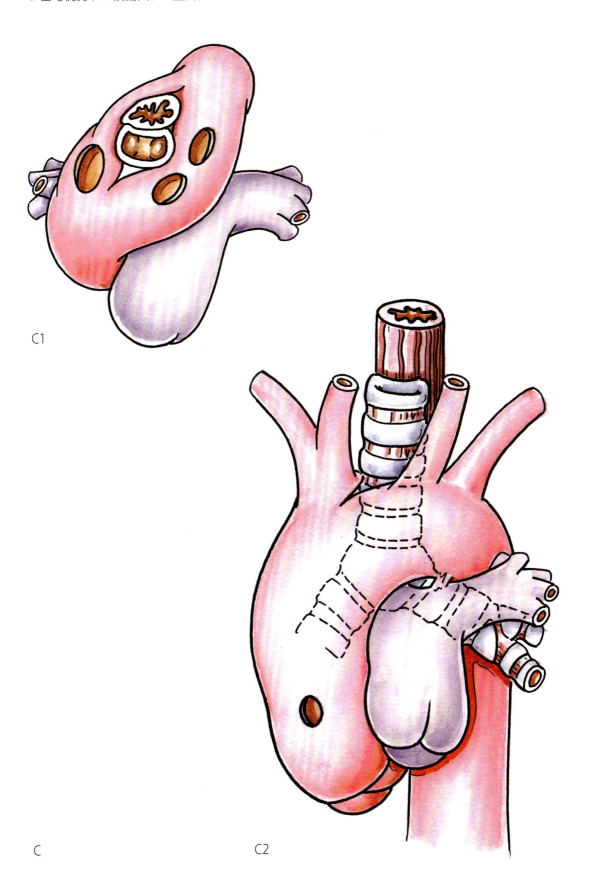

C1

C

C2

图 10-1 (续)

Figure 10-1 cont'd

D. 手术通常采用左后外侧第 4 肋间隙进胸(左弓优势的患者则采用右后外侧切口)。

D. The surgeries are routinely performed through a left posterolateral thoracotomy, and the thorax is accessed through the fourth intercostal space (in patients with left arch dominant, the right posterolateral incision is the approach of choice).

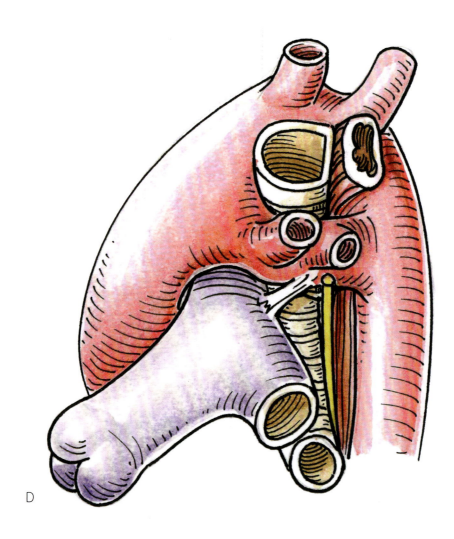

D

图 10-1（续）

E、F. 将次弓在和降主动脉连接处离断缝合。

Figure 10-1 cont'd

E, F. The lesser of two arches is dissected and then sutured at the junction with the descending aorta.

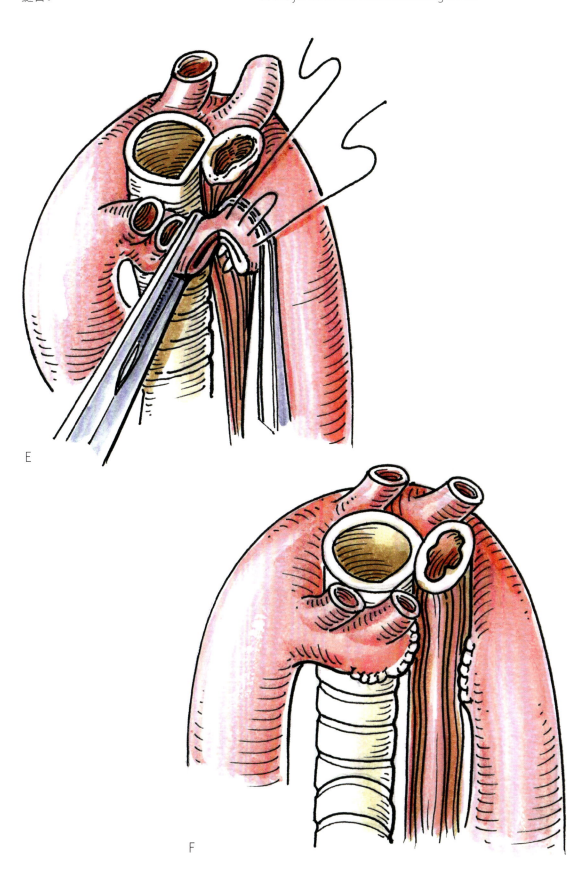

E

F

目前,国内一些医院采用胸腔镜下开展此类手术,创伤小恢复快,取得较好效果。

At present, some hospitals in China use thoracoscopes to carry out this kind of operation, with a small wound, rapid recovery, and good effect.

2. 右位主动脉弓合并左位动脉导管韧带(图 10-2)

2. Right aortic arch with left-sided ligamentum arteriosum (Figure 10-2)

图 10-2　右位主动脉弓合并左位动脉导管韧带

A. 左后外侧第 3 或第 4 肋间隙进胸,分离主动脉弓。

Figure 10-2　Right aortic arch with left arterial ligament
A. Left posterolateral thoracotomy is performed, and the thorax is accessed through the third or fourth intercostal space. The aortic arch is dissected.

Continued

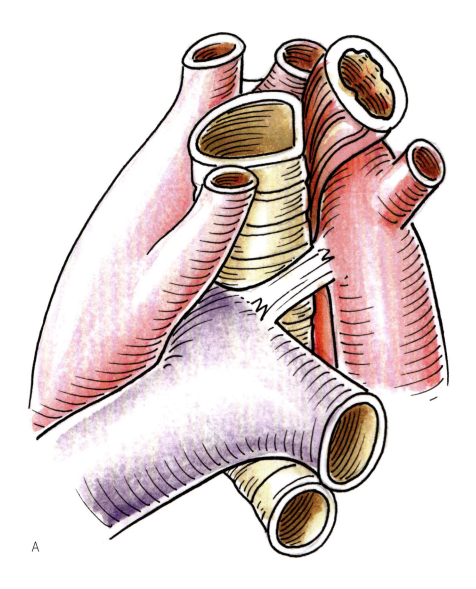

A

图 10-2（续）
B. 鉴别出动脉导管韧带，给予双道结扎并离断。

Figure 10-2 cont'd
B. The ligamentum arteriosum is identified, the ligamentum is doubly ligated and resected.

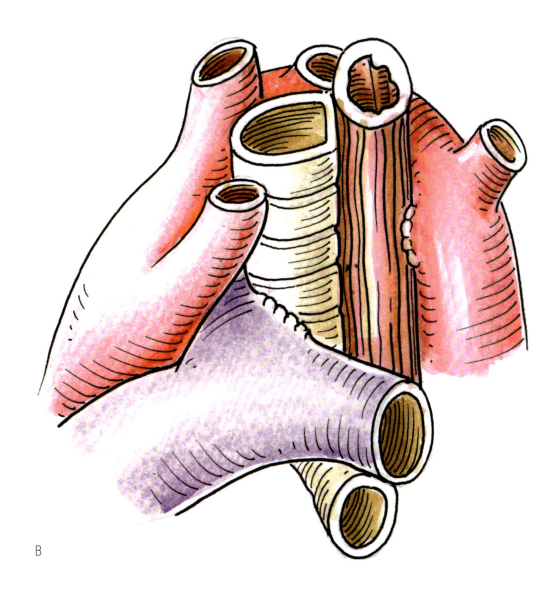

B

图 10-2（续）

C. 这类患者有时会在左锁骨下动脉自降主动脉起始部有 Kommerell 憩室，该憩室增大会造成食管和气管的压迫。

Figure 10-2 cont'd

C. These patients sometimes have Kommerell diverticulum at the origin of the left subclavian artery from the descending aorta. This enlarged diverticulum causes compression of the esophagus and trachea.

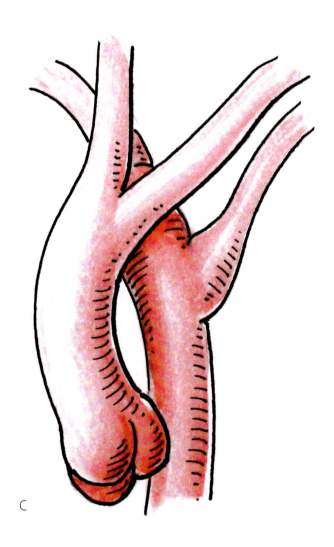

C

图 10-2（续）

Figure 10-2 cont'd

D. 需将憩室和动脉瘤样扩张的部分切除。

D. In this case, the diverticulum and aneurysmal dilatation should be excised.

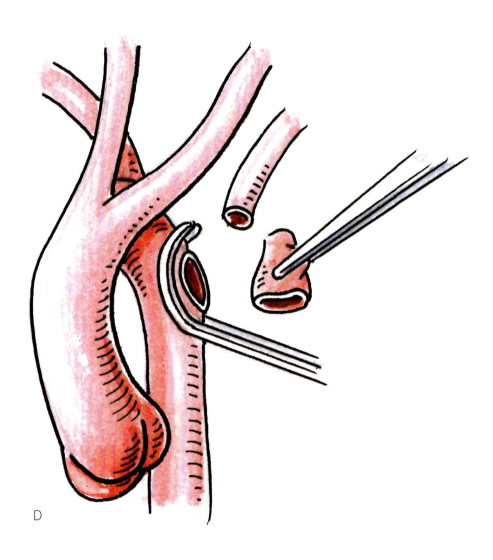

D

图 10-2（续）

E. 将左锁骨下动脉转移至左颈总动脉上。

Figure 10-2 cont'd

E. The left subclavian artery should be transferred to the left common carotid artery.

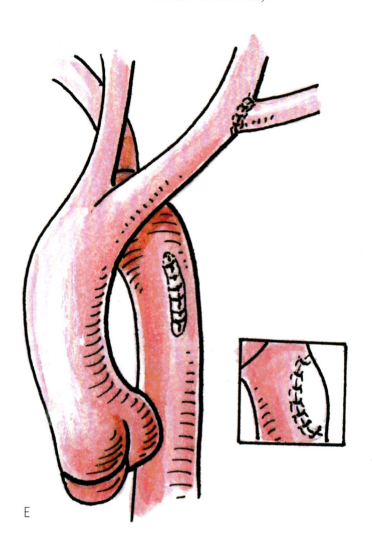

E

3. 无名动脉压迫综合征 通常选择右前侧第 3 肋间隙进胸，便于暴露，需将大部分右侧胸腺组织切除，用带垫片涤纶线将无名动脉固定在胸骨骨膜上，将无名动脉从气管上提起免除压迫。通常需缝合 2~3 针。在悬吊后实施气管镜检查，以确定气管受压解除（图 10-3）。

3. Innominate artery compression syndrome Right anterolateral thoracotomy is usually performed, and exposure is through the third intercostal space. Most of the right thymic tissues need to be excised. The innominate artery is fixed with pledget-supported polyester sutures to the sternum periosteum. The innominate artery is lifted away from the trachea to release pressure. Two or three stitches are routinely required. Tracheoscopy is performed after suspension to confirm the relief of tracheal compression (Figure 10-3).

图 10-3　无名动脉压迫综合征
A. 无名动脉压迫气管。

Figure 10-3　Innominate artery compression syndrome
A. Innominate artery compression of trachea.

Continued

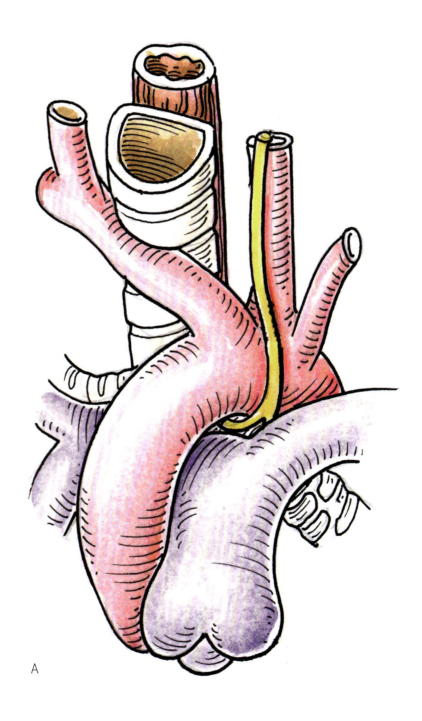

A

图 10-3（续）

B. 将无名动脉从气管上提起，悬吊缝合至胸壁。

Figure 10-3 cont'd

B. The innominate artery lifted from the trachea and fixed with pledget-supported polyester sutures to the sternum periosteum.

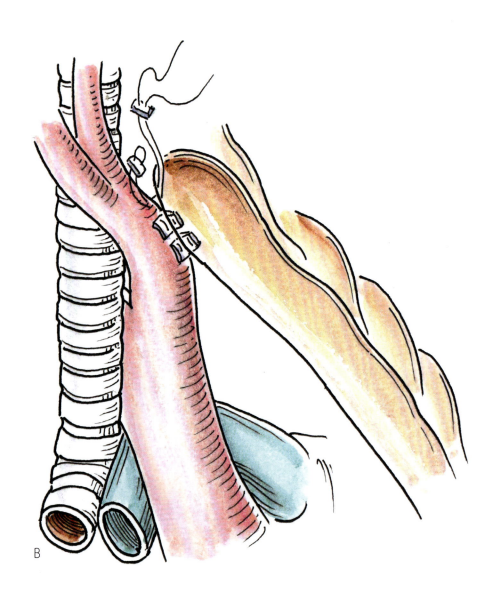

4. 肺动脉吊带　这是一种较为常见的导致气管受压的先天性心脏畸形,其左肺动脉起源于右肺动脉,并绕过右支气管主干,在气管和食管之间走行,形成一个压迫气管的"吊带"。常伴有气管软骨形成O形环(图10-4)。

手术采用胸骨正中切口。心肺转流术下,将左肺动脉完全离断,近端缝合关闭,远端左肺动脉从气管后方游离拖曳出后,重新种植在主肺动脉上。根据气管压迫的程度和患儿的临床症状决定是否需处理狭窄的气管。对短段的气管狭窄可采用狭窄段切除,气管直接端端吻合。对长段伴有O形环的气管狭窄,目前大多采用滑行法气管成形术(Slide技术)。

4. Pulmonary artery sling　Pulmonary artery sling is a relatively common congenital cardiac anomaly resulting in tracheal compression. In pulmonary artery sling, the left pulmonary artery anomalously originates from a normally positioned right pulmonary artery. The left pulmonary artery bypasses the main right bronchus and courses between the trachea and the esophagus, forming a "sling" that compresses the trachea. It is often associated with the formation of an O-shaped ring in the tracheal cartilage (Figure 10-4).

The procedure is performed through a median sternotomy. With the assistance of cardiopulmonary bypass, the left pulmonary artery is completely detached, the proximal part is closed, and the distal part of the left pulmonary artery is freed from the posterior aspect of the trachea and reimplanted into the main pulmonary artery. Whether a stenotic trachea is managed depends on the degree of tracheal compression and the patient's clinical symptoms. For short-segment tracheal stenosis, resection of tracheal stenosis and end-to-end anastomosis are performed. For long-segment tracheal stenosis with an O-shaped ring, a resection technique called "slide tracheoplasty" is often employed.

图 10-4　肺动脉吊带

A. 左肺动脉起源于右肺动脉。

Figure 10-4　Pulmonary artery sling

A. The left pulmonary artery anomalously originates from a normally positioned right pulmonary artery.

Continued

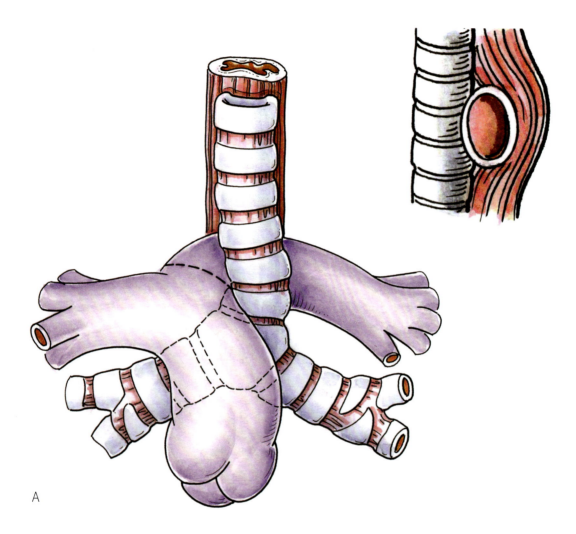

A

图 10-4（续）
B. 将左肺动脉远端从气管后方游离拖曳出后，重新种植在主肺动脉上。

Figure 10-4 cont'd
B. The distal part of the left pulmonary artery is freed from the posterior aspect of the trachea and reimplanted into the main pulmonary artery.

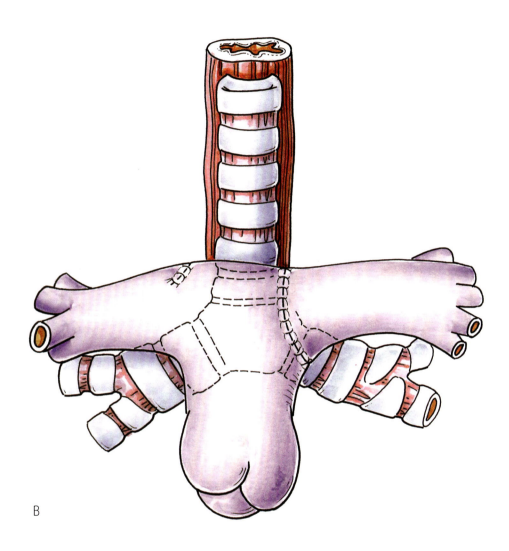

B

5. 左主动脉弓伴迷走右锁骨下动脉 位于锁骨下动脉和颈动脉之间的右侧第四弓退化,形成左主动脉弓伴迷走右锁骨下动脉。右锁骨下动脉起自左锁骨下动脉远端的降主动脉,并在食管后方向右走行,形成一个不完全的血管环,还通常造成食管受压性吞咽困难,大多不需要手术治疗(图10-5)。

5. Left aortic arch with aberrant right subclavian artery The right fourth arch between the subclavian artery and carotid arteries regresses, resulting in the left aortic arch with aberrant right subclavian artery. The right subclavian artery originates from the descending aorta at the distal end of the left subclavian artery and courses behind the esophagus to the right to form an incomplete vascular ring. It usually causes esophageal compression dysphagia, and most of them do not require surgical intervention (Figure 10-5).

图 10-5　左主动脉弓伴迷走右锁骨下动脉

Figure 10-5　Left aortic arch with aberrant right subclavian artery

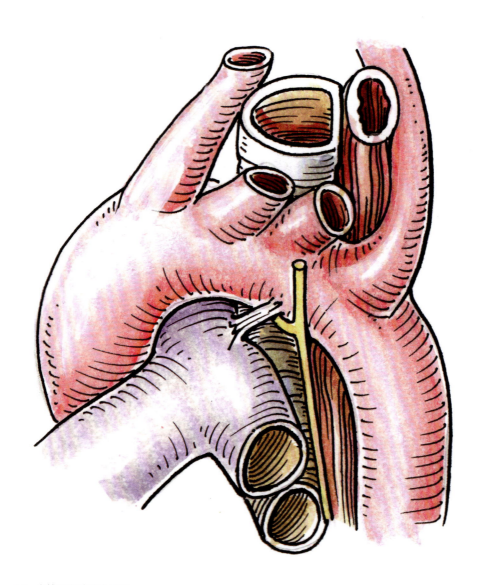

6. 气管狭窄成形术

（1）直接吻合技术：适用于短段狭窄（1~1.5cm）但狭窄程度严重的患儿，用可吸收缝线做直接端端吻合。

（2）补片扩大技术：主要用于长段的气管狭窄。将狭窄段气管切开，用心包补片连续缝合扩大狭窄段气管。该手术因很容易导致气管内肉芽增生、气管再狭窄，所以现在已很少应用。

（3）滑行法气管成形术：这是目前临床上应用最多的气管狭窄扩大技术。在狭窄气管的中间横断气管，两端分别向上、向下剪开直至正常气管组织。稍作修整，将两端气管滑行缝合。一般采用PDS可吸收缝线（图10-6）。

6. Stenotic Tracheoplasty

(1) Direct anastomosis technique: It is indicated for infants with short-segment tracheal stenosis (within 1-1. 5 cm), but the stenosis degree is severe. Direct end-to-end anastomosis is performed using absorbable suture.

(2) Patch tracheoplasty: It is mainly indicated for long-segment tracheal stenosis. A long-segment tracheal stenosis is incised, and a pericardial patch is sutured continuously to enlarge the stenotic segment of the trachea. This technique is rarely used because it can easily cause intratracheal granulation and restenosis of the trachea.

(3) Tracheal slide tracheoplasty technique: It is the most common technique for expanding tracheal stenosis in clinical practice. The trachea is transected in the middle of the stenotic trachea, with both ends cut through superiorly and inferiorly to normal tracheal tissue. After a little tidying, the trachea is sutured at both ends by sliding. PDS absorbable sutures are routinely used (Figure 10-6).

图 10-6　气管狭窄成形术

A. 直接吻合技术适用于短段狭窄患儿。

B. 切除狭窄段,直接端端吻合。

Figure 10-6　Stenotic tracheoplasty

A. Direct anastomosis technique is indicated for infants with short-segment tracheal stenosis.

B. The stenosed segment is resected and direct end-to-end anastomosis is performed.

Continued

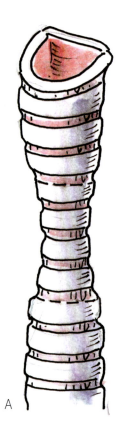

A

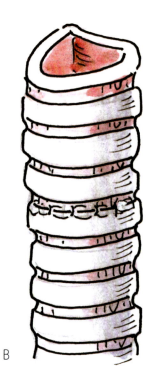

B

图 10-6(续)

C. 补片扩大技术主要用于长段的气管狭窄。

D. 将狭窄段气管切开，用心包补片连续缝合扩大狭窄段气管。

Figure 10-6 cont'd

C. Patch tracheoplasty is indicated for the long-segment tracheal stenosis.

D. A long-segment tracheal stenosis is incised, and a pericardial patch is sutured continuously to enlarge the stenotic segment of the trachea.

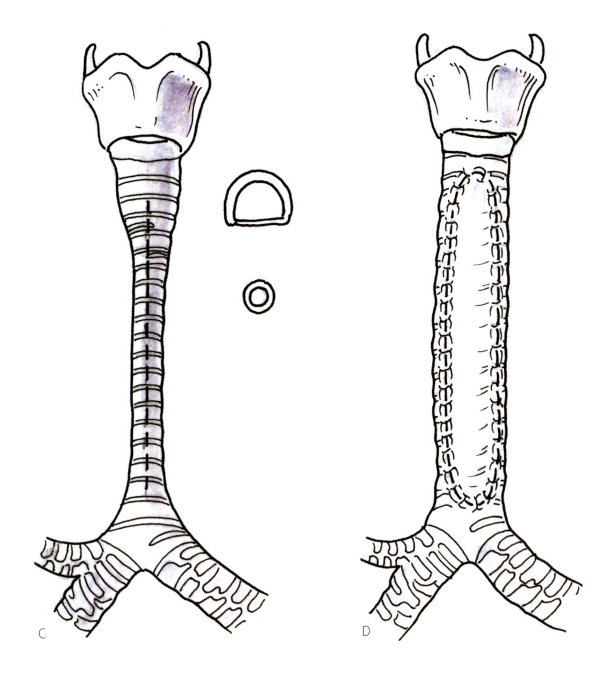

图 10-6（续）

E. 在狭窄气管的中间横断气管，两端分别向上、向下剪开直至正常气管组织。

Figure 10-6 cont'd

E. The trachea is transected in the middle of the stenotic trachea, with both ends cut through superiorly and inferiorly to normal tracheal tissue.

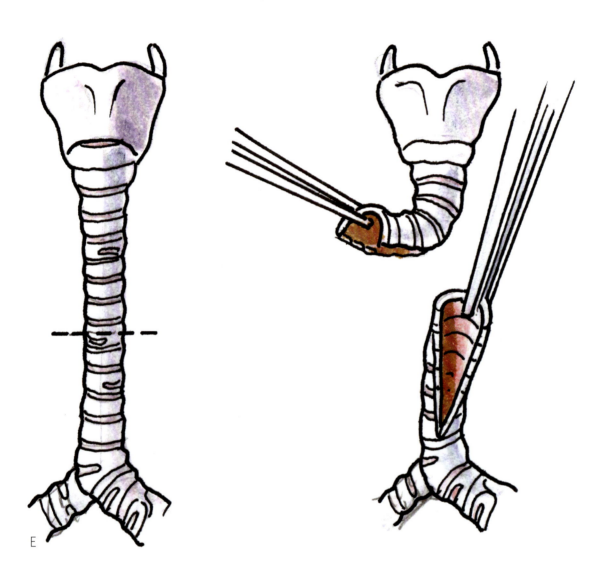

E

图 10-6(续)

F. 将两端气管滑行缝合。一般采用
PDS 可吸收缝线。

Figure 10-6 cont'd

F. The trachea is sutured at both ends by sliding. PDS absorbable sutures are routinely used.

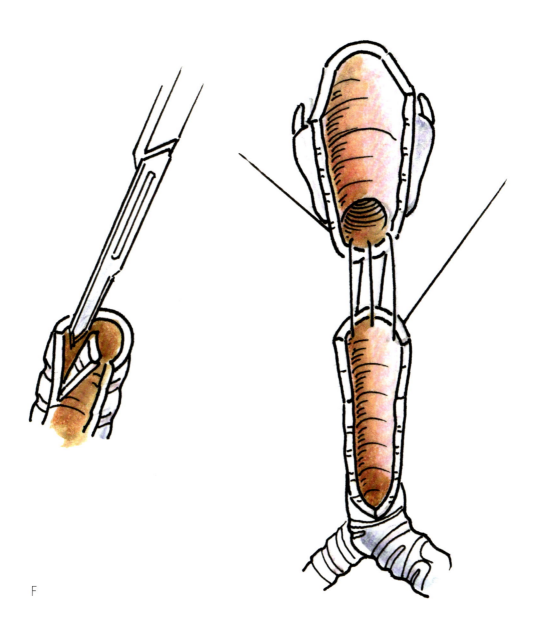

F

图 10-6(续)

G. 缝合后气管的正、侧面图示。

Figure 10-6 cont'd

G. Side and the front view of the trachea after the suture is illustrated.

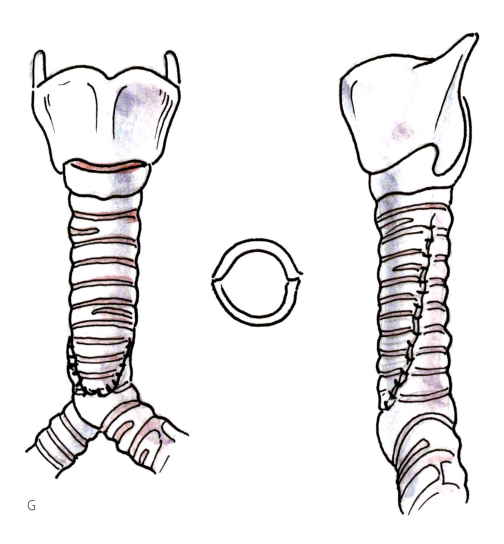

G

11 主动脉瓣上狭窄

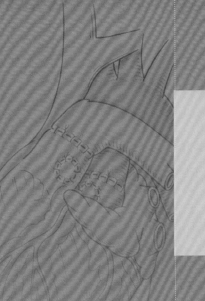

11 Supravalvular Aortic Stenosis

一、解剖分型

主动脉瓣上狭窄（supravalvular aortic stenosis，SVAS）是指主动脉瓣膜以上的主动脉管腔狭窄，按病理解剖特点可分为局限型和广泛型（图 11-1）。

I. Anatomical Typing

Supravalvular aortic stenosis (SVAS) refers to the stenosis of aortic luminal stenosis above the aortic valve. It can be classified as limited and extensive types based on pathological and anatomic features (Figure 11-1).

图 11-1　主动脉瓣上狭窄解剖分型
A. 局限型主动脉瓣上狭窄。
B. 广泛型主动脉瓣上狭窄。

Figure 11-1　Anatomical typing of supravalvular aortic stenosis
A. Limited SVAS.
B. Extensive SVAS.

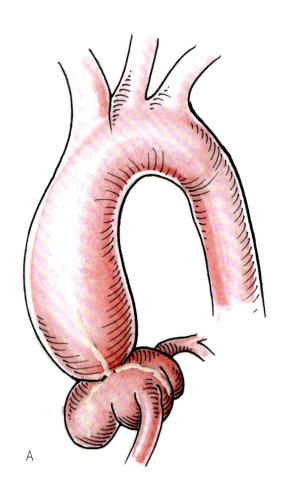
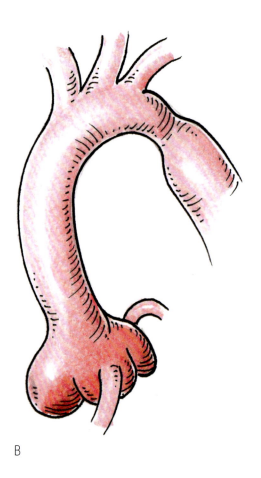

A

B

二、手术方法

1. 一块补片修补方法　取牛心包补片或人工材料补片（ePTFE），剪成泪滴状。将升主动脉狭窄处剪开，朝无冠窦方向延伸。若最狭窄处有明显的纤维嵴，可将其切除。用 5-0 或 6-0 Prolene 缝线将补片扩大缝合。对狭窄较严重的，也可将补片剪成倒三角形。术中将升主动脉最狭窄处剪开，并向无冠窦和右冠窦方向剪开，特别是在向右冠窦方向剪开时需注意右冠状动脉开口，避免损伤（图 11-2）。

II. Surgical Methods

1. Single-patch repair technique　Bovine pericardial patch or artificial patch (usually ePTFE) is cut into a teardrop shape. The stenosis of the ascending aorta is cut open and extended toward the noncoronary sinus. Obvious fibrous ridges at the narrowest position are to be excised. The patch is sutured with a 5-0 or 6-0 Prolene suture to enlarge the sinuses. For those with severe stenosis, the patch can be cut into an inverted triangle. During the operation, the maximal stenosis of the ascending aorta is cut towards the noncoronary sinus and right coronary sinus. Special attention should be paid to avoiding injuries to the ostium of the right coronary artery when cutting towards the right coronary sinus (Figure 11-2).

图 11-2　一块补片修补方法

A. 将升主动脉狭窄处剪开,朝无冠窦方向延伸。

Figure 11-2　Single-patch repair technique

A. The narrowing of the ascending aorta is cut open and extended toward the noncoronary sinus.

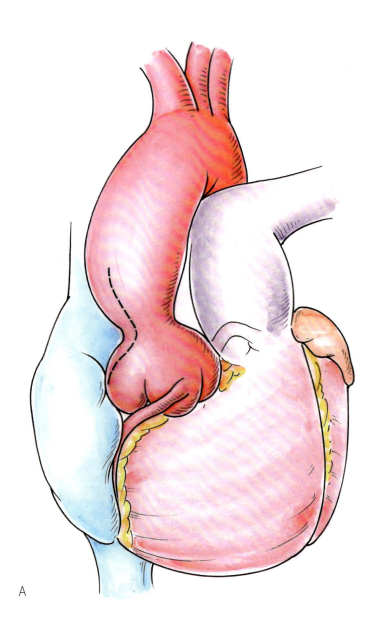

A

Continued

图 11-2（续）

B. 若最狭窄处有明显的纤维嵴，可将其切除。

Figure 11-2 cont'd

B. Obvious fibrous ridges at the narrowest position are to be excised.

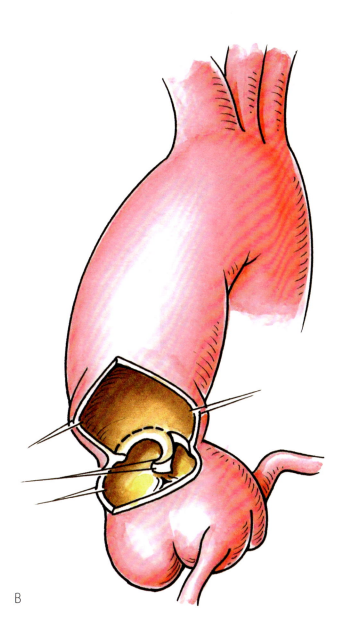

B

图 11-2（续）

C、D. 补片剪成泪滴状，用 5-0 或 6-0
Prolene 缝线将补片扩大缝合。

Figure 11-2 cont'd

C, D. A patch is cut into a teardrop shape and sutured with a
5-0 or 6-0 Prolene suture to enlarge the sinuses.

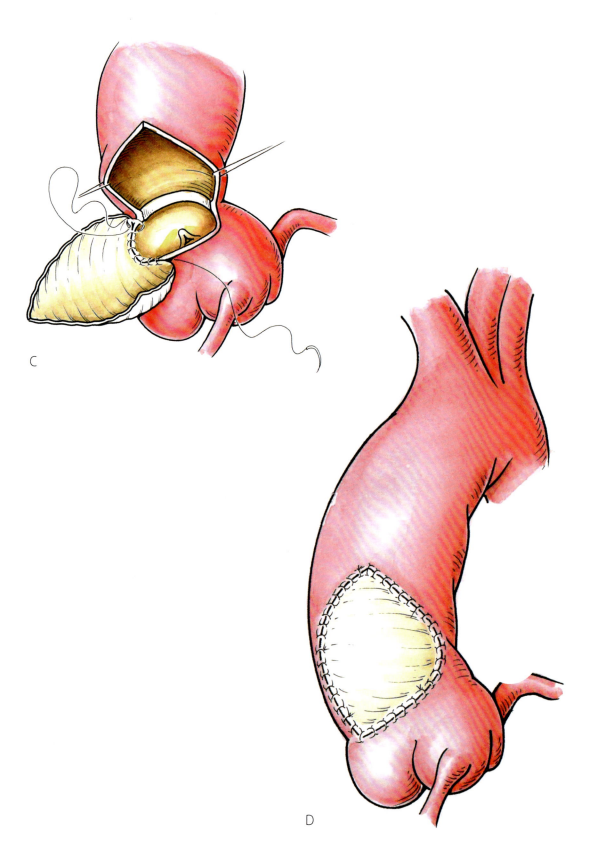

C

D

图 11-2（续）

E. 对较严重的狭窄，术中将升主动脉最狭窄处剪开，并向无冠窦和右冠窦方向剪开。

Figure 11-2 cont'd

E. For those with severe stenosis, the maximal stenosis of the ascending aorta is cut towards the noncoronary sinus and right coronary sinus.

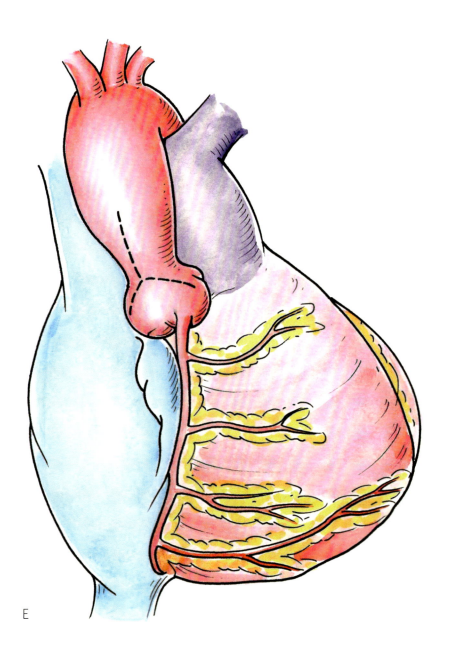

E

图 11-2（续）

F. 向右冠窦方向剪开时需注意右冠状动脉开口，避免损伤。

Figure 11-2 cont'd

F. Special attention should be paid to avoiding injuries to the ostium of the right coronary artery when cutting towards the right coronary sinus.

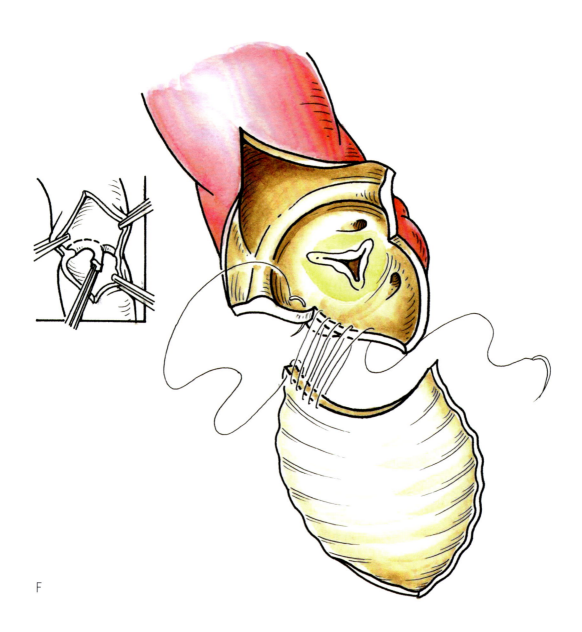

F

图 11-2 (续)

G. 将补片剪成倒三角形,用 Prolene 缝线缝合补片。

Figure 11-2 cont'd

G. The patch can be cut into an inverted triangle and sutured with Prolene sutures.

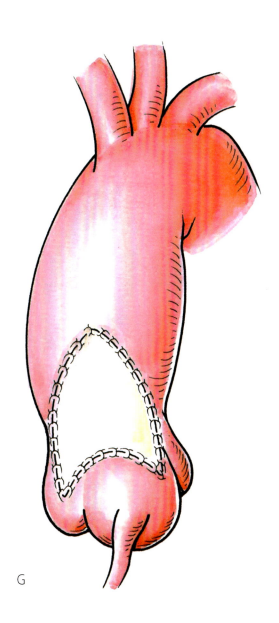

G

2. 三块补片修补方法　对严重主动脉瓣上狭窄的患者，采用三块补片分别扩大，即术中先将升主动脉最狭窄处横断，然后将三个瓣窦分别剪开扩大。用三块补片分别扩大主动脉窦，再与升主动脉远端连接。若升主动脉远端偏小，可再用一块三角形补片扩大（图 11-3）。

2. Three-patch technique　In patients with severe SVAS, three tailored patches can respectively be used to enlarge each sinus. Transect the maximal stenosis of the ascending aorta first, incise and augment the three sinuses by inserting three patches, and attach the patches to the distal ascending aorta. If the distal end of the ascending aorta is too small, an additional triangular patch may be used to enlarge it (Figure 11-3).

图 11-3　三片补片修补方法
A. 将升主动脉最狭窄处横断。

Figure 11-3　Three-patch technique
A. Transect the maximal stenosis of the ascending aorta.

Continued

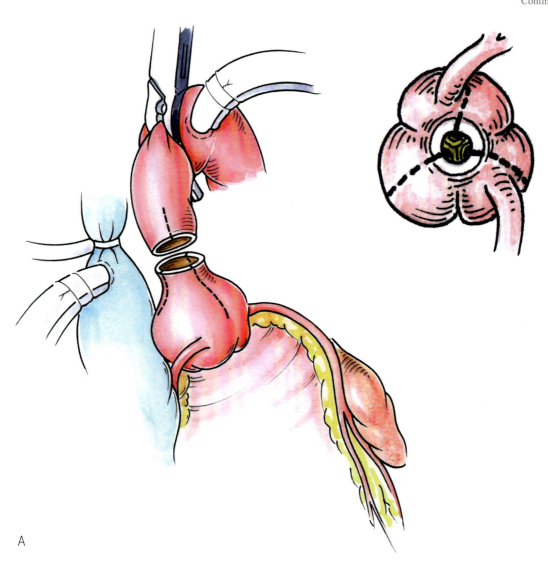

A

图 11-3（续）

B. 三个瓣窦分别剪开扩大。

Figure 11-3 cont'd

B. Incise and augment the three sinuses.

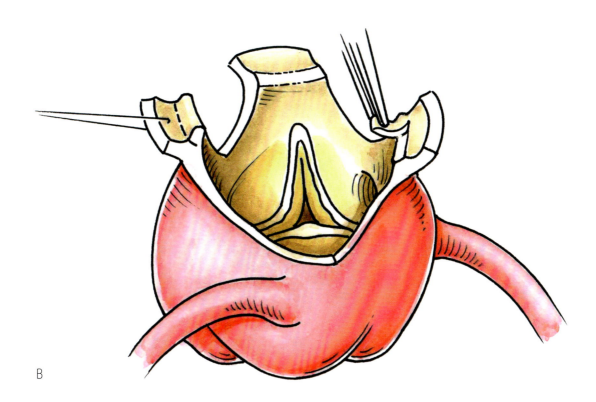

B

图 11-3（续）

Figure 11-3 cont'd

C. 用三块补片分别扩大主动脉窦。

C. Insert three patches into the sinuses to enlarge them.

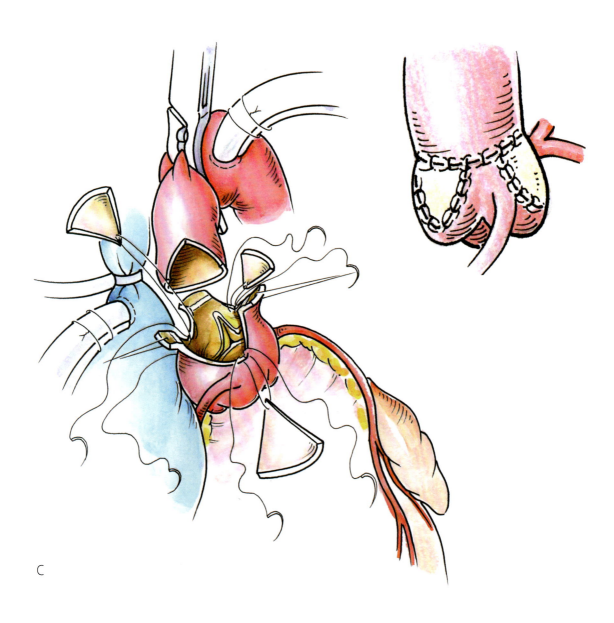

C

图 11-3（续）

D. 若升主动脉远端偏小，可再用一块三角形补片扩大。

Figure 11-3 cont'd

D. If the distal end of the ascending aorta is too small, an additional triangular patch may be used to enlarge it.

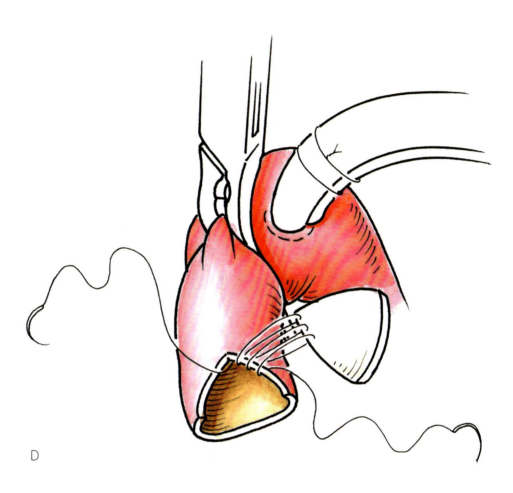

D

图 11-3(续)

Figure 11-3 cont'd

E. 与升主动脉远端连接。

E. Attach the patches to the distal ascending aorta.

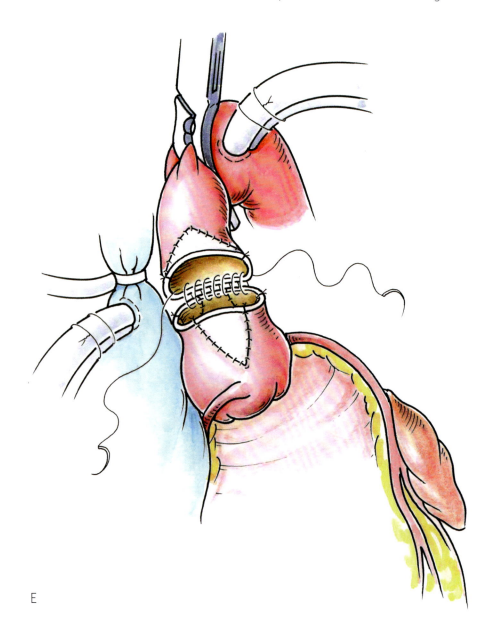

E

3. 滑动主动脉成形术 其瓣上切口的做法和普通三片法切口相同。该手术的优点是用自身组织扩大狭窄段,而不需使用人工或生物材料(图 11-4)。

3. Sliding aortoplasty The incision of sliding aortoplasty is the same as that of three-patch repair. This approach has the advantage of enlarging the narrowing with autologous tissues instead of artificial or biological materials (Figure 11-4).

图 11-4　滑动主动脉成形术
A. 在离断的升主动脉远端做三个对应切口。

Figure 11-4　Sliding aortoplasty
A. The three corresponding incisions are made in the position distal to the transected ascending aorta.

Continued

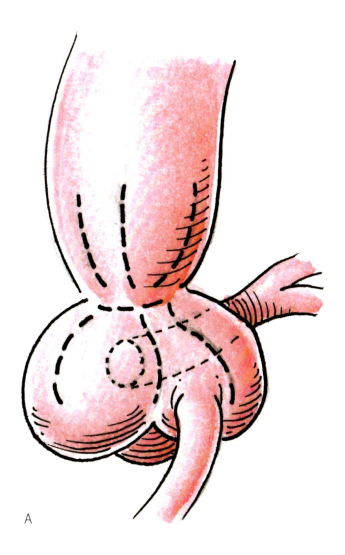

A

图 11-4（续）

B、C. 将切开的升主动脉组织滑入近端主动脉凹口内。

Figure 11-4 cont'd

B, C. The aorta tissue is slid into the proximal aortic notch.

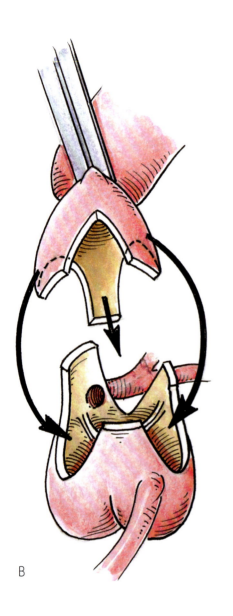

B

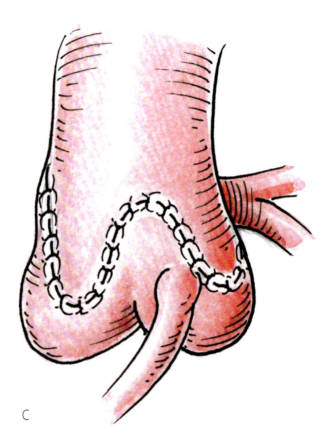

C

4. 升主动脉和主动脉弓成形术 伴有升主动脉和主动脉弓发育不良的患者,除了扩大主动脉瓣上狭窄外,还需用一块较大的牛心包补片或 ePTFE 补片剪成一段较长的三角形补片,扩大主动脉弓和升主动脉。此时,心肺转流术需采用深低温脑灌注技术或深低温停循环技术(图 11-5)。

4. Ascending aorta and aortic arch plasty In patients with dysplastic ascending aorta and aortic arch, apart from widening the supravalvular aortic stenosis, an extended triangular patch made from a large bovine pericardial patch or ePTFE patch can be used to enlarge the aortic arch and ascending aorta. This procedure requires cardiopulmonary bypass with a hypothermic cerebral perfusion technique or deep hypothermic circulatory arrest (Figure 11-5).

图 11-5　升主动脉和主动脉弓成形术

A. 主动脉瓣上及升主动脉切口。

Figure 11-5　Ascending aorta and aortic arch plasty
A. The supravalvular aortic incision extending to the ascending aorta.

Continued

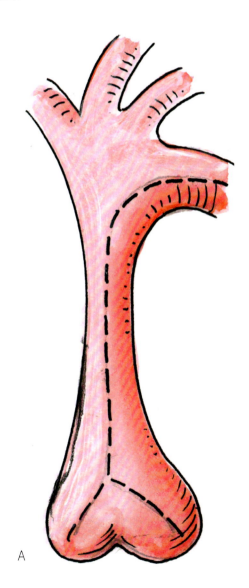

A

图 11-5（续）

B. 补片扩大主动脉弓和升主动脉。

Figure 11-5 cont'd

B. A patch is used to enlarge the aortic arch and ascending aorta.

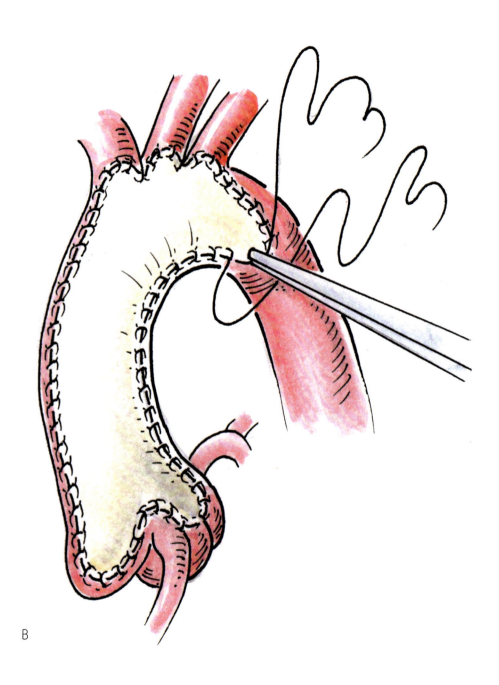

B

12 主动脉瓣病变

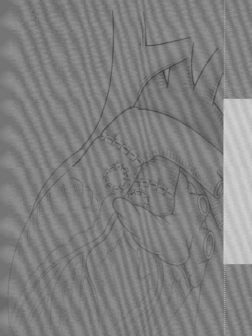

12 Aortic Valve Leision

一、解剖分型

主动脉瓣病变包括两大类，主动脉瓣狭窄和主动脉瓣反流。而主动脉瓣反流通常是由其他先天性心脏病引起的继发性改变，如：球囊扩张后反流、瓣下型室间隔缺损合并反流、瓣下狭窄导致反流和主动脉根部扩张合并反流。原发性主动脉瓣反流极为罕见。关于主动脉瓣狭窄将在《主动脉瓣及瓣下狭窄》一章详细介绍。

I. Anatomical Typing

Aortic valve leision falls into two broad categories: aortic stenosis and aortic regurgitation. Aortic regurgitation is usually an acquired leision caused by other congenital heart diseases, such as regurgitation after balloon dilation, subvalvular VSD with regurgitation, regurgitation caused by subvalvular stenosis, and aortic root dilatation with regurgitation. Primary aortic regurgitation is extremely rare. Aortic stenosis is described in detail in the chapter *"Aortic & Subaortic Stenosis"*.

二、手术方法

1. 球囊扩张术后的主动脉瓣反流修补（图 12-1）

II. Surgical Methods

1. Repair the aortic regurgitation after balloon dilatation (Figure 12-1)

图 12-1　球囊扩张术后的主动脉
　　　　　瓣反流修补

Figure 12-1　Repair the aortic regurgitation after
　　　　　　　balloon dilatation

A. 常规升主动脉 "倒冰球棍" 形切口，向无冠瓣延伸来暴露主动脉瓣。

A. Inverted hockey stick-shaped incision is made in ascending aorta and extended toward the non-coronary cusp, exposing the aortic valve.

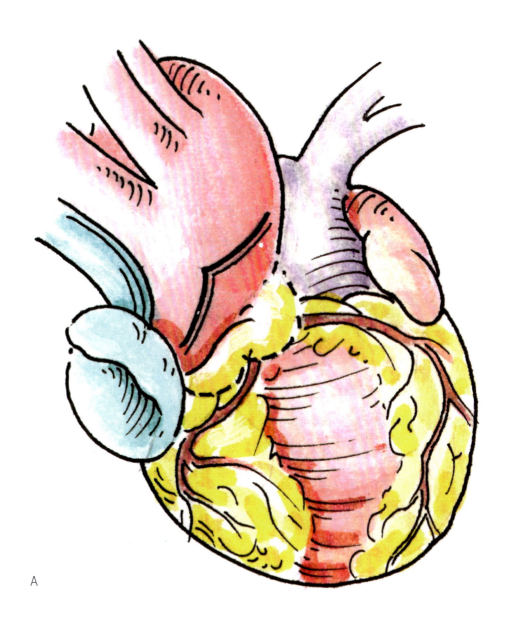

A

Continued

图 12-1（续）
B. 狭窄的主动脉瓣常为双叶瓣，球囊扩张后导致交界撕脱。

Figure 12-1 cont'd
B. Aortic valve stenosis is usually bileaflet, and balloon dilation causes junctional avulsion.

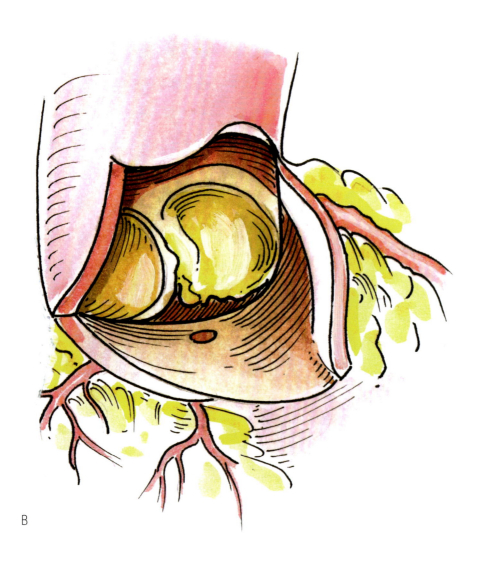

B

图 12-1（续）

C、D. 用自身心包补片对撕脱且脱垂的瓣叶做修补和交界缝合，必要时对脱垂的瓣叶做悬吊。

Figure 12-1 cont'd

C, D. Repair and commissural suture is made to the torn and prolapsed leaflets with the autogenous pericardial patch, and the prolapsed leaflets are to be suspended if necessary.

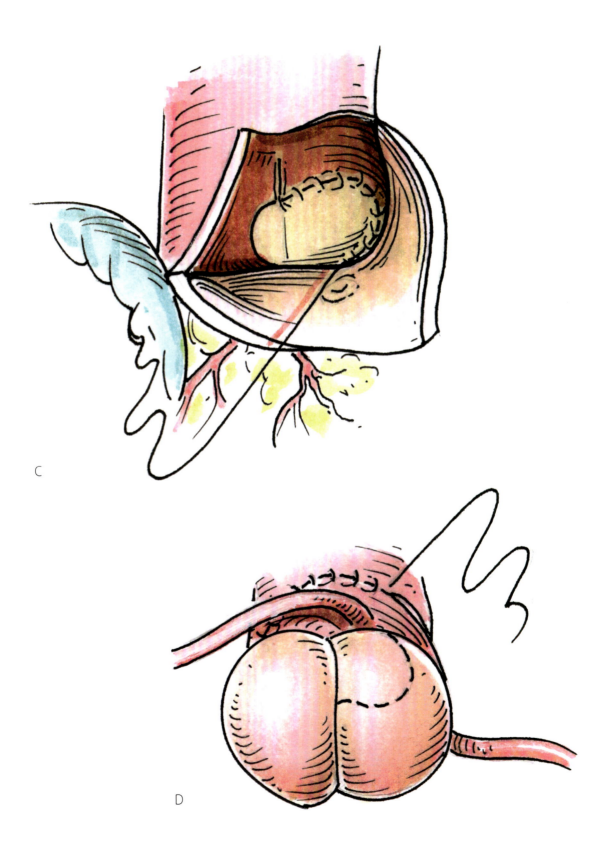

C

D

2. 瓣下型室间隔缺损合并主动脉瓣反流 瓣下型 VSD 紧邻主动脉右冠瓣下方,由于 VSD 分流导致文丘里效应,造成右冠瓣脱垂。所以对这类 VSD,要求在 2 岁以内完成手术修补(图 12-2)。

2. Subvalvular VSD with aortic regurgitation Subvalvular VSD is right below the right coronary valve of the aorta and causes prolapse of the right coronary valve due to the Venturi effect caused by the VSD shunt. Therefore, for this type of VSD, surgical repair is required under the age of two (Figure 12-2).

图 12-2　瓣下型室间隔缺损合并主动脉瓣反流

A. VSD 分流导致文丘里效应。
B. 体循环压力直接加重主动脉瓣叶脱垂,脱垂之右冠瓣会造成 VSD 几乎闭合。
C. VSD 闭合后,主动脉瓣被托起,反流减轻。

Figure 12-2　Subvalvular VSD with aortic regurgitation
A. Venturi effect due to VSD shunt.
B. Aortic leaflet prolapse is aggravated directly by systemic pressure. The prolapsed right coronary valve may cause a completely closed VSD.
C. After the closure of the VSD, the aortic valve is lifted, and regurgitation is reduced.

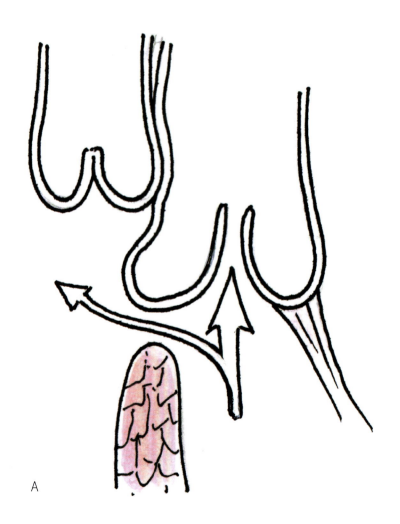

A

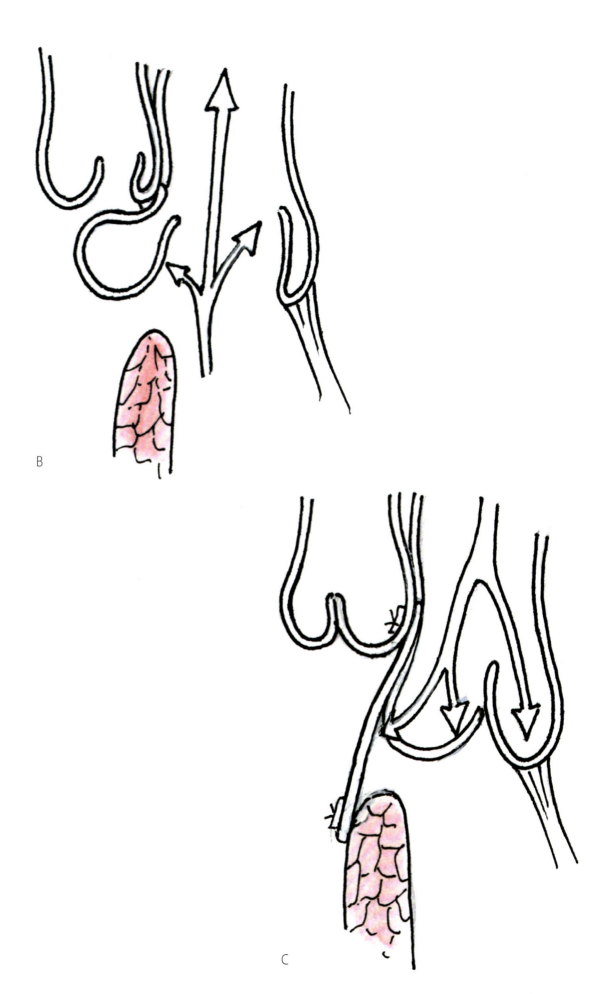

B

C

3. 主动脉瓣下狭窄造成主动脉瓣反流　主动脉瓣下隔膜或纤维环狭窄会造成湍流，可损伤主动脉瓣并导致主动脉瓣反流。湍流造成纤维组织增生，延伸到主动脉心室面，造成瓣叶增厚扭曲。主动脉瓣反流逐步加重，瓣叶边缘增厚卷曲，瓣叶对合差，反流加重形成恶性循环（图 12-3）。

3. Aortic regurgitation caused by subaortic aortic stenosis　Stenosis of the subaortic septum or annulus can cause turbulence, which can damage the aortic valve and result in aortic regurgitation. Turbulence causes fibrous tissue to proliferate, which will extend to the ventricular surface of the aorta, causing thickening and distortion of the valve leaflets. Progressive aggravation of aortic regurgitation, the thickening and curling of leaflet edge, and poor alignment of valve leaflets increase regurgitation to form a vicious circle (Figure 12-3).

图 12-3　**主动脉瓣下狭窄造成主动脉瓣反流**

A. 湍流造成纤维组织增生，主动脉瓣叶增厚扭曲。

Figure 12-3　Aortic regurgitation caused by subaortic stenosis

A. Turbulence causes fibrous tissue to proliferate, causing thickening and distortion of the aortic valve leaflets.

Continued

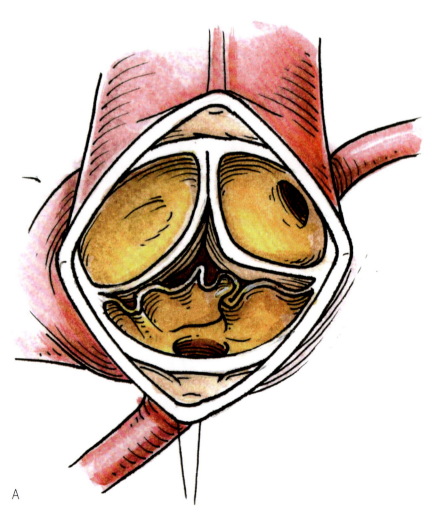

A

图 12-3（续）

B. 用带垫缝线褥式缝合，将脱垂之瓣叶折叠悬吊。

Figure 12-3 cont'd

B. The prolapsed leaflets are plicated and suspended using a pledget-supported mattress suture.

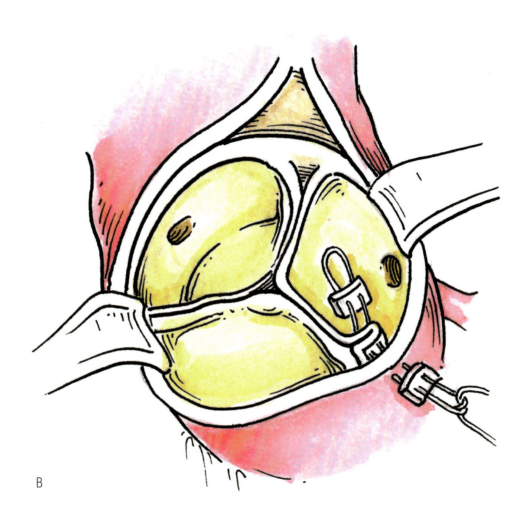

B

图 12-3（续）

Figure 12-3 cont'd

C. 部分脱垂严重的患者需在瓣叶两侧都做折叠悬吊。

C. Some patients with severe prolapse require folding and suspension on both sides of the valve leaflets.

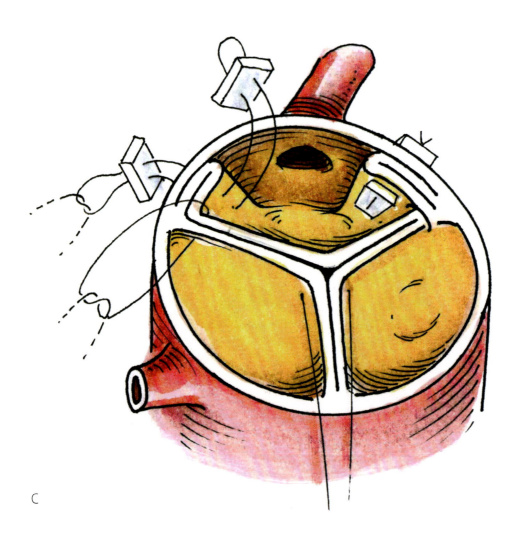

C

图 12-3（续）

D. 为确保瓣叶对合良好,可在两片主动脉瓣叶之间用心包垫片 U 形加固缝合。

Figure 12-3 cont'd

D. To ensure good leaflet apposition, a U-shaped pericardial pledget-supported suture can be used between the two aortic valve leaflets.

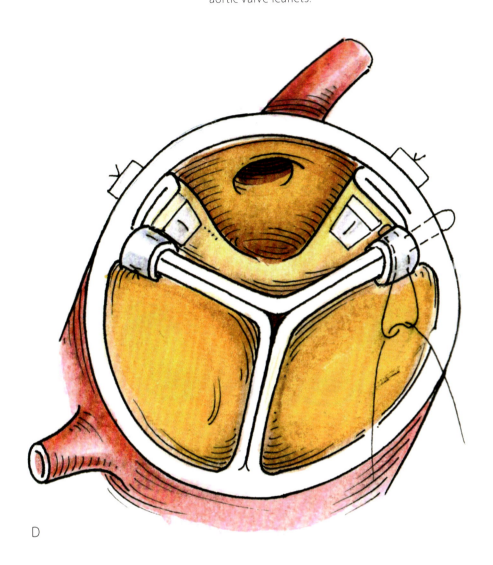

D

4. 主动脉根部扩张导致主动脉瓣反流 诸如马方综合征等结缔组织病,导致主动脉瓣根部扩张致主动脉瓣反流。有时大年龄手术的法洛四联症或肺动脉闭锁患儿也可见主动脉根部扩张(图 12-4)。

4. Aortic regurgitation caused by aortic root dilation Connective tissue diseases, such as Marfan syndrome, can cause aortic regurgitation due to dilatation of the aortic root. Sometimes, aortic root dilatation is also seen in elder children undergoing surgery with tetralogy of Fallot or pulmonary artery atresia (Figure 12-4).

图 12-4　主动脉根部扩张导致主
　　　　动脉瓣反流

A. 主动脉根部扩张,主动脉瓣交界的顶部受到牵拉,导致中央性反流。楔形切除部分扩张的主动脉壁。

B. 5-0 Prolene 缝线连续缝合缩小扩张的主动脉根部。

Figure 12-4　Aortic regurgitation caused by aortic root dilation

A. Central regurgitation caused by aortic root dilatation with traction on the top of the aortic commissure. Wedge resection of the partially dilated aortic wall.

B. Reduce the dilated aortic root with 5-0 Prolene running suture.

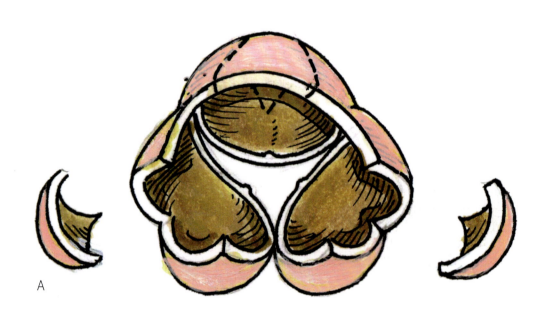

A

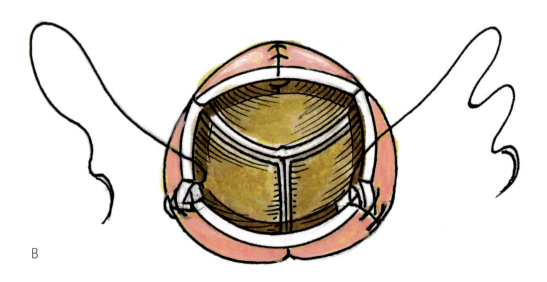

B

5. 主动脉瓣置换术 严重的主动脉瓣病变或多次整形效果不佳的儿童患者,则需做瓣膜置换手术。儿童瓣膜置换手术多选用机械瓣。一般采用带垫 U 形间断缝合(图 12-5)。

5. Aortic valve replacement For children with severe aortic valve lesions or poor results of repeated valvuloplasty, valve replacement surgery is required. Mechanical valves are the most common choice in valve replacement for children, and U-shaped interrupted sutures with pledget are generally applied (Figure 12-5).

图 12-5　**主动脉瓣置换术**
A. 缝合时垫片可放在左室面。

Figure 12-5　Aortic valve replacement
A. The pledget may be placed on the left ventricular surface.

Continued

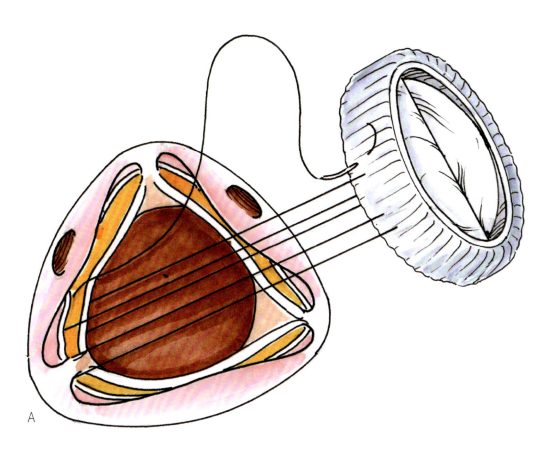

图 12-5（续）

B. 垫片也可放在主动脉面，缝合时位置不宜过高，避免影响冠状动脉开口。

C. 也可采用连续缝合，一般先缝合三个点。连续缝合后用神经拉钩帮助收紧缝线，再三根缝线互相打结。

Figure 12-5 cont'd

B. The pledget may also be placed on the aortic surface when suturing. The suture should not be too high so as not to affect the coronary ostium.

C. Running sutures are also applied in surgery, with three points sutured first. After running suturing, nerve hooks are used to help tighten the sutures, and three sutures are knotted to each other.

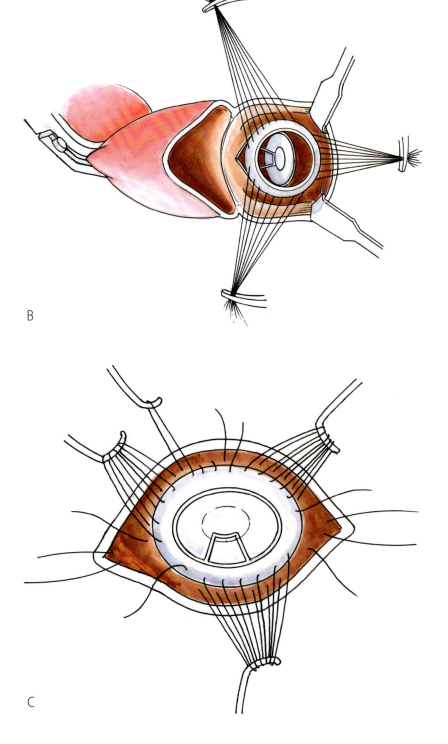

B

C

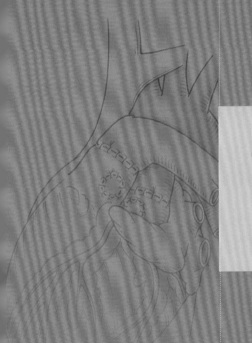

13 主动脉瓣及瓣下狭窄

13 Aortic Valve Stenosis and
Subaortic Stenosis

一、解剖分型

I. Anatomical Typing

在儿童先天性左心室流出道梗阻性疾病中，主动脉瓣狭窄是常见的类型。其临床症状取决于狭窄的程度，有些二叶主动脉瓣轻度狭窄可以没有任何症状，但有些重症狭窄患者则必须在新生儿期干预。主动脉瓣下狭窄的最常见类型是左心室流出道中异常存在的纤维肌性结构造成的固定性梗阻，另一组则是肥厚型心肌病，大多在学龄期出现症状。

Aortic stenosis represents one of the most common lesions in children with congenital left ventricular outflow tract obstruction. The clinical symptoms depend on the degree of stenosis, patients with bicuspid aortic and mild stenosis may be asymptomatic, but for some patients with severe stenosis, intervention in the neonatal period is necessary. The most common type of subvalvular aortic stenosis is fixed obstruction due to an abnormal fibromuscular structure present in the left ventricular outflow tract. The other group is hypertrophic cardiomyopathy, which is routinely symptomatic during school age.

二、手术方法

II. Surgical Methods

1. 危重型新生儿主动脉瓣狭窄球囊扩张 在不少心脏中心，球囊扩张已成为治疗危重型新生儿主动脉瓣狭窄的首选方法。通常由配合默契、技术娴熟的小儿心脏内外科医生共同完成。血管入路是这种操作的一个重要考虑因素。在新生儿，脐动脉是首选，而年长儿童患者则考虑使用股动脉进入（图 13-1）。

1. Balloon dilatation in neonates with severe aortic stenosis In many cardiac centers, balloon valvuloplasty has become the first choice for neonates with severe aortic stenosis. It is usually performed by skilled pediatric cardiac physicians and surgeons with cooperation. Vascular access is an important consideration for this procedure. In neonates, the umbilical artery is the first choice, while the femoral artery is frequently used for access in elder patients (Figure 13-1).

图 13-1　球囊扩张示意图　　　　　　Figure 13-1　Diagram of balloon valvuloplasty

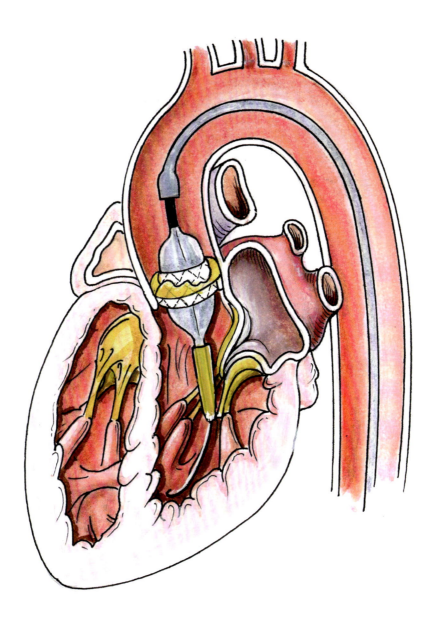

2. 新生儿和婴儿主动脉瓣狭窄切开术 主动脉瓣交界切开对瓣膜狭窄的解除比球囊扩张更精准彻底(图 13-2)。

2. Open surgical aortic valvotomy in neonates and infants The opening of the aortic valve junction can relieve valve stenosis more accurately and thoroughly than balloon valvuloplasty does (Figure 13-2).

图 13-2　**主动脉瓣狭窄切开术**
A. 心肺转流术插管略偏高,便于暴露主动脉切口。

Figure 13-2　Open surgical valvotomy
A. The cardiopulmonary bypass cannula is slightly higher for a clear exposure of the aortic incision.

Continued

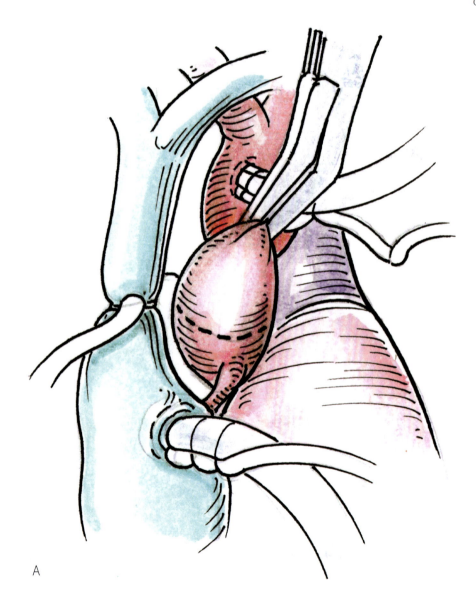

A

图 13-2 (续)

B. 主动脉根部以上 1cm 横切口, 显示
狭窄之主动脉瓣。

Figure 13-2 cont'd

B. Transverse aortotomy is performed at 1cm above the
root of the aorta to expose the stenotic aortic valve.

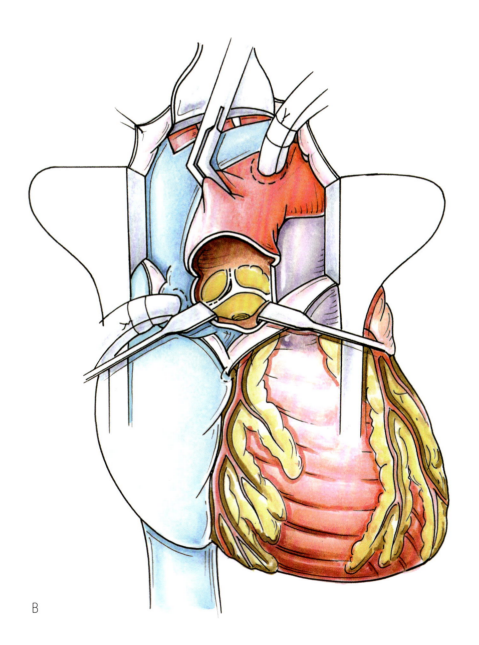

B

图 13-2（续）

C. 用三角刀切开交界融合的主动脉
瓣叶,不宜切除过度,易导致主动脉瓣
反流。

Figure 13-2 cont'd

C. A lancet is utilized to cut the fused aortic valve leaflets at the commissures. It is not advisable to over-excise, as it will easily lead to aortic regurgitation.

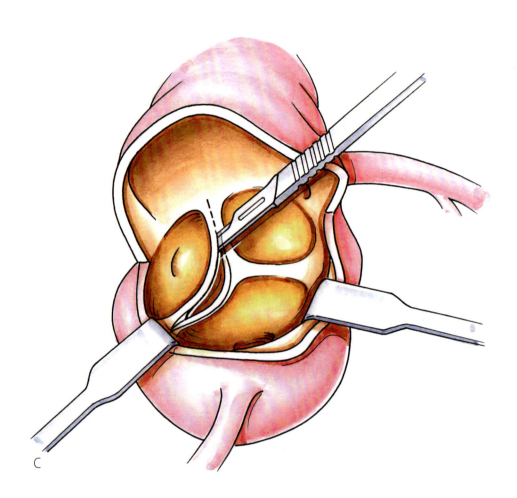

C

图 13-2 (续)

Figure 13-2 cont'd

D. 瓣叶切开术完成后,缝合主动脉切口。

D. The aortic incision is sutured when valvotomy is completed.

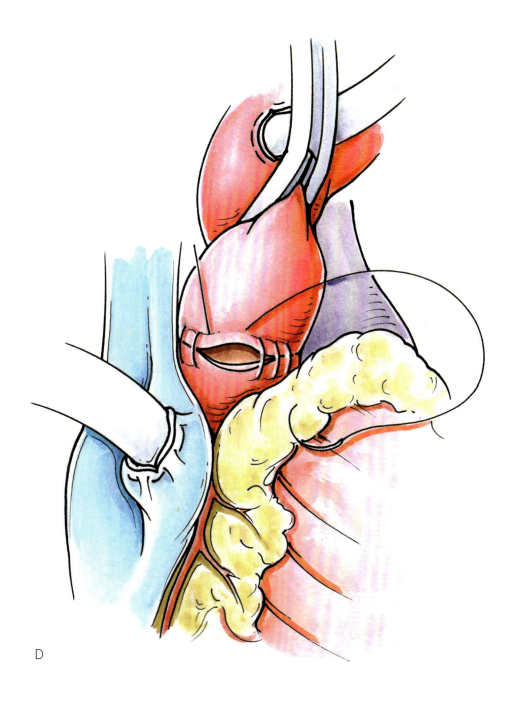

D

3. 主动脉瓣下狭窄切开术 主动脉瓣下狭窄可有许多不同类型,可为原发性的主动脉下隔膜,也可形成一个长管状纤维肌性隧道,故手术切除方法不同(图 13-3)。

3. Subvalvular aortic stenosis repair There are many different types of subvalvular aortic stenosis. It can be a primary subaortic septum, or it can form a long tubular fibromuscular tunnel. Therefore, surgical management is different (Figure 13-3).

图 13-3　**主动脉瓣下狭窄切开术**
A. 主动脉瓣下隔膜的切除:通过"倒冰球棍"形切口向无冠瓣延伸,显露主动脉瓣下隔膜。

Figure 13-3　Subvalvular aortic stenosis repair
A. Subaortic septum resection: extend through the inverted hockey stick-shaped incision to the non-coronal valve to expose the subaortic septum.

Continued

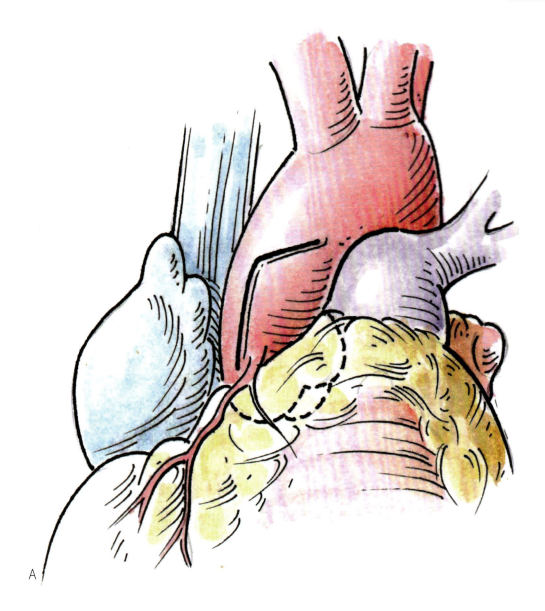

A

图 13-3（续）

B. 主动脉瓣下隔膜通常位于主动脉瓣下方数毫米，有时会延伸到二尖瓣前瓣的心室面。

Figure 13-3 cont'd

B. Subaortic septum is usually a few millimeters below the aortic valve and sometimes extends to the ventricular surface of the anterior mitral valve.

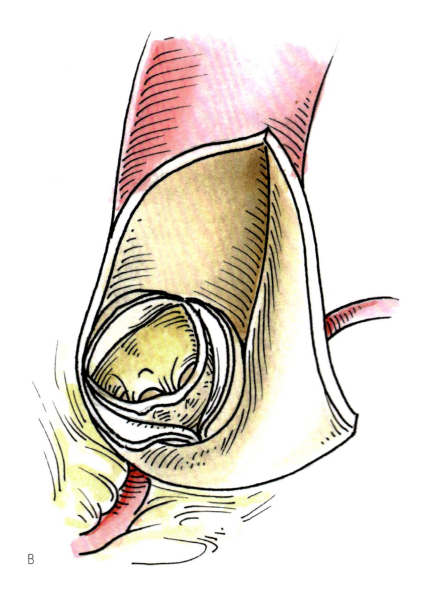

B

图 13-3（续）

C. 用镊子夹住隔膜组织,用三角刀贴着左心室面将隔膜完整切除。

Figure 13-3 cont'd

C. Clamp the septum tissue with forceps and use a lancet against the surface of the left ventricle to completely excise the septum.

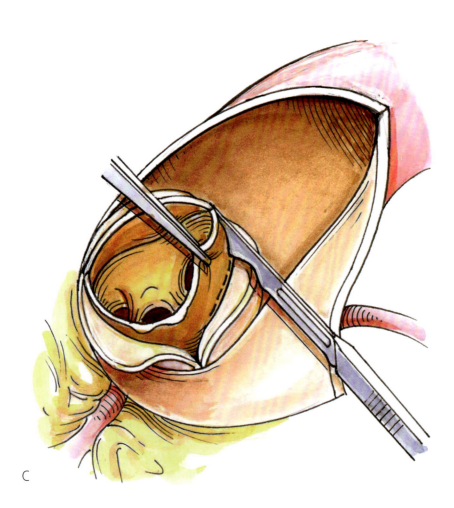

C

图 13-3（续）

Figure 13-3 cont'd

D. 隧道样主动脉瓣下狭窄须通过更大范围的手术操作进行处理，又可称为改良 Konno 手术：经朝向冠窦交界的主动脉切口和右心室漏斗部横切口。

D. Tunnel-like subaortic stenosis must be managed by surgery on a larger scale, also known as a modified Konno procedure: Konno procedure is performed via an aortic incision directed toward the coronary sinus junction and a transverse incision into the right ventricular infundibulum.

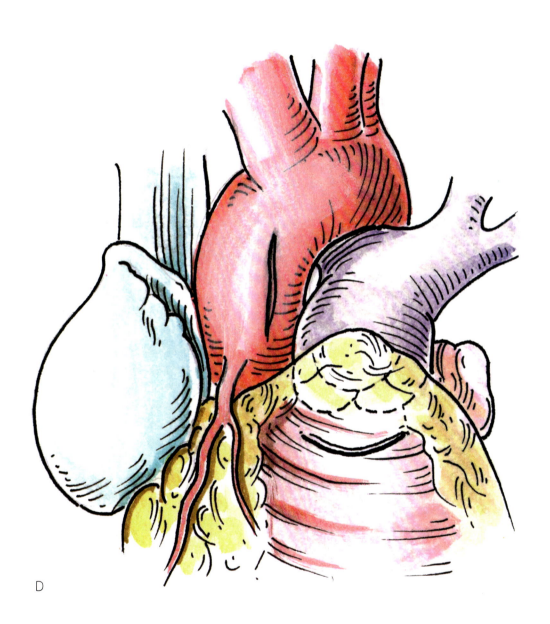

D

图 13-3（续）

E. 用主动脉切口暴露左心室流出道。经漏斗部切口来暴露左心室流出道和右心室面。朝着主动脉瓣的冠窦交界做室间隔切口。必要时可切除部分肥厚之肌肉。

Figure 13-3 cont'd

E. The aortic incision is made to expose the left ventricular outflow tract. The right ventricular incision is made to expose the left ventricular outflow tract and the right ventricular surface. A septal incision is made toward the coronary sinus junction of the aortic valve. If necessary, hypertrophic muscles may be partially excised.

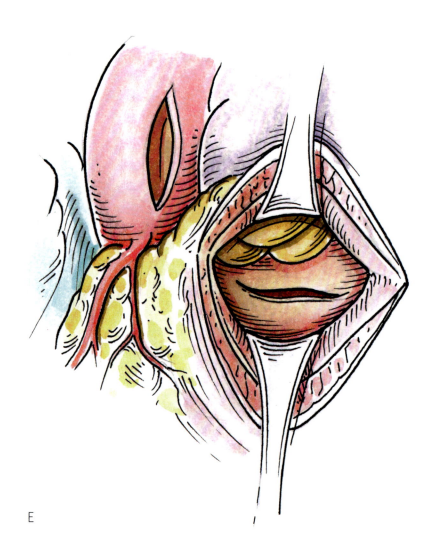

E

图 13-3 (续)

F. 取 ePTFE 补片关闭切开的室间隔右室面，同时扩大左心室流出道。

Figure 13-3 cont'd

F. The ePTFE patch is used to close the right ventricular surface of the incised ventricular septum and enlarge the left ventricular outflow tract.

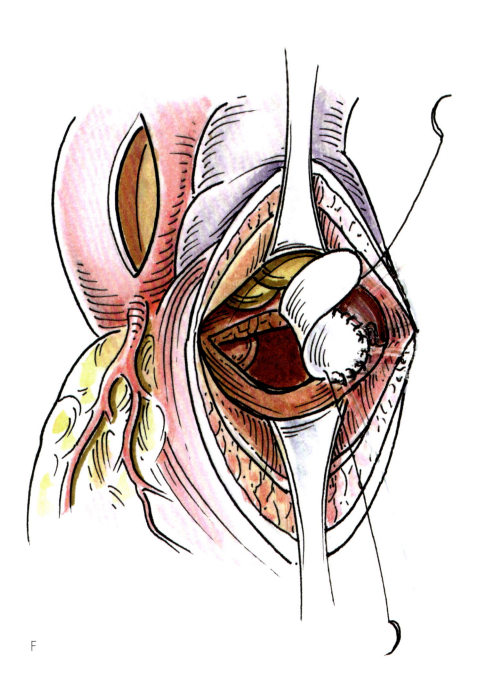

F

4. 肥厚型心肌病手术 通常指特发性肥厚性主动脉瓣下狭窄（idiopathic hypertrophic subaortic stenosis，IHSS），其特征为不对称的室间隔肥厚导致左心流出道梗阻。可以是室间隔增厚形成的一种固定性狭窄，也可以是二尖瓣前瓣的收缩期前向运动造成的动力性梗阻。现主要使用 Morrow 手术方法（图13-4）。若术后仍有残留梗阻，应考虑应用改良 Konno 手术（方法见前述）。

4. Hypertrophic cardiomyopathy scurgery It is often referred to as idiopathic hypertrophic subaortic stenosis (IHSS), which is mainly characterized by asymmetrical ventricular septal hypertrophy leading to obstruction of the left cardiac outflow tract. It can be fixed stenosis resulting from the thickening of the interventricular septum or a dynamic obstruction caused by the systolic anterior motion of the anterior mitral valve. Morrow procedure is commonly used these days (Figure 13-4). If there is still residual obstruction, a modified Konno procedure should be considered (see above surgical procedures).

图 13-4　Morrow **手术方法**
A. 心脏停搏后，主动脉根部斜切口，向无冠窦延伸。

Figure 13-4　Morrow procedure
A. After cardiac arrest, the aortic root is obliquely incised, and the incision is extended towards the noncoronary sinus.

Continued

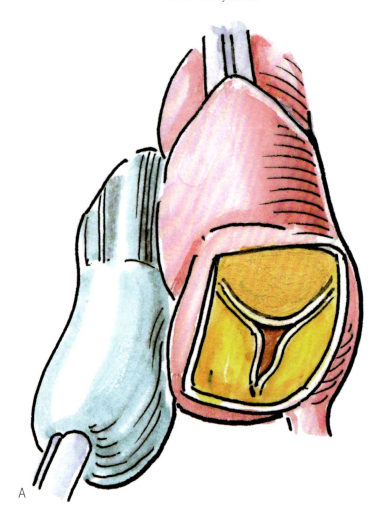

A

图 13-4（续）
B. 用直角小拉钩牵开右冠瓣，暴露肥厚心室间隔。

Figure 13-4 cont'd
B. The right coronary valve is retracted with a right-angled small retractor to expose the hypertrophic interventricular septum.

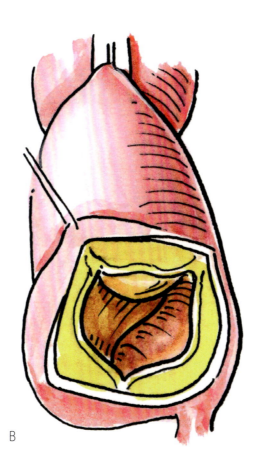

B

图 13-4（续）

C. 在右冠瓣下方肥厚肌肉上做两条平行切口，深度可依据术前超声心动图评估局部心肌厚度。注意避免损伤主动脉瓣和二尖瓣前乳头肌。

D. 紧靠主动脉瓣环下方，用尖刀或解剖剪刀切除两条切口间的肥厚心肌组织。剪除时可用手指轻压右室前壁和室间隔前方，这样有助于肥厚肌肉组织显露和切除。避免切穿室间隔。

E. 缝合主动脉切口。

Figure 13-4 cont'd

C. Two parallel incisions are made in the hypertrophic muscle below the right coronary valve, and the depth of the incision can be determined based on the local myocardial thickness, which is assessed by the preoperative echocardiographic assessment. Care should be taken to avoid injuries to the aortic valve and anterior papillary muscle of the mitral valve.

D. Immediately below the aortic valve annulus, a sharp knife or dissecting scissors are used to excise the hypertrophic myocardial tissue between the two incisions. When dissecting, the anterior wall of the right ventricle and the front of the ventricular septum can be gently pressed with fingers, which helps to expose and excise the hypertrophic muscle tissue. Care should be taken to avoid cutting through the interventricular septum.

E. The aortic incision is sutured.

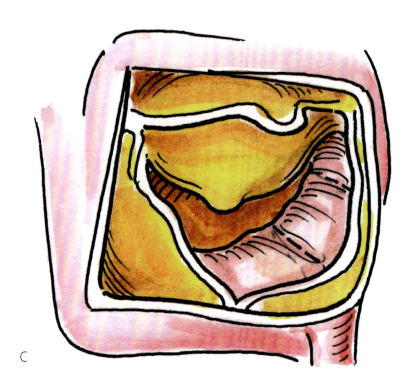

C

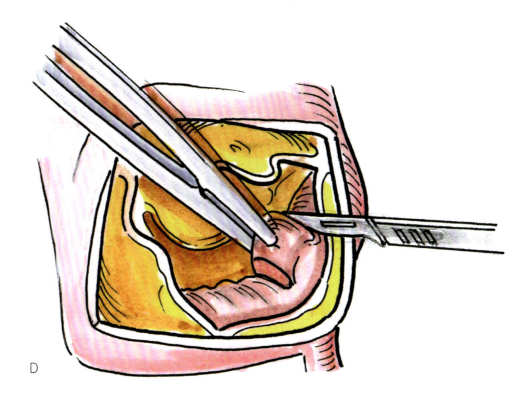

D

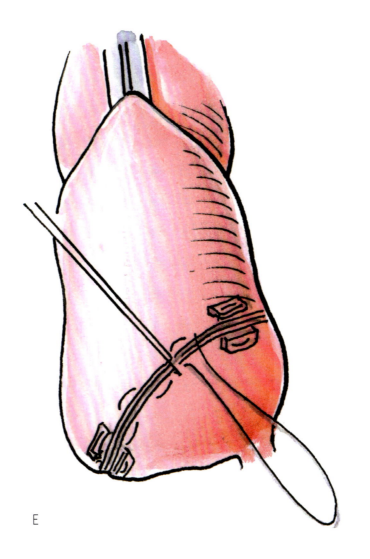

E

图 13-4 (续)

Figure 13-4 cont'd

F. 心脏复跳后做左心室测压,评估梗阻解除情况。

F. Left ventricular pressure is measured after the heartbeats again to assess relief of the obstruction.

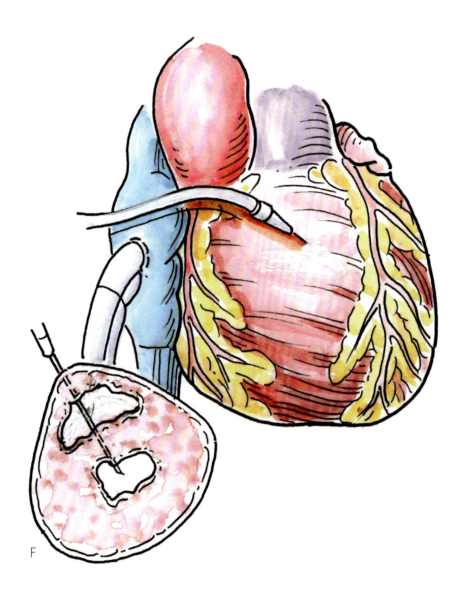

5. Ross 手术　儿童主动脉瓣病变常采用 Ross 手术,该手术是用患者自身的肺动脉瓣来替换病变主动脉瓣,再用同种异体带瓣管道或异种带瓣管道(牛颈静脉或人工管道)来替换肺自身肺动脉瓣。其优点是使用患者自己的肺动脉瓣,存在生长潜能,使用时间长,并无须抗凝治疗(图 13-5)。

5. Ross procedure　In children with aortic valve disease, Ross procedure is usually performed, in which the diseased aortic valve is replaced by the patient's pulmonary valve, and the native pulmonary valve is replaced by valved homograft conduit or valved heterologous conduit (bovine jugular vein or artificial conduit). The advantage is the use of the patient's pulmonary valve, which has the ability of potential growth to provide a durable valve and no need for anticoagulation therapy (Figure 13-5).

图 13-5　Ross 手术方法

A. 心脏停搏后取自身肺动脉瓣,肺动脉瓣上 1cm 处横断主肺动脉。用一把直角钳来确定肺动脉瓣的位置,在瓣下 0.5cm 做右心室切口,注意避免损伤左冠状动脉。

Figure 13-5　Ross procedure

A. The autologous pulmonary valve is harvested after cardiac arrest. The pulmonary artery is transected 1 cm above the pulmonary valve. A right-angled clamp is used to locate the pulmonary valve, and a right ventricular incision is made 0. 5 cm below the valve, taking care to avoid damaging the left coronary artery.

Continued

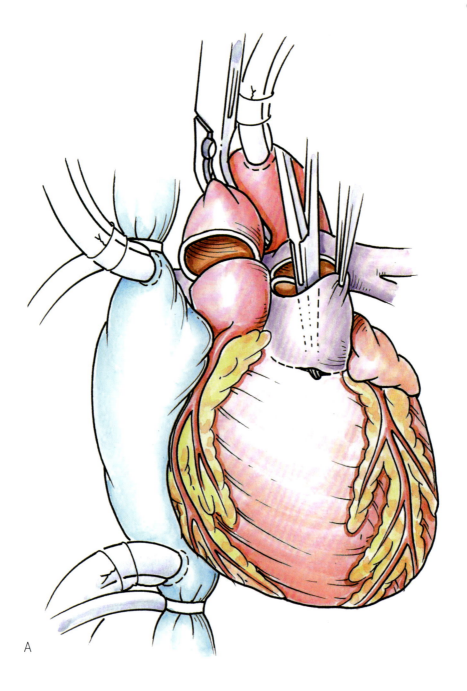

图 13-5 (续)
B. 切取带瓣肺动脉, 横断升主动脉, 取下左右冠状动脉开口的纽片, 并松解获取最大的活动度。

Figure 13-5 cont'd
B. Cut the valved pulmonary artery, transect the ascending aorta, remove the buttons of the left and right coronary artery openings, and loosen them for maximum mobility.

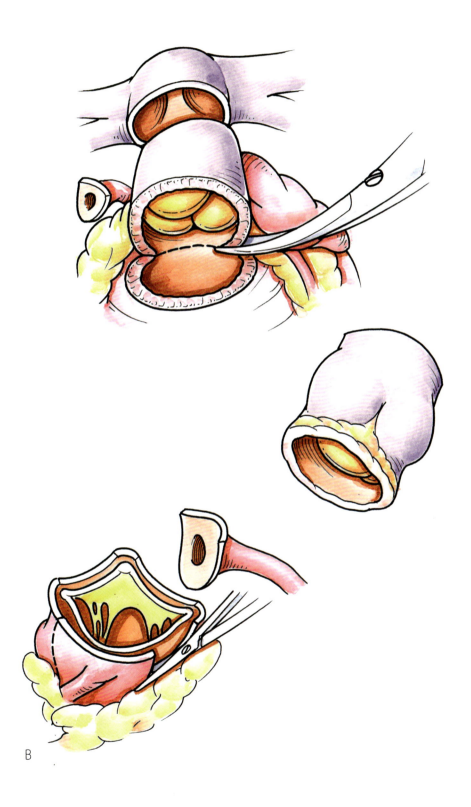

B

图 13-5（续）

C. 将自体肺动脉移植到左心室流出道，常用 6-0 Prolene 缝线连续缝合。必要时可采用带垫片针来缩小主动脉瓣环。

Figure 13-5 cont'd

C. The pulmonary autograft is implanted into the left ventricular outflow tract using a 6-0 Prolene running suture. If necessary, the pledget-supported sutures can be used to make the aortic annulus smaller.

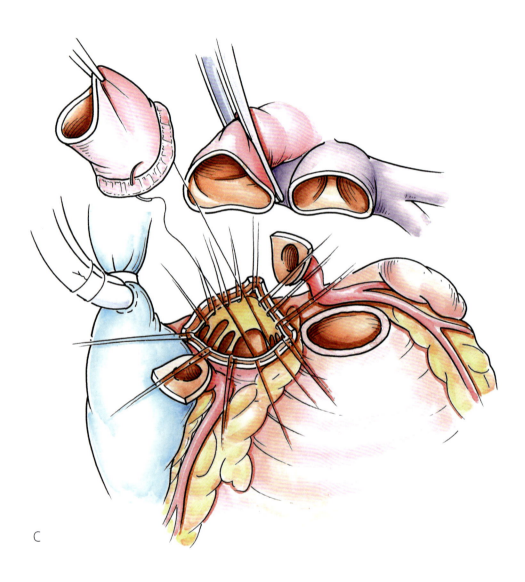

C

图 13-5（续）

Figure 13-5 cont'd

D. 移植左、右冠状动脉至新的主动脉根部，并将升主动脉缝合。

D. The left and right coronary arteries are implanted to the new aortic roots, and the ascending aorta is sutured.

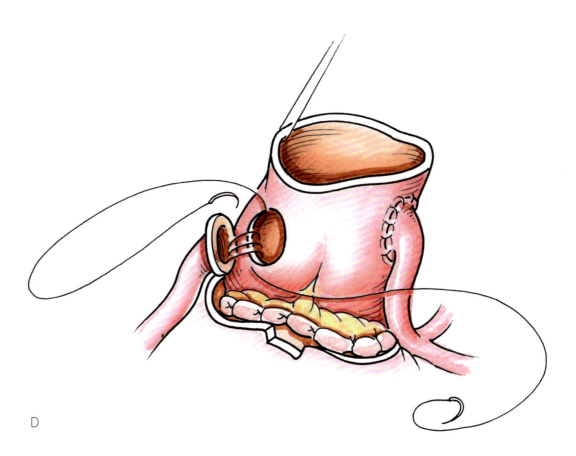

D

图 13-5（续）

Figure 13-5 cont'd

E、F. 取同种异体带瓣管道移植在原肺动脉处。

E, F. The homograft valved conduit is implanted into the original pulmonary artery.

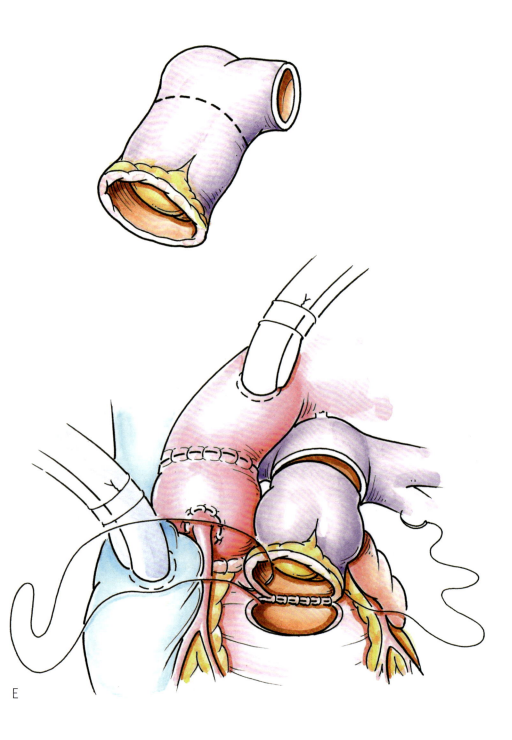

E

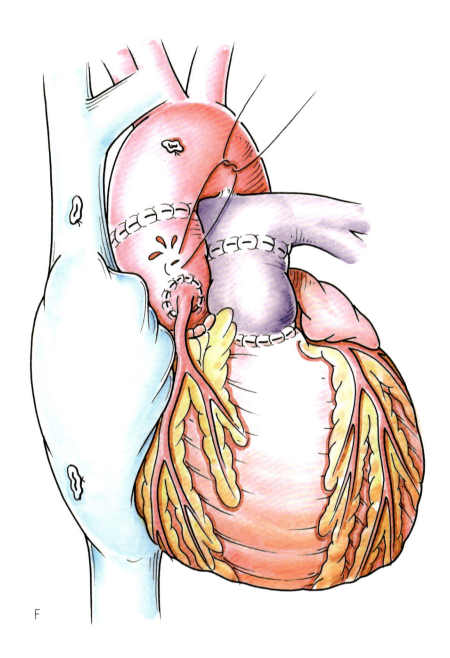

F

6. Ross-Konno 手术 该手术适用于主动脉瓣和瓣下同时存在狭窄的患者。与单纯 Ross 手术不同，需同时扩大左心室流出道（图 13-6）。

6. Ross-Konno procedure The Ross-Konno procedure is indicated for patients with both aortic and subvalvular aortic stenosis. Unlike the Ross procedure alone, the left ventricular outflow tract needs to be expanded at the same time (Figure 13-6).

图 13-6 **Ross-Konno 手术**

A. 取自体肺动脉瓣时，需适当延长右心室前壁组织用作修补切开的室间隔。

Figure 13-6 **Ross-Konno procedure**

A. When the autologous pulmonary valve is harvested, the tissue of the anterior wall of the right ventricle needs to be appropriately extended to repair the incised ventricular septum.

Continued

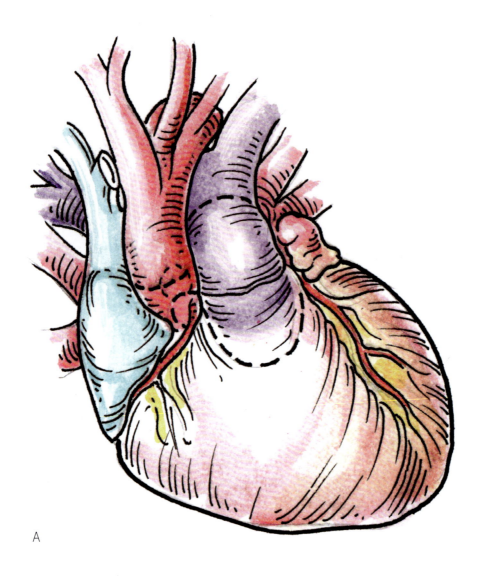

A

图 13-6（续）

B. 在左、右冠瓣之间，沿主动脉根部向室间隔方向做一个纵行切口。前方延伸至右心室流出道，后方向室间隔左心室面延伸，扩大左心室流出道。

Figure 13-6 cont'd

B. A longitudinal incision along the aortic root toward the interventricular septum is made between the left and right coronary valves. It extends anteriorly to the right ventricular outflow tract and posteriorly to the left ventricular surface of the ventricular septum, expanding the left ventricular outflow tract.

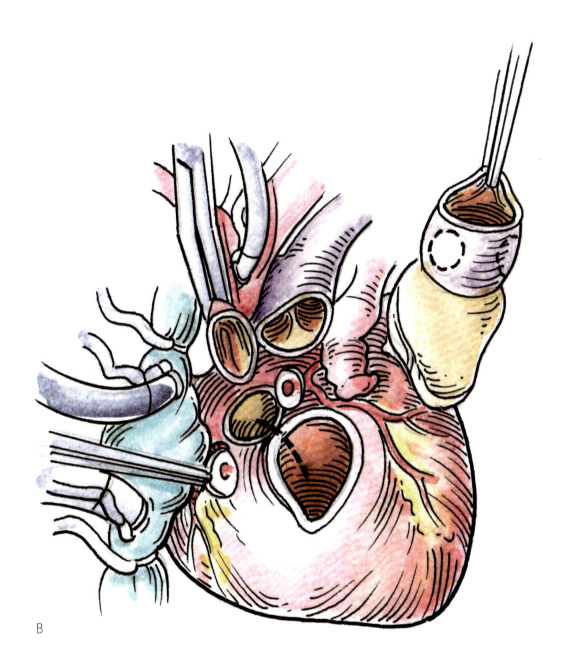

B

图 13-6 (续)

C. 也可采用 ePTFE 或 Dacron 补片修补扩大的室间隔, 更彻底地解除左心室流出道梗阻。

Figure 13-6 cont'd

C. ePTFE or Dacron patch can also be used to repair the enlarged ventricular septum, allowing for more complete relief of left ventricular outflow tract obstruction.

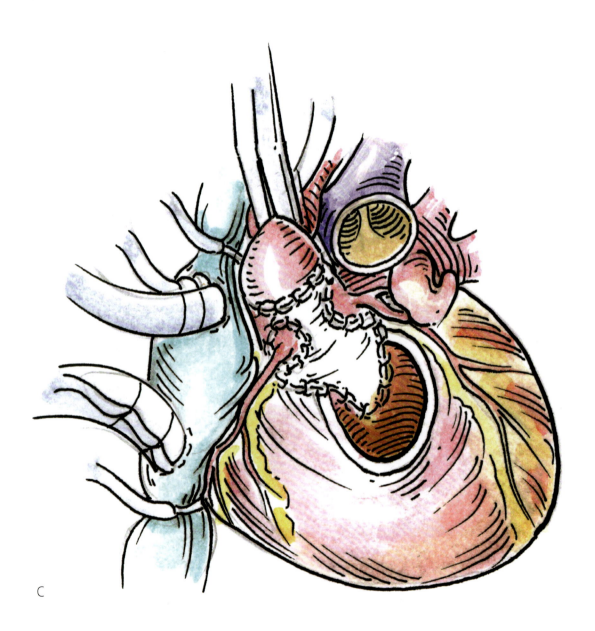

C

图 13-6 (续)

Figure 13-6 cont'd

D. 其余部分与 Ross 手术相同。

D. The rest of the Ross-Konno procedure is the same as the Ross procedure.

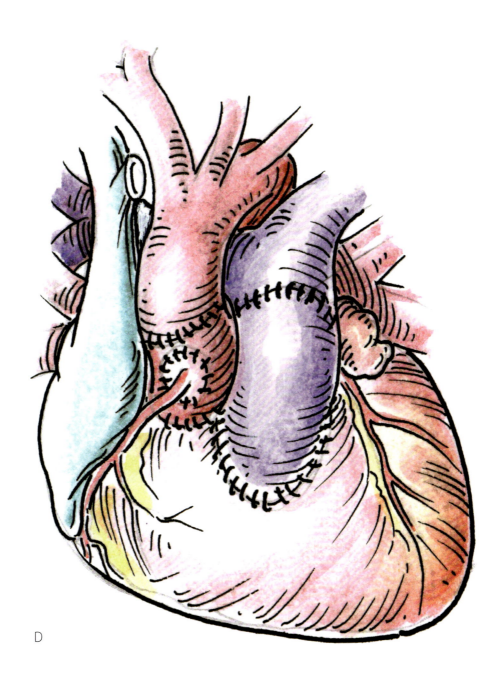

D

7. Konno-Rastan 手术 该手术主要适用于主动脉瓣置换同时扩大左心室流出道（图 13-7）。

7. Konno-Rastan operation This operation is mainly used for aortic valve replacement while expanding the left ventricular outflow tract (Figure 13-7).

图 13-7　Konno-Rastan 手术
A. 虚线显示主动脉、右心室联合切口，并将室间隔切开，扩大左心室流出道。

Figure 13-7　Konno-Rastan operation
A. The dotted line shows the combined incision of the aorta and the right ventricle, and the ventricular septum is incised to expand the left ventricular outflow tract.

Continued

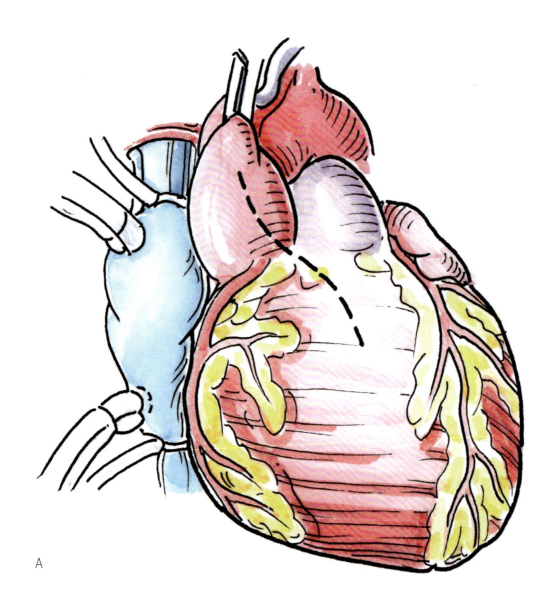

A

图 13-7（续）

Figure 13-7 cont'd

B. 儿童通常选用机械瓣膜置换主动脉瓣。

B. A mechanical valve is usually chosen to replace the aortic valve in children.

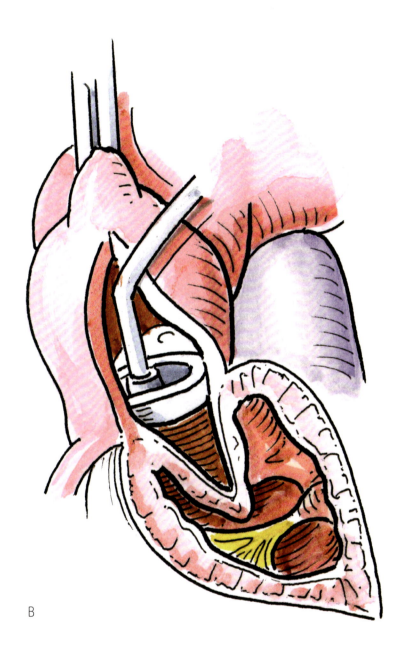

B

图 13-7 (续)

Figure 13-7 cont'd

C. 取两块牛心包或 ePTFE 补片,一块修补切开的室间隔。

C. Two bovine pericardial or ePTFE patches were taken. One was used to repair the ventricular septum.

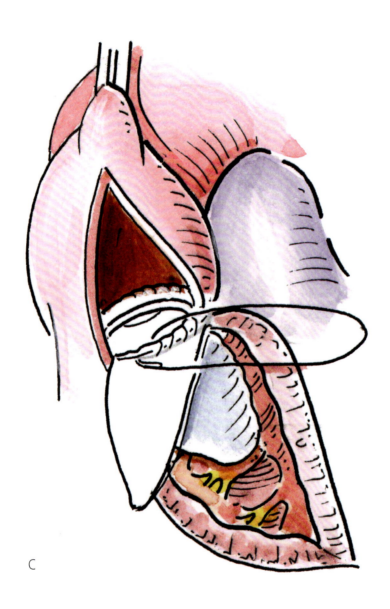

C

图 13-7 (续)

D. 另取一块补片扩大主动脉根部。

Figure 13-7 cont'd

D. Another patch was to enlarge the aortic root.

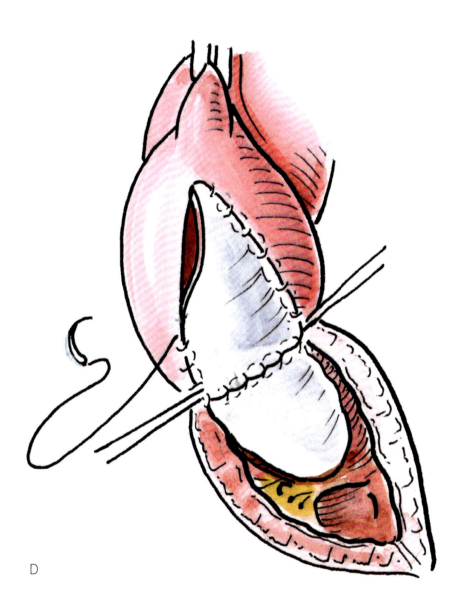

D

图 13-7（续）

Figure 13-7 cont'd

E. 最后再用一块牛心包补片关闭右心室流出道切口。靠近主动脉根部处可将补片缝在之前的补片上。注意避免损伤冠状动脉。

E. Finally, a bovine pericardial patch was used to close the right ventricular outflow tract incision. The patch can be sutured to the previous patch near the root of the aorta. Take care to avoid damage to the coronary arteries.

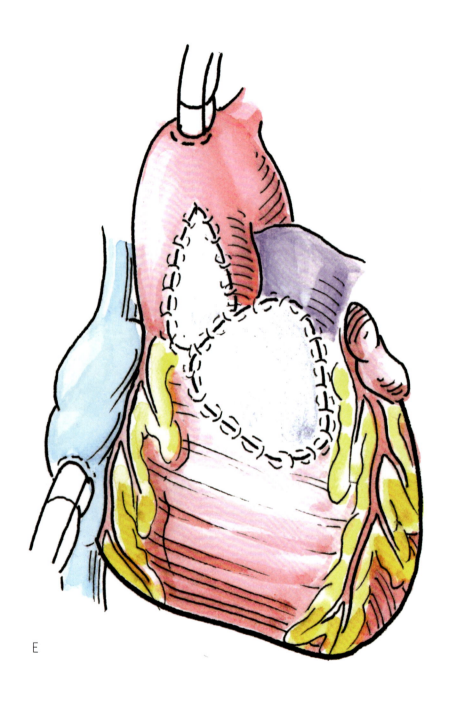

E

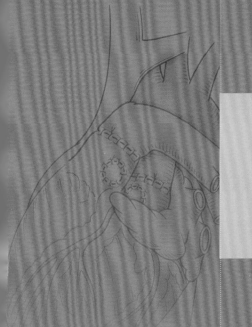

14　冠状动脉起源异常

14　Anomalies of Coronary
Artery Origin

先天性冠状动脉畸形的分类包括：①左冠状动脉或右冠状动脉起源于肺动脉，最常见是前者；②冠状动脉的主动脉起源异常；③冠状动脉瘘。继发性冠状动脉病变主要是川崎病导致的冠状动脉瘤和狭窄，极少数是心导管经皮介入治疗导致的冠状动脉损伤。

The classification of congenital coronary artery anomalies includes: ① Anomalous origin of the left coronary artery from the pulmonary artery (ALCAPA) or anomalous origin of the right coronary artery originating from the pulmonary artery (ARCAPA), with the former being the more common type; ② Anomalous aortic origin of a coronary artery (AAOCA); ③ Coronary artery fistulas. Secondary coronary artery lesions include primarily coronary artery aneurysms and stenosis caused by Kawasaki disease in most cases or iatrogenic injuries to the coronary artery caused by percutaneous invasive procedures with cardiac catheters on rare occasions.

一、左冠状动脉起源于肺动脉

I. Anomalous Origin of the Left Coronary Artery from the Pulmonary Artery

1. 冠状动脉直接移植　左冠状动脉开口自肺动脉右后瓣窦，靠主动脉侧较近（图 14-1）。

1. Direct coronary implantation　The left coronary ostium originates from the right posterolateral sinus of the pulmonary artery and is near the aortic side (Figure 14-1).

图 14-1　**冠状动脉直接移植**

A. 体外循环建立后，圈套左右肺动脉，横断主肺动脉，取下纽扣状左冠状动脉开口组织，游离松解。

Figure 14-1　Direct coronary implantation

A. After establishment of extracorporeal circulation, constrict the left and right pulmonary arteries, transect the main pulmonary artery, and dissociate the left coronary and separate the coronary button.

Continued

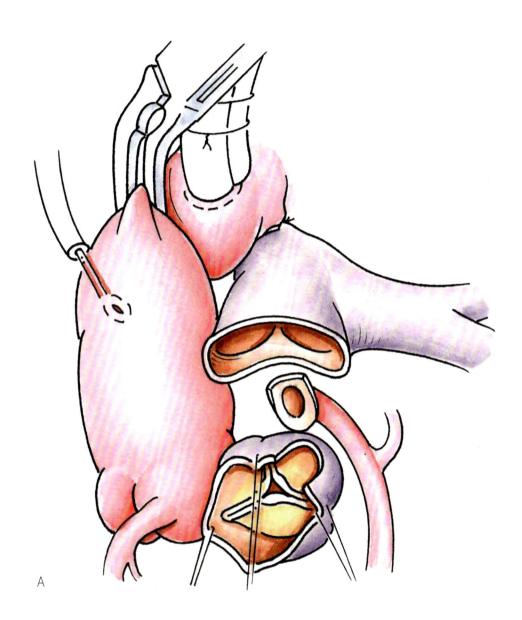

A

图 14-1（续）

B. 将左冠状动脉开口直接种植在升主动脉侧壁。

Figure 14-1 cont'd

B. The left coronary ostium is implanted directly into the lateral wall of the ascending aorta.

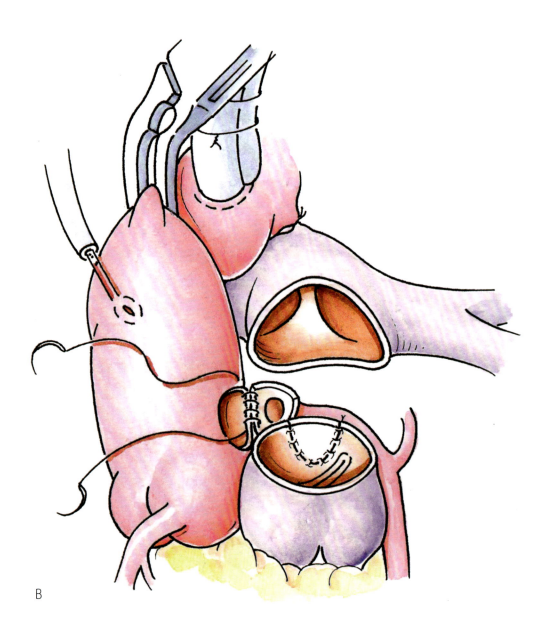

B

图 14-1（续）

C. 肺动脉缺口用自身心包补片扩大缝合，主肺动脉端端吻合。

Figure 14-1 cont'd

C. The pulmonary artery opening is enlarged and sutured with an autologous pericardial patch, and end-to-end anastomosis is performed at the main pulmonary artery.

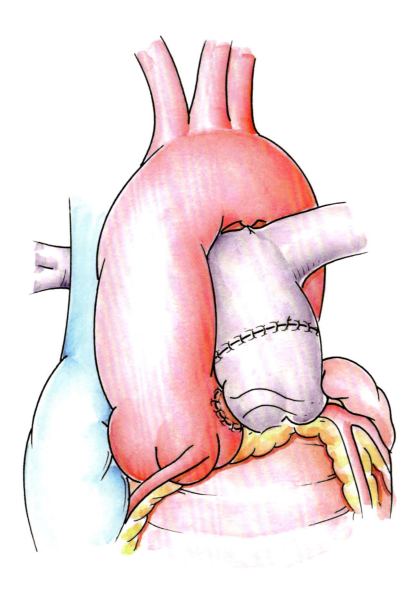

C

图 14-2　**血管壁皮瓣方法**
A. 左冠状动脉异常起源于肺动脉常见位置在肺动脉根部的左后侧瓣窦。在右心室漏斗部表面常可见冠状动脉侧支血管建立。

Figure 14-2　Vascular wall flap methods
A. ALCAPA often originates from the left posterior sinus at the root of the pulmonary artery. The establishment of coronary collateral vessels is often seen on the infundibular surface of the right ventricle.

Continued

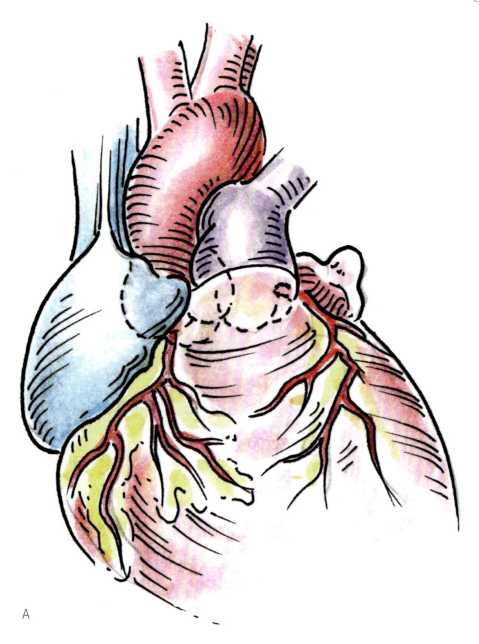

A

图 14-2（续）

B. 在转流开始后立刻圈套收紧左右肺动脉，防止冠状动脉窃血，也可防止左心室过度膨胀，并尽快放置左心室引流管。

Figure 14-2 cont'd

B. As the bypass starts, the left and right pulmonary arteries are constricted to avoid coronary steal and left ventricular over-distension, and then the left heart drainage tube is inserted as soon as possible.

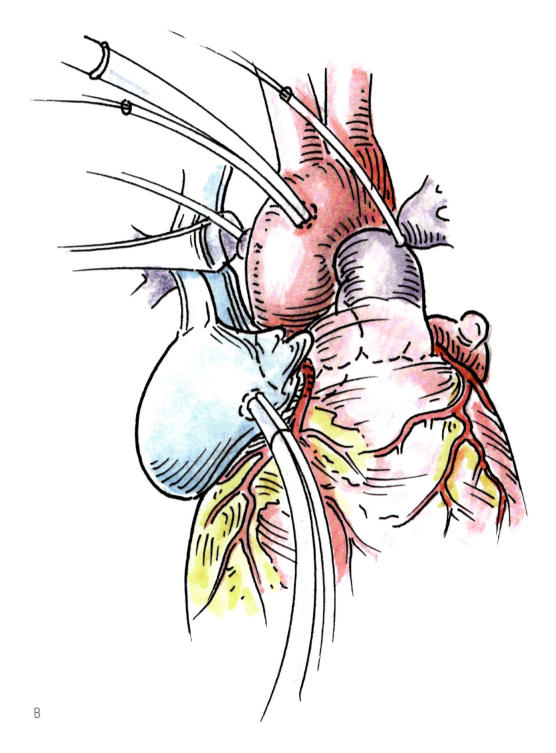

B

图 14-2（续）

C. 为避免移植冠状动脉张力过大，可使用主肺动脉前壁和升主动脉前壁部分组织作为"皮瓣"延长冠状动脉长度。

Figure 14-2 cont'd

C. In order to avoid excessive coronary tension, the tissues from the anterior wall of the main pulmonary artery and ascending aorta are taken as a "flap" to prolong the length of the coronary artery.

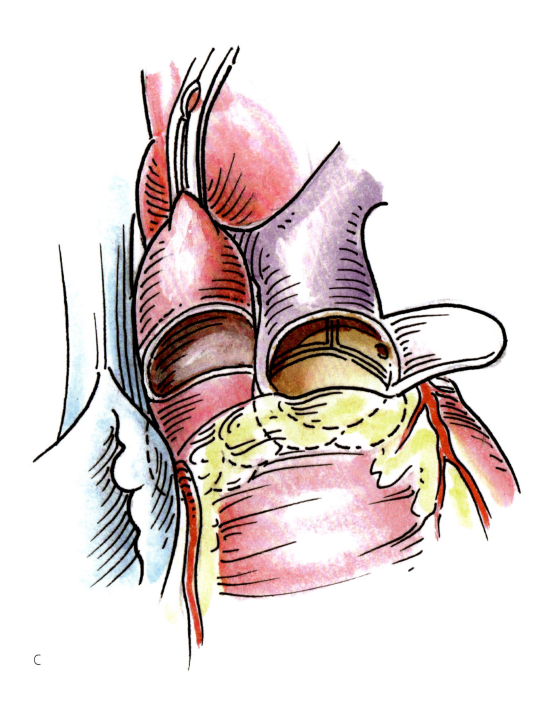

C

图 14-2（续）

D. 通常将主动脉壁作为冠状动脉后壁，肺动脉壁作为冠状动脉的前壁。

Figure 14-2 cont'd

D. Generally, the aortic wall is considered as the posterior wall of the coronary artery and the pulmonary wall as the anterior wall.

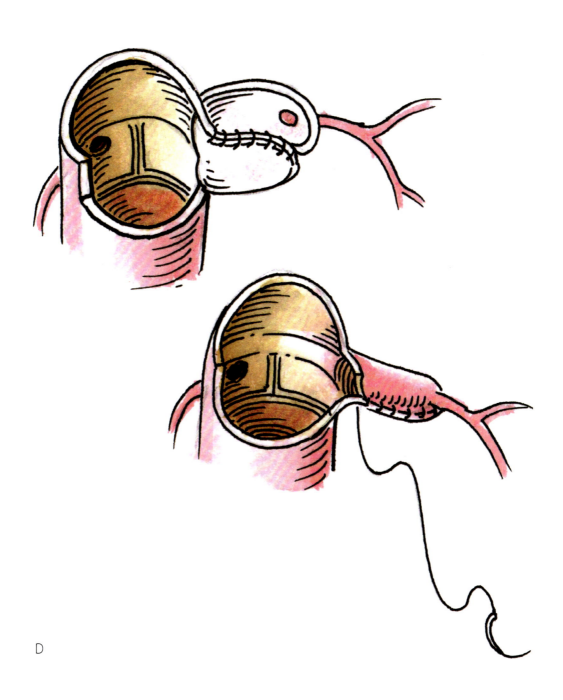

D

图 14-2（续）

E. 主肺动脉充分游离松解后可直接缝合。升主动脉须取自体心包补片扩大缝合。

Figure 14-2 cont'd

E. The main pulmonary artery can be fully dissociated and then directly sutured, but the ascending aorta is enlarged and sutured with an autologous pericardial patch.

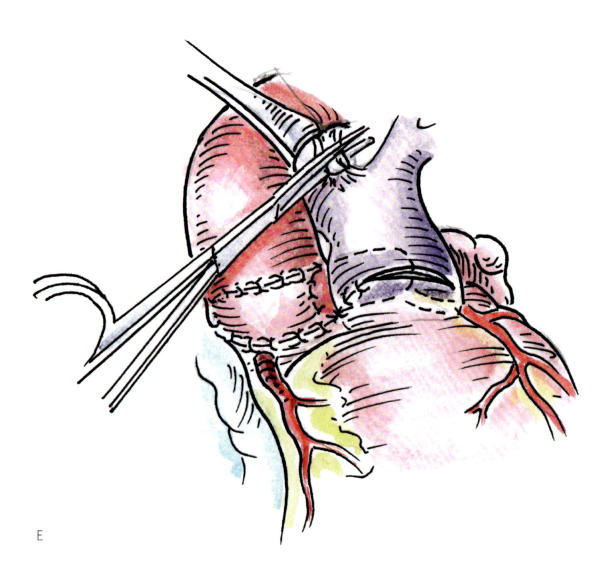

E

3. 内隧道方法（Takeuchi 手术） 即将肺动脉前壁剪下一条"血管瓣"覆盖在左冠状动脉开口处，在主动脉与肺动脉侧壁开孔，后壁直接缝合，前壁用自体血管瓣缝合，肺动脉前壁再用自身心包补片扩大。该手术优点是取自体组织材料，有生长的潜力，但易导致肺动脉瓣上狭窄。现在临床较少应用（图 14-3）。

3. Internal tunneling methods (Takeuchi operation) A vascular flap is cut from the anterior wall of the pulmonary artery to cover the left coronary ostium. Perforate the wall of the aorta and pulmonary artery and directly suture the posterior wall. The anterior wall is sutured with an autologous vascular flap. The anterior wall of the pulmonary artery is augmented with an autologous pericardial patch. Takeuchi operation offers the advantages of using an autologous graft, which has the growth potential, but it predisposes to supravalvular pulmonary stenosis and hence is rarely used clinically (Figure 14-3).

图 14-3　内 隧 道 方 法（Takeuchi 手术）

Figure 14-3　Internal tunneling methods (Takeuchi operation)

A. 打开肺动脉前壁。

A. Make an incision on the anterior wall of the pulmonary artery.

Continued

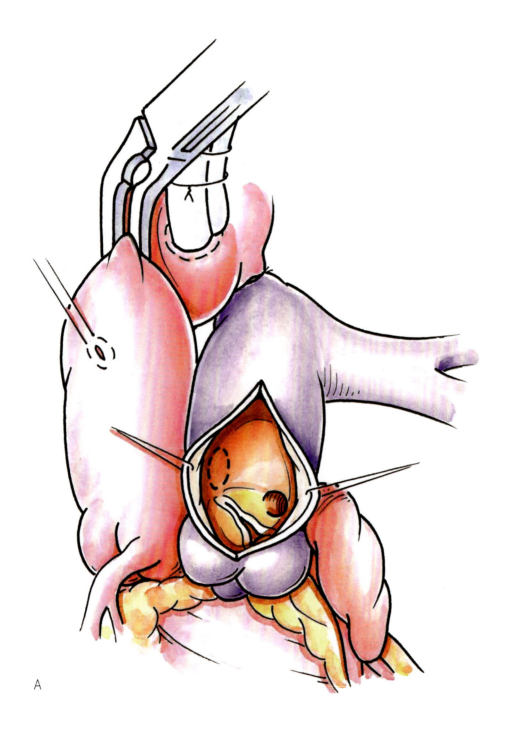

A

图 14-3(续)

B. 在主动脉与肺动脉侧壁开孔,后壁直
接缝合。

Figure 14-3 cont'd

B. Perforate the wall of the aorta and pulmonary artery and directly suture the posterior wall.

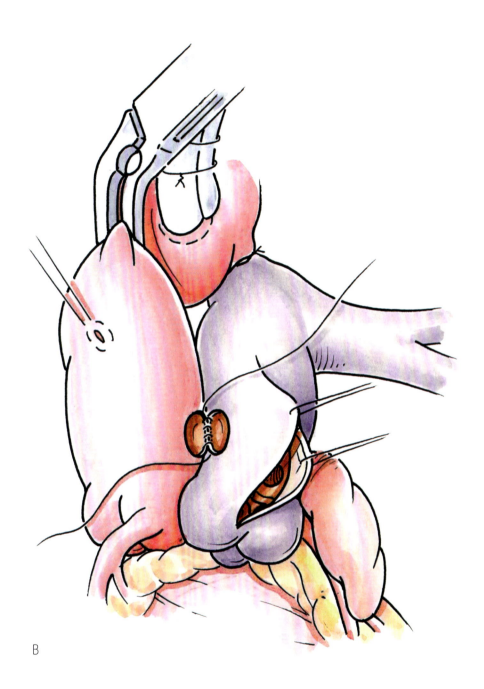

B

图 14-3（续）

C. 将肺动脉前壁剪下一条"血管瓣"覆盖在左冠状动脉开口处。

Figure 14-3 cont'd

C. A vascular flap is cut from the anterior wall of the pulmonary artery to cover the left coronary ostium.

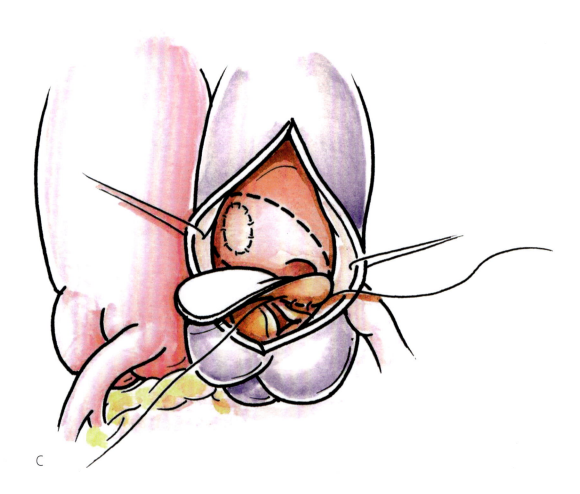

C

图 14-3（续）

D. 肺动脉前壁用自身心包补片扩大。

Figure 14-3 cont'd

D. The anterior wall of the pulmonary artery is augmented with an autologous pericardial patch.

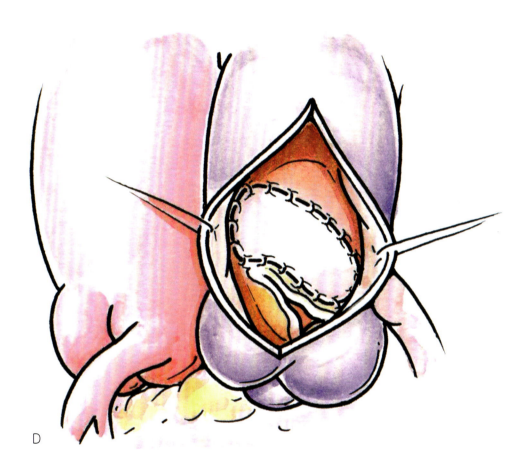

D

二、冠状动脉的主动脉起源异常

II. Anomalous Aortic Origin of a Coronary Artery

常见两大类,左冠状动脉起源于右冠窦或右冠状动脉起源于左冠窦。有一段冠状动脉走行在主动脉壁内,容易在青少年期发生猝死。

Generally, AAOCA is a congenital abnormality in which the left coronary artery arises from the right coronary sinus or the right coronary artery from the left coronary sinus. It is often associated with the intramural course of the coronary artery within the aortic wall. Patients with AAOCA are prone to sudden death in adolescence.

1. 右冠状动脉开口异常(图 14-4)

1. Anomalous right coronary ostium (Figure 14-4)

图 14-4　右冠状动脉开口异常
A. 横断升主动脉,暴露冠状动脉开口。可见右冠状动脉开口在左冠窦内,并有一段右冠状动脉走行在主动脉壁内。

Figure 14-4　Anomalous right coronary ostium
A. Transect the ascending aorta to expose the coronary ostium. The right coronary ostium will be found at the left aortic sinus, and a segment of the right coronary artery traverses intramurally within the aortic wall.

Continued

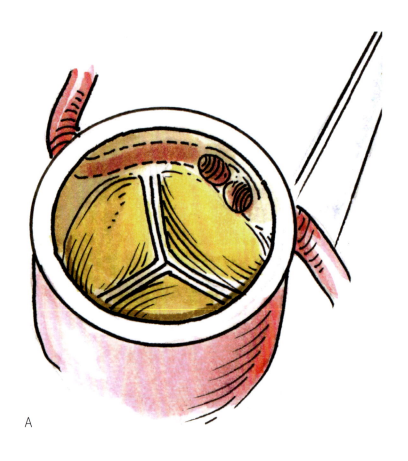

A

图 14-4（续）

B. 沿着冠状动脉走行长度，剪开主动脉内壁，实施去顶手术。

C. 在新的冠状动脉开口上用 7-0 或 8-0 Prolene 缝线间断缝合，将内膜层重新固定在冠状动脉开口处，以防血栓形成和血管壁夹层。

Figure 14-4 cont'd

B. Cut open the aortic wall along the length of the intramural coronary artery and perform the unroofing procedure.

C. Interrupted sutures are applied to the coronary ostium with 7-0 or 8-0 Prolene suture, and the intimal layer is refixed to the coronary ostium to avoid thrombosis and dissection.

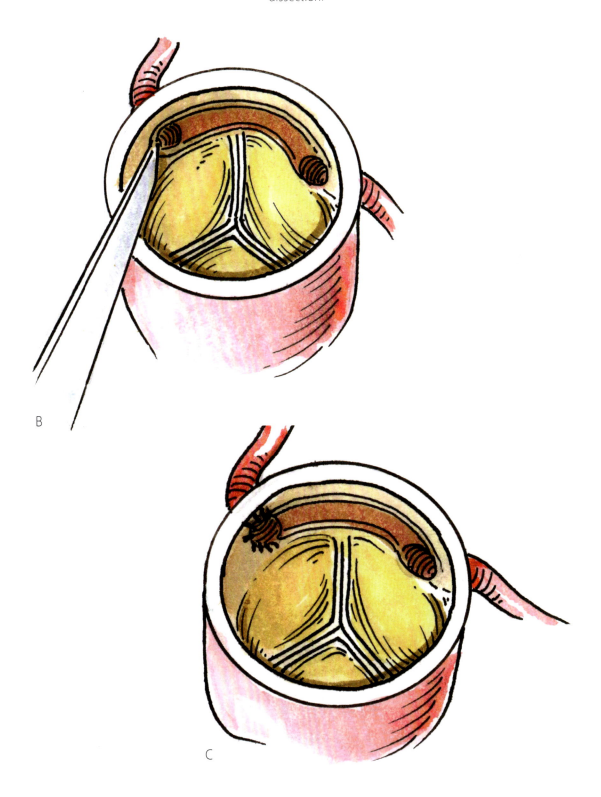

B

C

2. 左冠状动脉开口异常（图 14-5）

2. Anomalous left coronary ostium(Figure 14-5)

图 14-5　左冠状动脉开口异常

A. 横断升主动脉，暴露冠状动脉开口。可见左冠状动脉开口在右冠窦内，并有一段左冠状动脉走行在主动脉壁内。

Figure 14-5　Anomalous left coronary ostium

A. Transect the ascending aorta to expose the coronary ostium. The left coronary ostium will be found inside the right aortic sinus, and a segment of the left coronary artery traverses intramurally within the aortic wall.

Continued

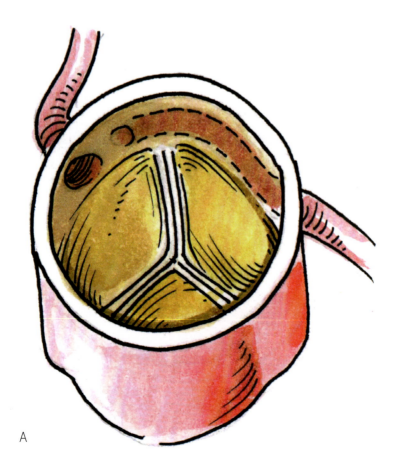

A

图 14-5（续）

Figure 14-5 cont'd

B、C. 手术方法与右冠状动脉开口异常处理相同。

B. C. The surgical approach is the same as that for anomalous right coronary ostium.

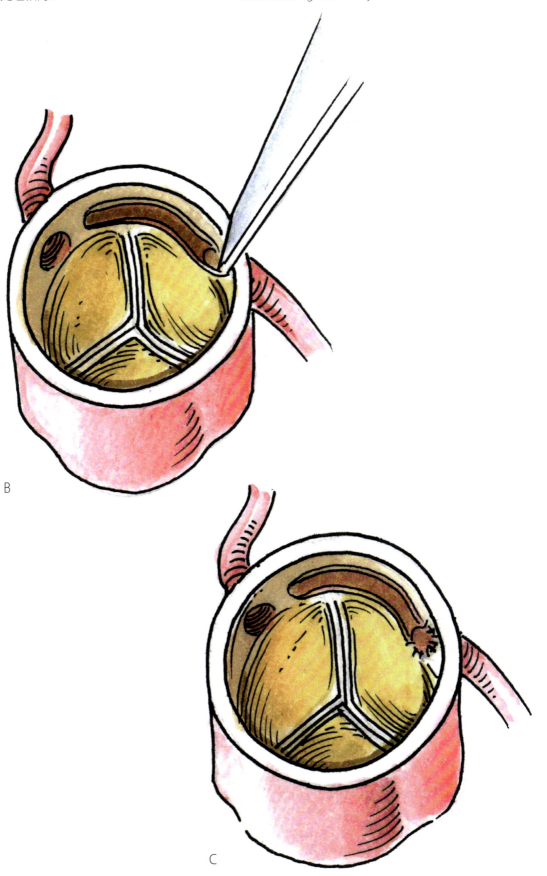

B

C

3. 构建左冠状动脉的新开口 （图 14-6）

3. Construction of a new ostium in the left coronary artery (Figure 14-6)

图 14-6　**构建左冠状动脉的新开口**

A. 有些患者左冠状动脉开口在右冠窦，左冠状动脉较长，并绕行在主动脉后壁，非壁内走行，但容易形成狭窄。

Figure 14-6　Construction of a new ostium in the left coronary artery

A. Some AAOCA patients have left coronary ostium in the right coronary sinus, but the stenosis is easily formed because of the long left coronary artery coursing around the posterior wall of the aorta rather than within the wall.

Continued

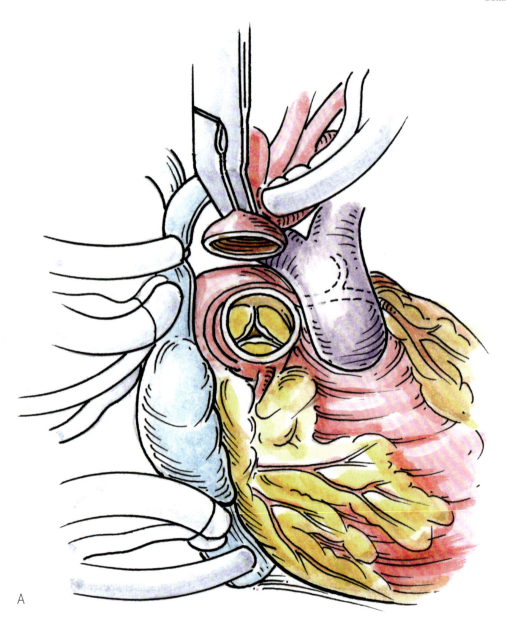

A

图 14-6（续）

B. 手术方法是在左冠状动脉靠近左冠窦处开孔，做侧侧吻合。

Figure 14-6 cont'd

B. Surgical methods: perforate on the left coronary artery near the left coronary sinus and perform the side-to-side anastomosis.

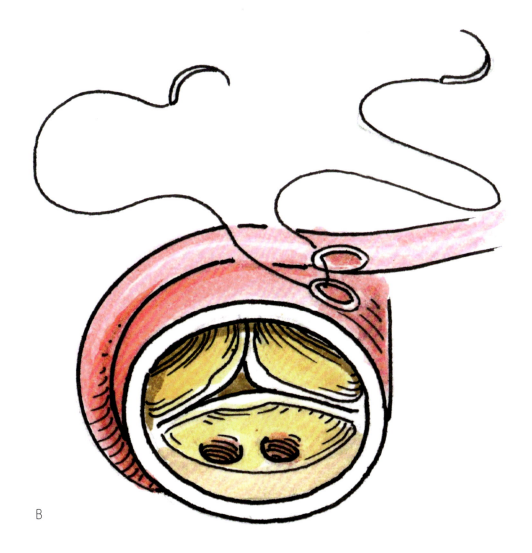

B

图 14-6（续）
C. 新建的冠状动脉开口更接近正常冠状动脉的解剖位置。

Figure 14-6 cont'd
C. New coronary ostium are closer to the anatomical location of normal coronary arteries.

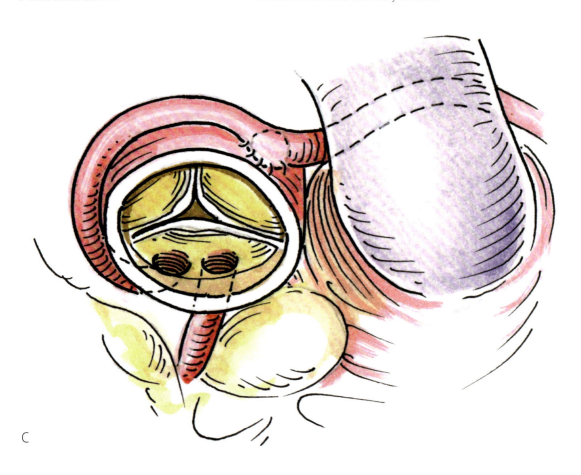

C

三、冠状动脉瘘

孤立性冠状动脉瘘常见起源于右冠状动脉和左冠状动脉，极少起源于回旋支。最常见终点位置为右心室和肺动脉，而流入左侧心腔很少见（8%）。随着心导管介入技术的提高，绝大多数患者可通过介入封堵技术处理。但一些大型的瘘口仍需通过手术治疗（图 14-7）。

III. Coronary Artery Fistulas

Isolated coronary fistulas mainly originate from the right and left coronary arteries and rarely from the circumflex artery. Drainage into the right ventricle and pulmonary artery is more prevalent, and drainage into the left chamber occurs rarely (accounting for 8%). With the advances in cardiac catheterization, most patients with coronary artery fistulas can be managed by interventional occlusion. However, some large fistulae need to be treated by surgery (Figure 14-7).

图 14-7　冠状动脉瘘

A、B. 对单一瘘口、比较靠近心脏表面，可不使用心肺转流术。可将冠状动脉瘘口游离出来，在进入心肌前给予结扎。

Figure 14-7　Coronary artery fistulas

A, B. Isolated fistula proximal to the surface of the heart can be treated without cardiopulmonary bypass. Free the coronary fistula and ligate it before draining into the myocardium.

Continued

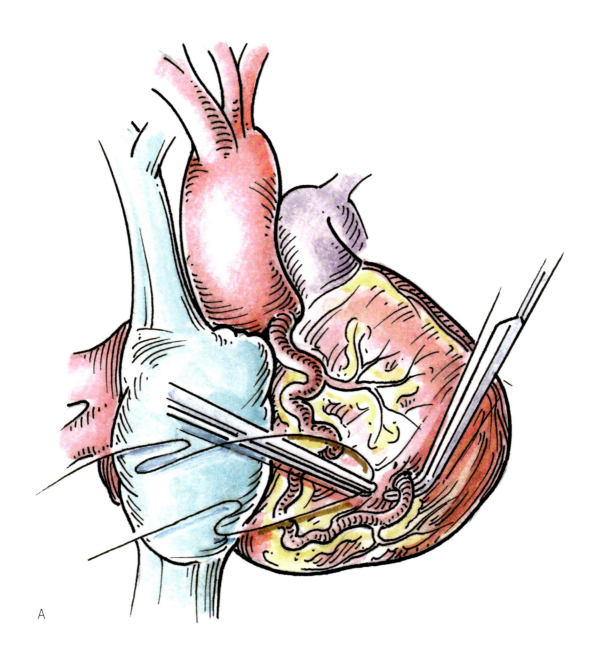

A

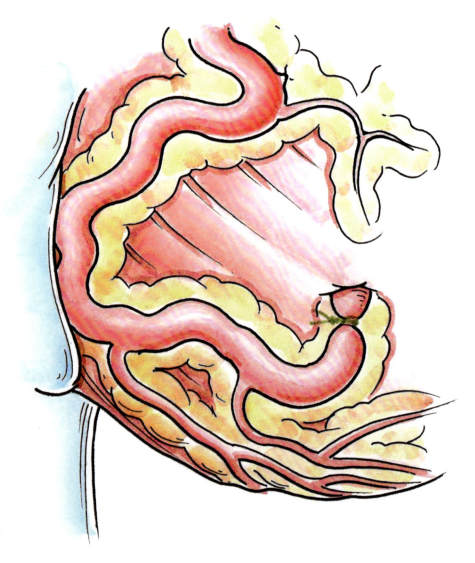

B

图 14-7（续）

C~E. 对右冠状动脉开口在右心室表面的多发瘘口，也可在非心肺转流术时，用带垫片缝线在冠状动脉下方做水平褥式缝合，必要时可加固，直到震颤完全消失。

Figure 14-7 cont'd

C-E. For multiple fistulae with the right coronary ostium on the right ventricular surface, horizontal mattress sutures with pledget are performed below the coronary artery without cardiopulmonary bypass and, if necessary, can be reinforced until the complete disappearance of tremor.

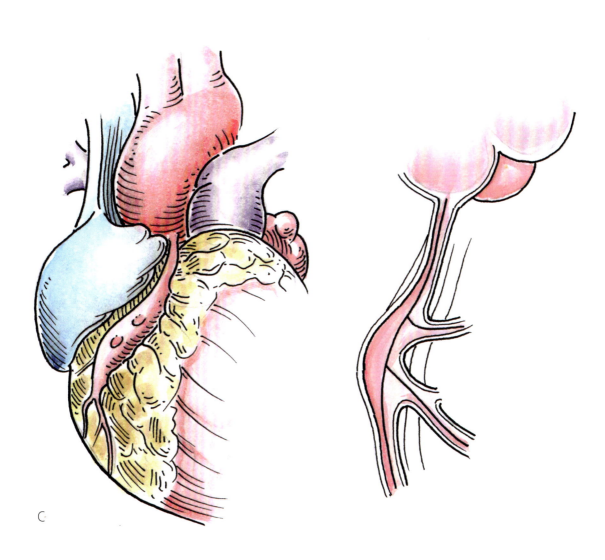

C

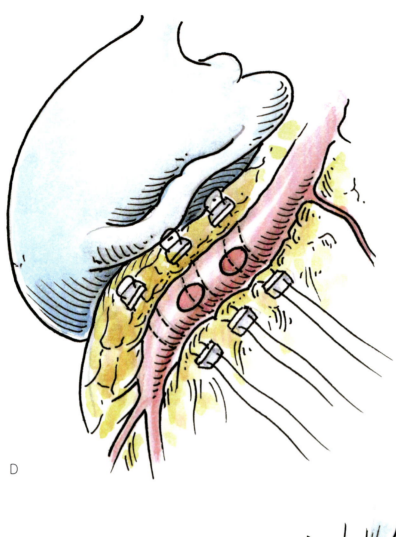

D

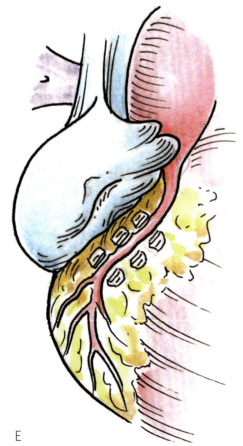

E

图 14-7（续）

F、G. 更为可靠方法是在心肺转流术时切开扩张的冠状动脉瘤，暴露瘘口，直接缝合或用心包补片修补。

Figure 14-7 cont'd

F, G. A more reliable method is to incise the dilated coronary artery aneurysm to expose the fistula and directly suture it or repair it with a pericardial patch under cardiopulmonary bypass.

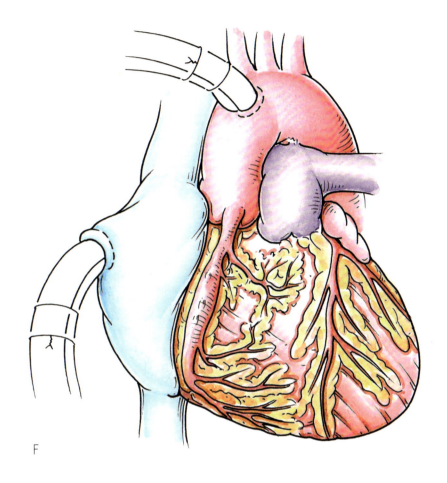

F

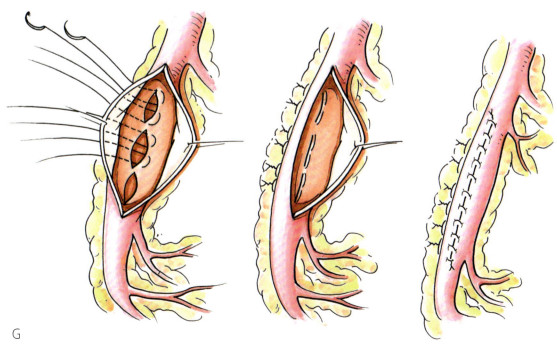

G

图 14-7 (续)

H. 对心室内的瘘口, 采用心脏停搏后, 主动脉根部继续灌注心肌保护液, 探查瘘口的位置, 再做心内缝合或补片修补。

Figure 14-7 cont'd

H. For intraventricular fistulae, after cardiac arrest, continuously perfuse the aortic root with cardioplegic solution to detect the position of fistulae, and then perform intracardiac suture or patch repair.

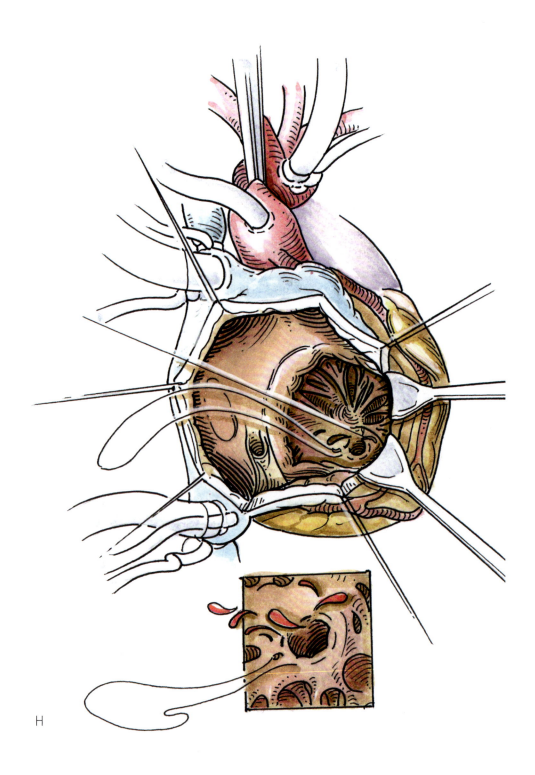

H

15 先天性二尖瓣疾病

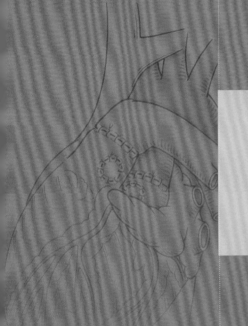

15 Congenital Mitral Valve Disease

一、解剖分型

1. 二尖瓣狭窄　先天性孤立性二尖瓣狭窄非常少见。常合并二尖瓣发育不全,是 Shone 综合征的一部分。二尖瓣狭窄可以是结构性的,如降落伞式二尖瓣、二尖瓣瓣上环(图 15-1),也可以是二尖瓣结构正常,但因瓣膜和瓣环发育不全而导致功能性二尖瓣狭窄。

I. Anatomical Typing

1. Mitral stenosis　Congenital isolated mitral stenosis is very rare. It is often associated with mitral dysplasia and is part of Shone's syndrome. Mitral stenosis may be structural, such as the parachute mitral valve, supramitral ring (Figure 15-1), or the mitral valve may be normal in structure, but functional mitral stenosis is caused by dysplasia of the valve and annulus.

图 15-1　**二尖瓣狭窄**
A. 降落伞式二尖瓣。

Figure 15-1　**Mitral stenosis**
A. Parachute mitral valve.

Continued

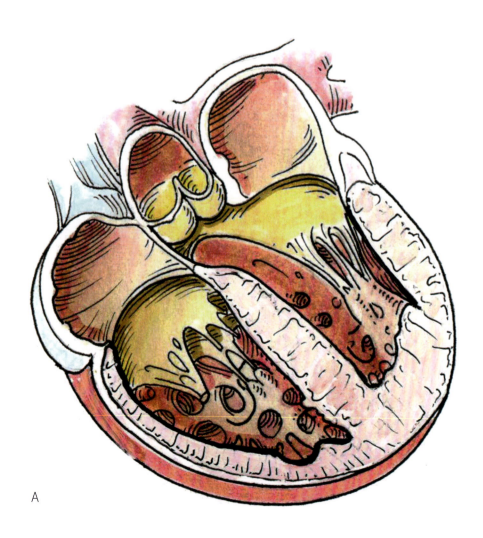

A

图 15-1（续）

B. 二尖瓣瓣上环。

Figure 15-1 cont'd

B. Supramitral ring.

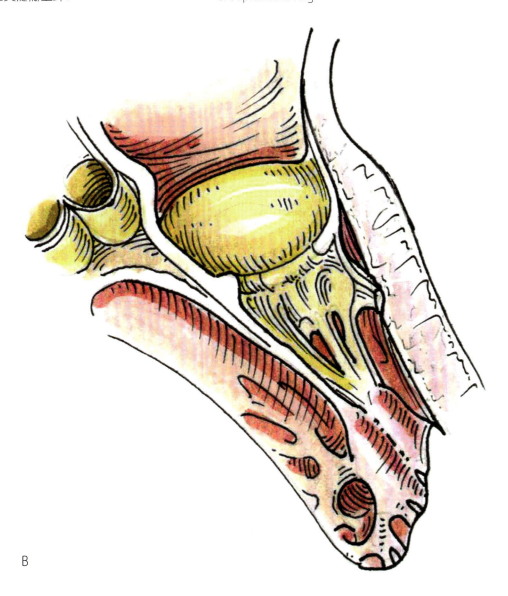

B

2. 二尖瓣反流　先天性二尖瓣反流比二尖瓣狭窄更常见，以二尖瓣裂缺为多见，大多出现在房室隔缺损患者（图 15-2），也可能是左心功能不全、左心室扩大、二尖瓣瓣环扩大导致二尖瓣反流。

2. Mitral regurgitation　Congenital mitral regurgitation is more common than mitral stenosis. The most common one is mitral valve cleft, which occurs often in patients with atrio-ventricular septal defect (Figure 15-2). Left ventricular dysfunction, left ventricular enlargement, and a mitral annular enlargement may also lead to mitral regurgitation.

图 15-2　二尖瓣裂缺

Figure 15-2　Mitral valve cleft

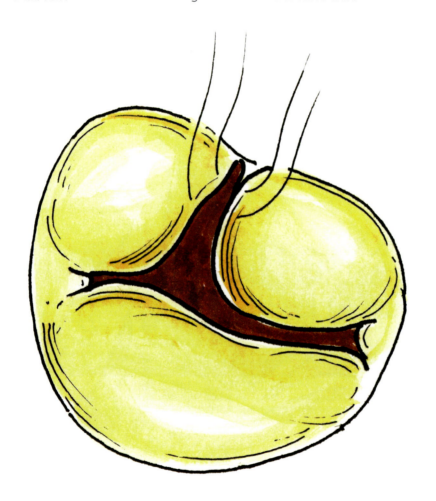

二、手术方法

先天性二尖瓣病变手术方法较多,主要包括以下几种。

针对二尖瓣狭窄的手术方法有交界切开术、瓣叶和腱索开窗术、二尖瓣瓣上环切除术、乳头肌劈开术等。针对二尖瓣反流为主手术方法有裂缺修补、瓣叶部分切除或瓣叶扩大术、瓣环成形术(O 形环或 C 形环)、腱索缩短或替代、瓣膜置换术。

II. Surgical Methods

There are many surgical methods for congenital mitral valve diseases, which mainly include the following types.

The main surgical methods for mitral stenosis include commissurotomy, leaflet and chordal fenestration, resection of supramitral ring, and splitting of papillary muscle. The surgical methods for mitral regurgitation are cleft repair, partial leaflet resection or leaflet enlargement, annuloplasty (O-shaped ring or C-shaped ring), chordal shortening or replacement, and mitral valve replacement.

1. 降落伞式二尖瓣（图 15-3）

1. Parachute mitral valve (Figure 15-3)

图 15-3　降落伞式二尖瓣

A. 单组乳头肌或乳头肌融合,常起源于左心室后壁。

Figure 15-3　Parachute mitral valve

A. Single papillary muscle or fused papillary muscles often arise from the posterior left ventricular wall.

Continued

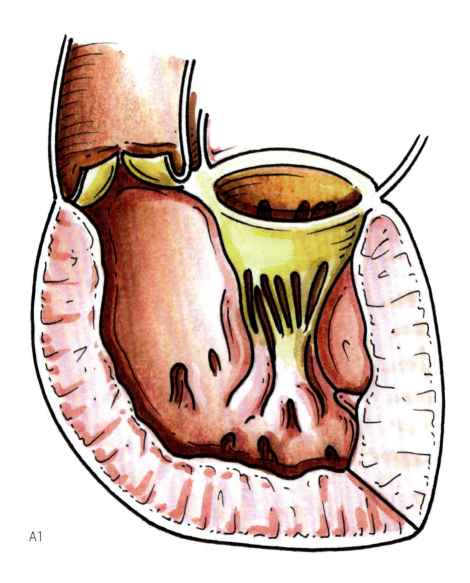

A1

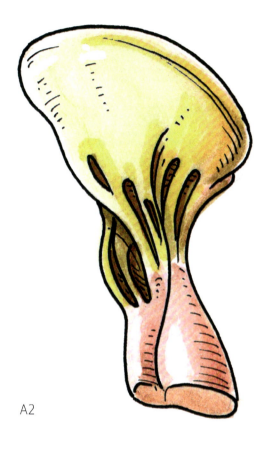

A2

A

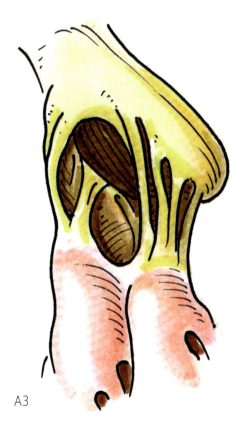

A3

图 15-3 (续)

B. 将瓣叶和乳头肌做部分切开，扩大心室开口面。

Figure 15-3 cont'd

B. The leaflets and papillary muscles are partially dissected to enlarge the ventricular inlet.

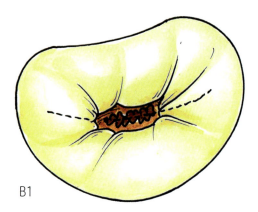

B1

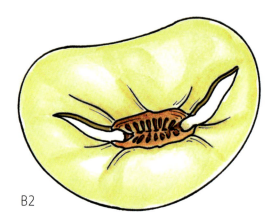

B2

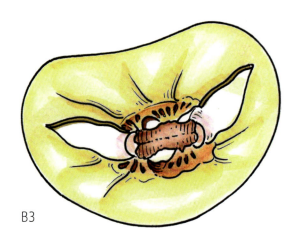

B3

B

图 15-3 (续)

C. 暴露粗大融合乳头肌,切开松解来增加瓣膜的活动度,有利舒张期血液回流和收缩期的瓣叶对合。

Figure 15-3 cont'd

C. Expose the fused coarse papillary muscles and dissect them to increase valve mobility and facilitate diastolic blood return, and systolic leaflet coaptation.

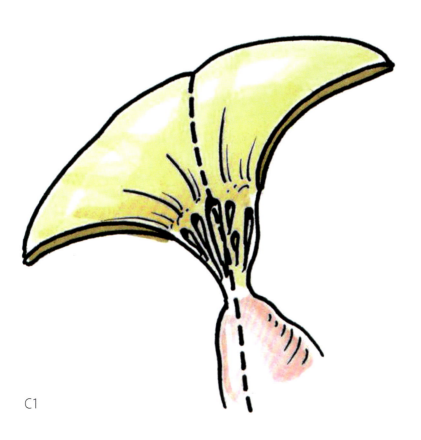

C1

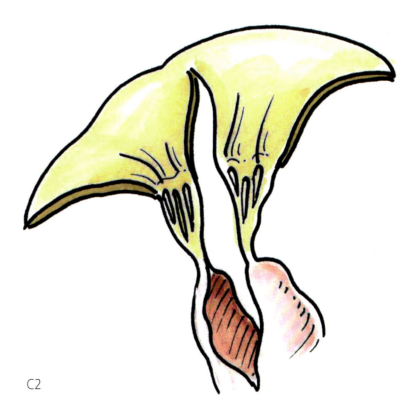

C

C2

2. 二尖瓣瓣上环（图 15-4）

2. Supramitral ring (Figure 15-4)

图 15-4　二尖瓣瓣上环

A. 经房间隔或房间沟左房处切口暴露二尖瓣,可清楚显示二尖瓣瓣上环纤维组织。

Figure 15-4　Supramitral ring

A. An incision is made through the atrial septum or left atrium near the atrial sulcus, and the mitral valve is exposed. A clear view of the fibrous tissue of the supramitral ring is achieved.

Continued

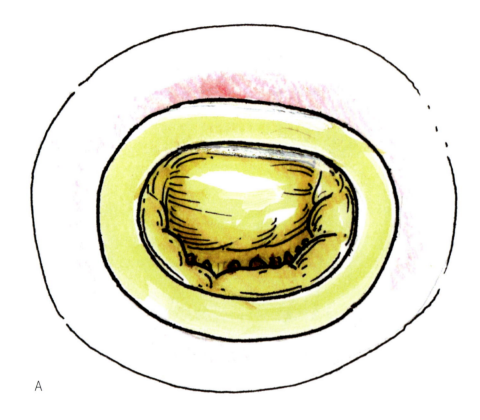

A

图 15-4（续）

B、C. 在纤维组织上缝置一根牵引线,沿着左房壁将二尖瓣瓣上环钝性分离,注意不要损伤瓣膜组织。

Figure 15-4 cont'd

B, C. With the help of a traction suture sewn to the fibrous tissue, the supramitral ring is bluntly separated along the left atrial wall. Take care not to damage the valve tissue.

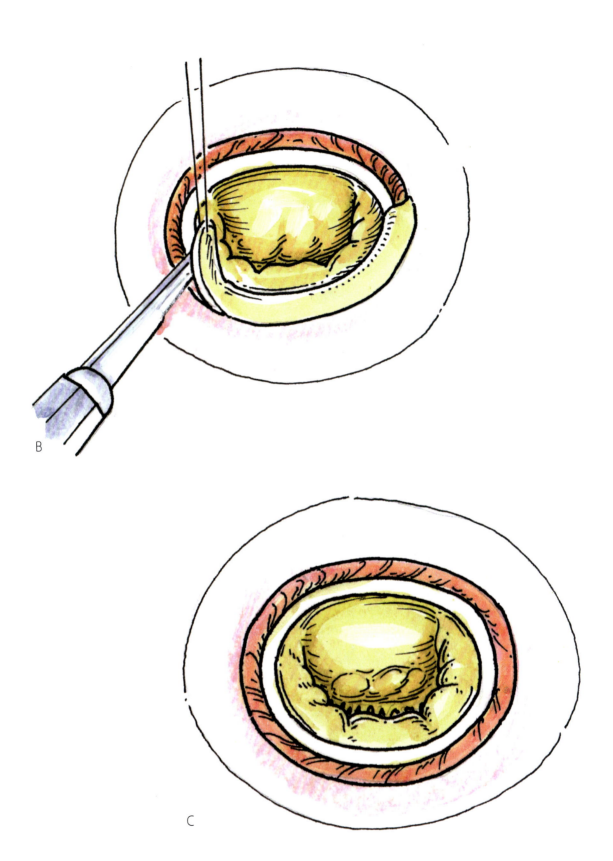

B

C

3. 二尖瓣裂缺修补术(图 15-5)

3. Mitral valve cleft repair (Figure 15-5)

图 15-5　二尖瓣裂缺修补术

A. 部分或完全房室隔缺损的患者常合并有二尖瓣裂缺。

B. 手术采用 5-0 Prolene 缝线加心包垫片间断 U 形缝合数针。

Figure 15-5　Mitral valve cleft repair

A. Mitral valve cleft is common in patients with partial or complete atrioventricular septal defect.

B. An interrupted U-shaped suture is made with 5-0 Prolene suture, and a pericardial patch is added.

Continued

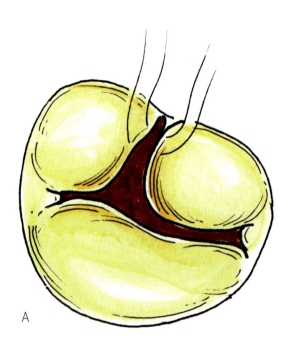

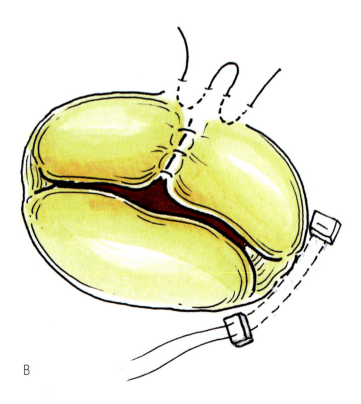

图 15-5（续）

C. 对同时有二尖瓣瓣环扩大产生二尖瓣中央反流者,可在两侧瓣膜交界处采用带垫片褥式缝合缩小二尖瓣瓣环。

Figure 15-5 cont'd

C. For patients with central mitral regurgitation due to mitral annulus enlargement, pledget-supported mattress sutures can be used at the junction of the two valves to reduce the mitral annulus.

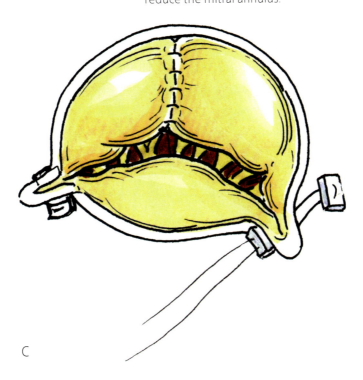

C

4. 瓣叶部分切除或瓣叶补片扩大术（图 15-6）

4. Partial leaflet resection or leaflet patch aortoplasty (Figure 15-6)

图 15-6　瓣叶部分切除或瓣叶补片扩大术

A. 对二尖瓣后瓣脱垂病变,可采用在瓣叶中心体做一矩形切口。

Figure 15-6　Partial leaflet resection or leaflet patch aortoplasty

A. For the posterior mitral valve prolapse, a rectangular incision can be made in the center of the valve leaflet.

Continued

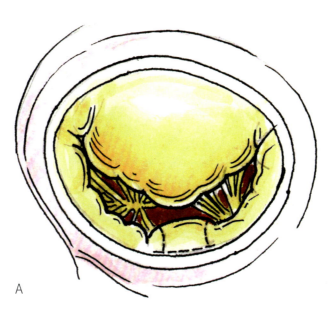

A

图 15-6（续）

B. 部分瓣叶切除后沿瓣环做部分切开。

C. 将后瓣瓣环做部分折叠缝合。

Figure 15-6 cont'd

B. Partial dissection along the annulus after partial resection.

C. The posterior annulus is partially plicated and sutured.

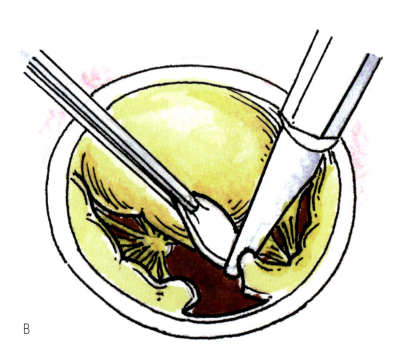

B

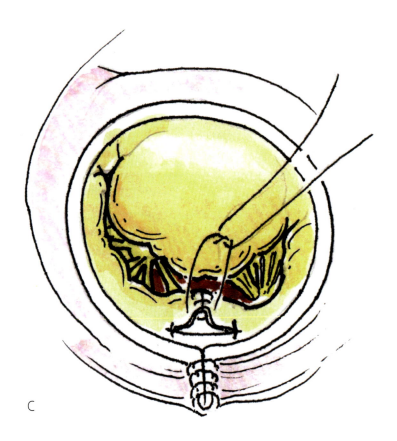

C

图 15-6（续）

D. 将剪开之瓣叶对合间断缝合，对年龄较大儿童可同时再上一个 C 形环。

Figure 15-6 cont'd

D. Then clipped leaflets are coapted and completed with interrupted sutures, and a C-shaped ring can be applied at the same time in elder children.

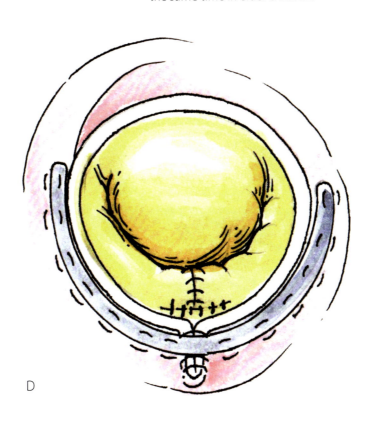

D

图 15-6（续）

E~G. 对二尖瓣后瓣僵硬发育不全,可采用心包补片扩大。将后瓣沿瓣环根部 1~2mm 切开,再用自身心包补片缝合扩大后瓣,以增加二尖瓣对合缘接触面。

Figure 15-6 cont'd

E-G. For posterior mitral valve stiffness and dysplasia, a pericardial patch can be used for enlargement. The posterior leaflet is incised along the root of the annulus at approximately 1-2 mm from the root, and the posterior valve is expanded with an autologous pericardial patch to increase the commissural contact surface of the mitral valve.

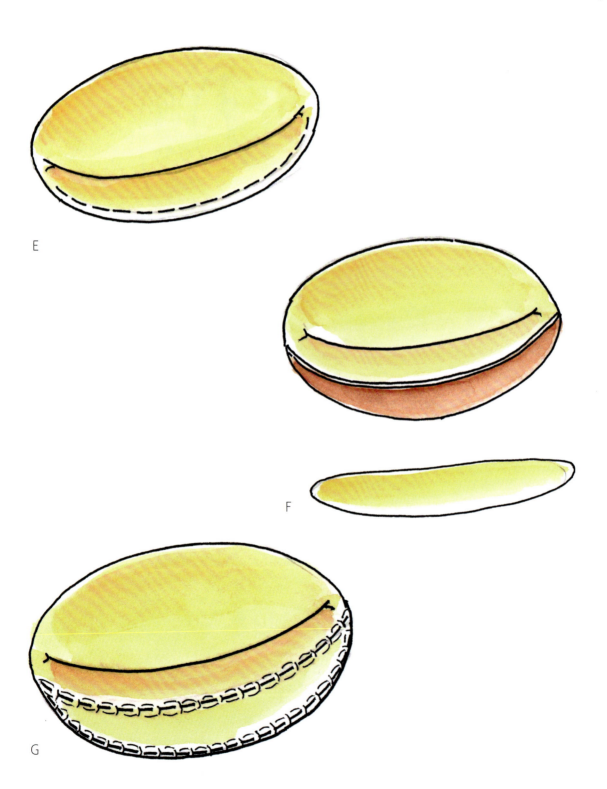

E

F

G

5. 二尖瓣腱索缩短或替代术 (图 15-7)

5. Shortening or replacement of the chordae tendineae of mitral valve (Figure 15-7)

图 15-7　二尖瓣腱索缩短或替代术
A. 先找出导致瓣叶假性脱垂的冗长腱索。
B. 将相应乳头肌顶端切开,形成凹槽。

Figure 15-7　Shortening or replacement of the chordae tendineae of mitral valve
A. Identify the elongated redundant chordae leading to false prolapse of the leaflet.
B. Cut the corresponding papillary muscles from the top to create a trough.

Continued

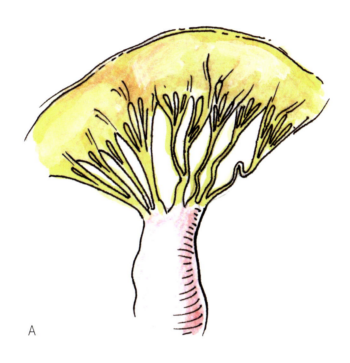

A

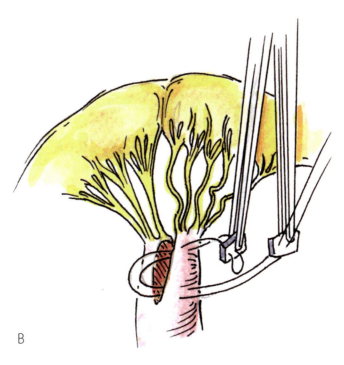

B

图 15-7（续）

Figure 15-7 cont'd

C. 用一针带垫片褥式缝线将腱索拉至槽内，将缝线收紧，再用另一针带垫褥式缝合加固。

C. The chordae can be drawn into the trough with a pledged mattress suture, and the suture is tightened. Then, the procedure is reinforced by a second mattress suture with pledget.

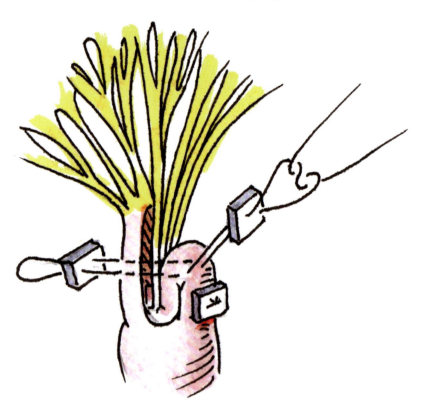

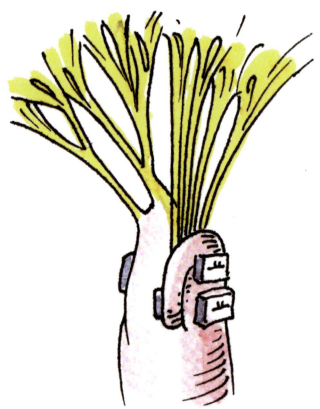

C

图 15-7 (**续**)

D. 对腱索断裂或缺失导致的瓣叶脱垂，可用 ePTFE 缝线做人造腱索。在瓣叶游离缘腱索缺失处缝置一针褥式缝线，然后将缝线向下缝到乳头肌顶端并加上垫片。

Figure 15-7 cont'd

D. For prolapsed leaflets caused by rupture or absence of chordae tendineae, artificial chordae can be used with ePTFE suture. A mattress suture is made through the free edge of the leaflet at the side where chordae tendineae are missing. Then the suture is brought down to the papillary muscle head, and a pledget is added.

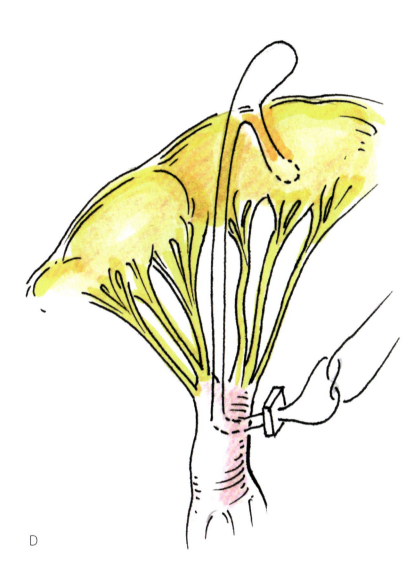

D

图 15-7 (续)

Figure 15-7 cont'd

E. 将脱垂之瓣叶拉至正常位置, 再将缝线打结固定。

E. Pull the prolapsed leaflet to the normal position and tie the suture to secure it with knots.

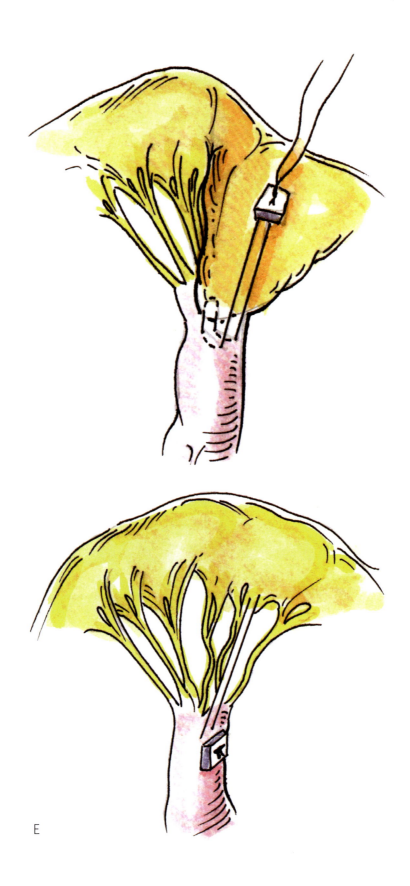

E

6. 二尖瓣瓣环成形术　当二尖瓣瓣环扩大导致反流加重,常需要缩小瓣环以减轻二尖瓣反流。常用方法有两种:带垫 U 形直接环缩或用人工瓣环做成形术(图 15-8)。

图 15-8　二尖瓣瓣环成形术
A. 用 5-0 或 4-0 带垫 Prolene 缝线沿瓣环交界处做间断缝合,一般不宜超过瓣环三分之一面积。
B. 将缝线收紧,注水测试反流状况,确认满意后再打结固定。

6. Mitral annuloplasty　When regurgitation is aggravated by mitral annular enlargement, it is often necessary to narrow the annulus to reduce mitral regurgitation. Two methods are commonly used: reducing the annulus with pledget-supported U-shaped sutures or applying annuloplasty with an artificial annulus (Figure 15-8).

Figure 15-8　Mitral annuloplasty
A. Pledget-supported 5-0 or 4-0 sutures are used for interrupted suturing along the annulus junction. It is not advisable to exceed one-third of the annulus area.
B. Tighten the suture, inject the cold saline to test the regurgitation condition, and confirm the condition before knot fixation.

Continued

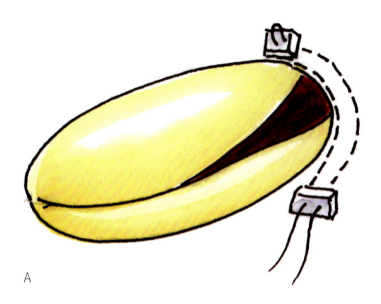

A

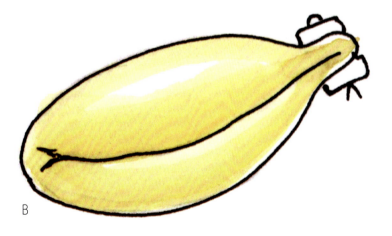

B

图 15-8（续）

C、D. 若患儿年龄超过 6 岁, 瓣环扩大严重可采用成形环。儿童多采用 C 形环（Carpentier-Edwords 环）。选择适合大小人工瓣环, 用带垫缝线 U 形间断缝合。全部缝线均匀缝合于成形环, 再将成形环推下至瓣环, 打结固定。

Figure 15-8 cont'd

C,D. Annuloplasty ring can be used if the valve ring is enlarged seriously and the child is over six years old. In children, the C-shaped ring (Carpentier-Edwords ring) is commonly used. A prosthetic annulus of proper size is selected, and U-shaped interrupted sutures with pledget are applied. All sutures are placed evenly to the ring, and then the ring is pushed down to the annulus and tied for fixation.

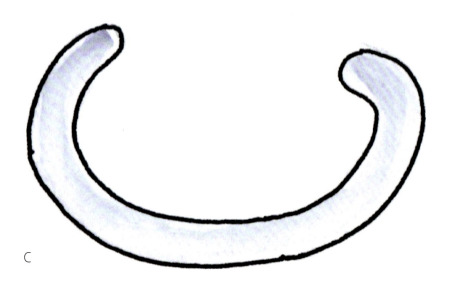

C

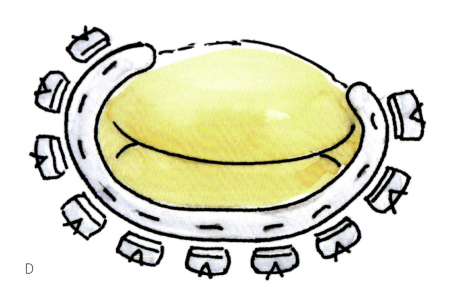

D

7. 二尖瓣置换术 儿童二尖瓣反流手术方法首选二尖瓣整形。但整形效果不佳或瓣膜病变严重无法做整形则考虑行瓣膜置换术。儿童大多选择机械瓣(图 15-9)。

7. Mitral valve replacement Mitral valve plasty is preferred in pediatric mitral regurgitation surgery. However, mitral valve replacement may be considered in cases of poor plastic effect or in which the valve lesion is too severe for plastic surgery. Mechanical valves are mostly used in children for valve replacement (Figure 15-9).

图 15-9 **二尖瓣置换术**
A~C. 将病变之瓣叶及附着的腱索等剪除,保留乳头肌等瓣下结构。

Figure 15-9 Mitral valve replacement
A-C. Remove the prolapsed leaflet and its attached chordae, and preserve the subvalvular structures such as papillary muscles.

Continued

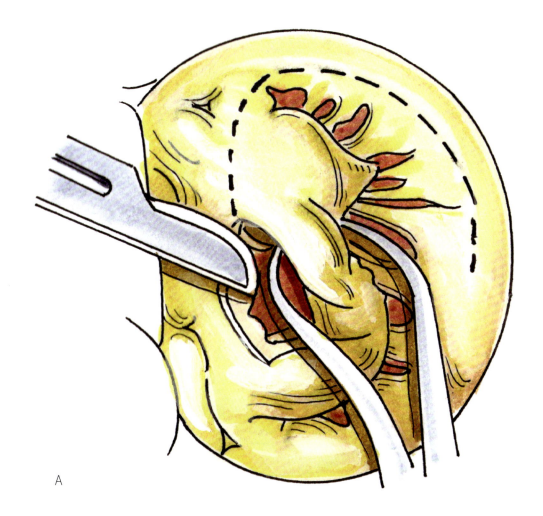

A

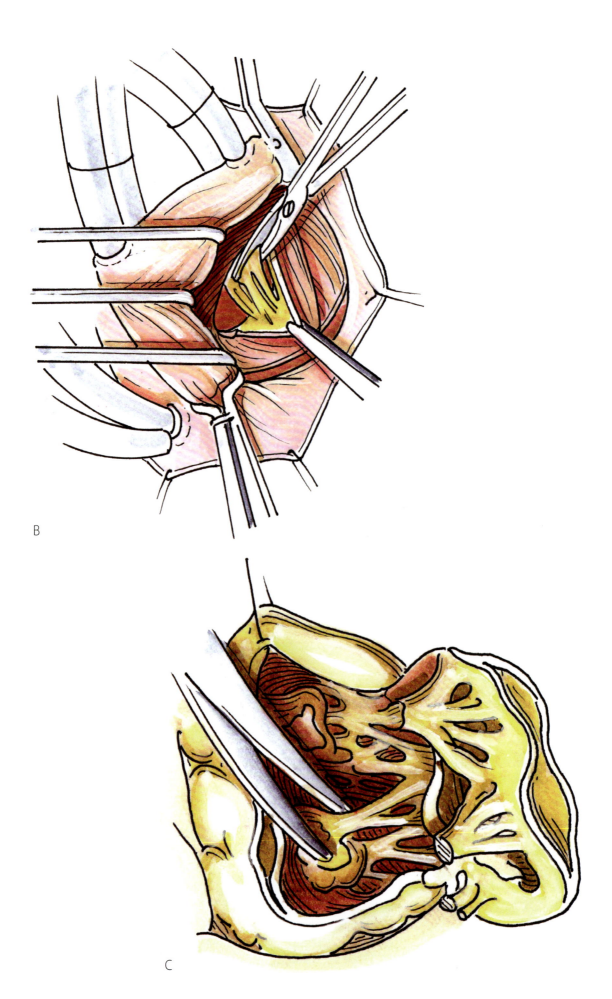

B

C

图 15-9(续)

D. 用测瓣器测量瓣环大小,选择相应尺寸的人工瓣膜。用带垫 U 形间断缝合在瓣膜涤纶环上,通常缝合 12 至 14 针,垫片放置在左房面。

Figure 15-9 cont'd

D. Measure the annulus size with the sizer. Select a prosthesis of appropriate size and U-shaped interrupted sutures with pledget are applied on the cuff of the valve. Usually, it requires 12 to 14 stitches. The pledget is placed on the left atrial surface.

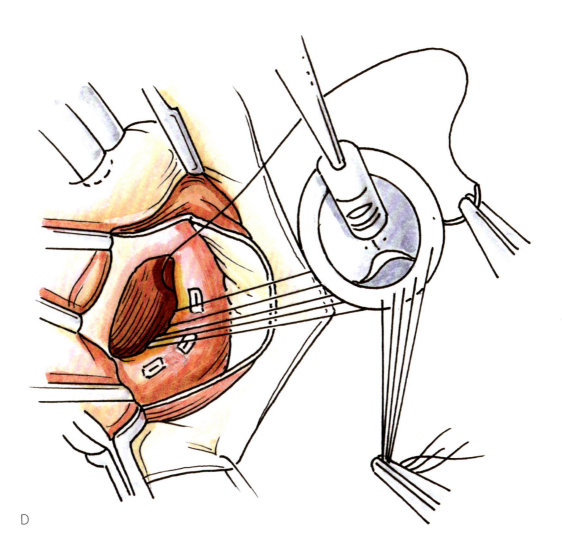

D

图 15-9（续）

E. 用持瓣器将瓣膜下推至二尖瓣环处，打结固定。

Figure 15-9 cont'd

E. The valve is pushed down to the mitral annulus using the valve holder and finally tied with a knot.

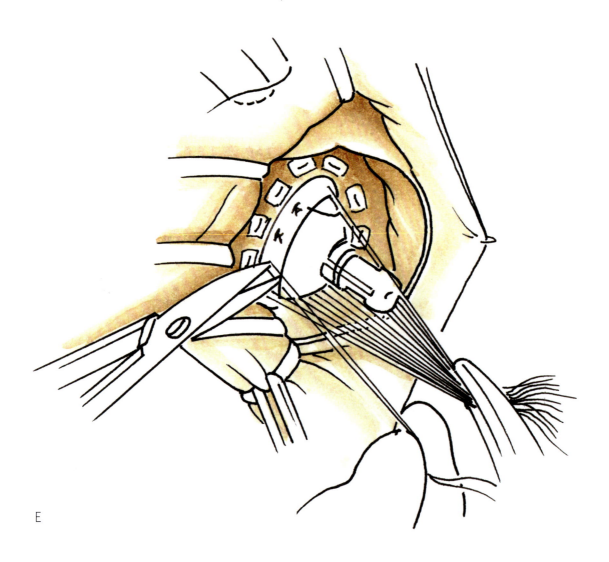

E

图 15-9（续）

F. 对瓣环发育较小，无法放置最小尺寸人工瓣膜，可采用瓣环上二尖瓣置换技术，即将瓣膜放置在左心房内位于下肺静脉开口和二尖瓣环之间。缝合技术同上。

Figure 15-9 cont'd

F. A supra-annular mitral valve replacement technique may be used in cases where the smallest size prosthetic valve cannot be placed because of poor development of the annulus. That is, the valve is placed in the left atrium between the inferior pulmonary vein opening and the mitral annulus. The suture technique is the same as above.

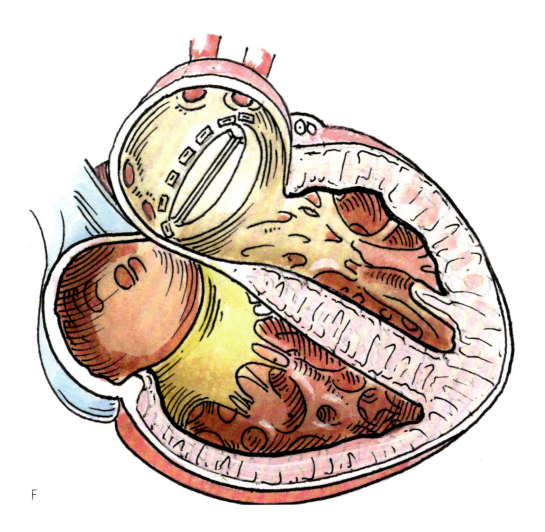

F

16 三尖瓣下移畸形

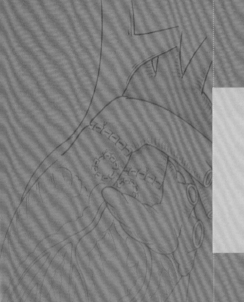

16 Ebstein's Anomaly

三尖瓣下移是一种较少见的心脏畸形，其病理特点是三尖瓣隔、后瓣下移，前瓣瓣叶冗长、穿孔、受牵拉。三尖瓣下移的瓣叶与其下方的心肌粘连，部分右心室"心房化"扩张。三尖瓣瓣环扩大，存在不同程度的三尖瓣反流（图16-1）。

Ebstein's anomaly is an uncommon cardiac abnormality. It is pathologically characterized by the downward displacement of the septal and posterior leaflets of the tricuspid valve as well as the perforated stretched larger anterior leaflets. The downward displaced leaflet of the tricuspid valve adheres to the underlying myocardium, and part of the right ventricle is atrialized and dilated. The tricuspid annulus is enlarged with varying degrees of tricuspid regurgitation (Figure 16-1).

图 16-1　三尖瓣下移畸形

Figure 16-1　Ebstein's anomaly

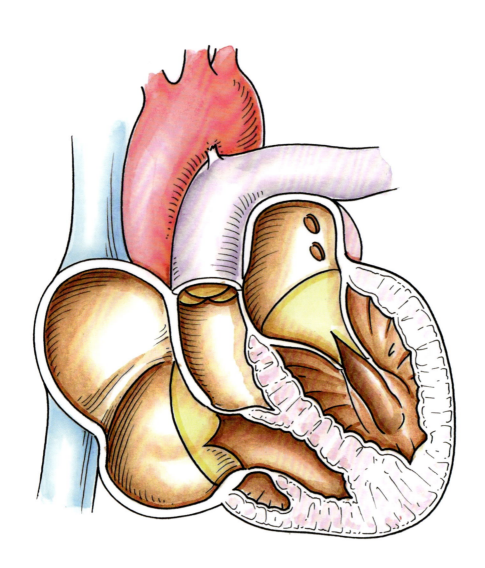

一、解剖分型

I. Anatomical Typing

Carpentier 医生将三尖瓣下移畸形分为四个类型（图 16-2）。

Dr. Carpentier classified Ebstein's anomaly into four types (Figure 16-2).

图 16-2　**三尖瓣下移解剖分型**

A. A 型：三尖瓣下移不严重，右心室的容积足够。

Figure 16-2　Anatomical typing

A. Type A: The tricuspid valve is not severely displaced downward with adequate right ventricle volume.

Continued

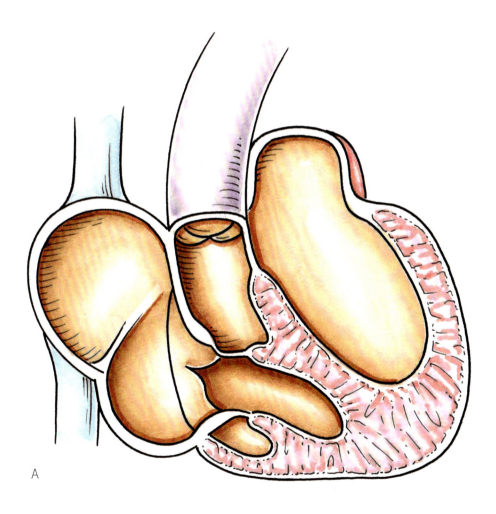

A

图 16-2（续）

B. B 型：右心室"心房化"部分扩大，但三尖瓣前瓣活动尚可。

Figure 16-2 cont'd

B. Type B: The atrialized part of the right ventricle is dilated, but the anterior tricuspid valve is still active.

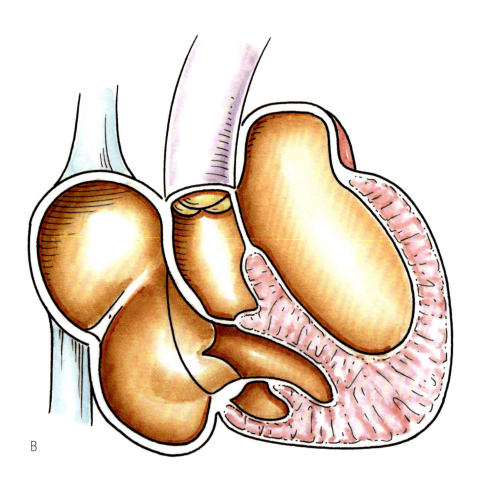

B

图 16-2（续）

C. C 型：三尖瓣前瓣活动受限，部分右心室流出道梗阻。

Figure 16-2 cont'd

C. Type C: The movement of the anterior tricuspid valve is limited, and the right ventricular outflow tract is partially obstructed.

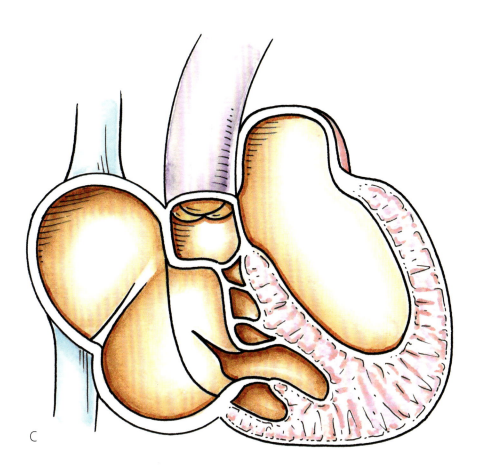

C

图 16-2（续）

Figure 16-2 cont'd

D. D 型：右心室几乎完全心房化，"囊袋样" 瓣叶组织黏附在扩张的右心室上。

D. Type D: The right ventricle is almost completely atrialized, and the pocket-like valve leaflet tissue adheres to the dilated right ventricle.

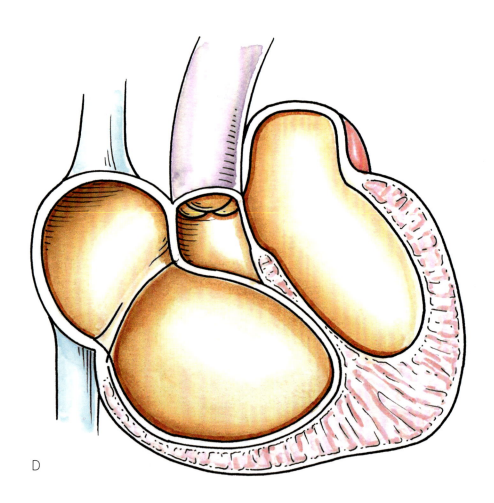

D

二、手术方法

II. Surgical Methods

1. 新生儿三尖瓣下移畸形 三尖瓣下移畸形症状明显的新生儿不论采用单心室或是双心室矫治,手术风险都很大,死亡率较高。

1. Neonates with Ebstein's anomaly Symptomatic neonates with Ebstein's anomaly are at high risk for surgery and have a high mortality rate regardless of single ventricle or biventricular repair.

（1）Knott-Craig 双心室修补手术（图 16-3）

(1) Knott-Craig biventricular repair (Figure 16-3)

图 16-3　Knott-Craig 双心室修补手术

A. 以三尖瓣前瓣构建一个单瓣,先将三尖瓣前瓣从根部游离,并将前瓣游离缘与右心室游离壁融合部分予以充分松解,使前瓣能自由活动。

Figure 16-3　Knott-Craig biventricular repair

A. The anterior tricuspid valve is used to construct a monocusp valve. The anterior tricuspid valve is first freed from the root part, and the fusion part of the leading edge of the anterior leaflet and the free wall of the right ventricle is fully delaminated so that the anterior leaflet can move freely.

Continued

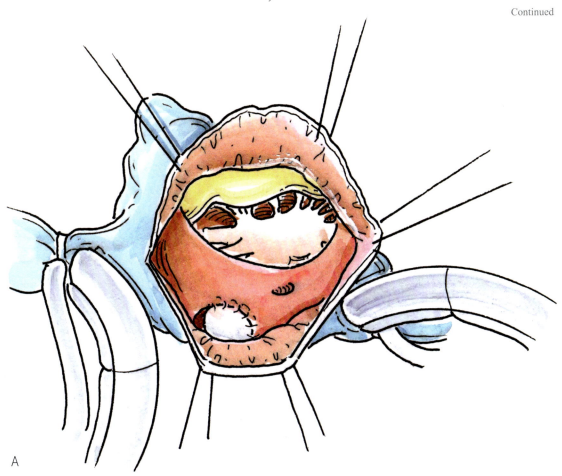

A

图 16-3（续）

B. 用带垫片 U 形缝合缩小扩张的三尖瓣瓣环。

Figure 16-3 cont'd

B. Reduce the dilated tricuspid annulus with pledget-supported U-shape sutures.

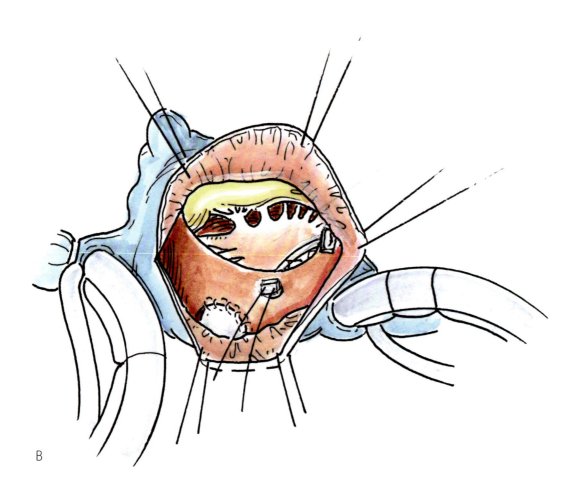

B

图 16-3（续）

Figure 16-3 cont'd

C. 对心房化右心室部分纵向折叠。

C. Fold the atrialized right ventricle longitudinally.

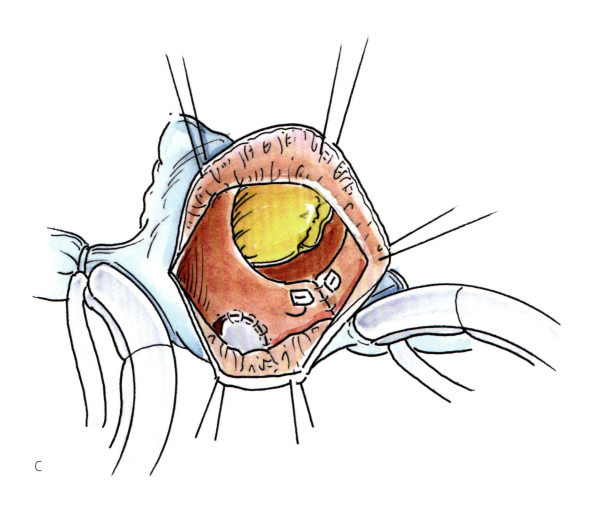

C

图 16-3（续）

D. 将游离的前瓣做部分顺时针转动,重新固定在三尖瓣瓣环上,形成一个大的单叶瓣。房间隔通常留 3~4mm 开口。

Figure 16-3 cont'd

D. Partially rotate the free anterior leaflet clockwise and refix it on the tricuspid valve annulus to create a large monocusp valve. Leave a 3-4 mm opening in the atrial septal defeat.

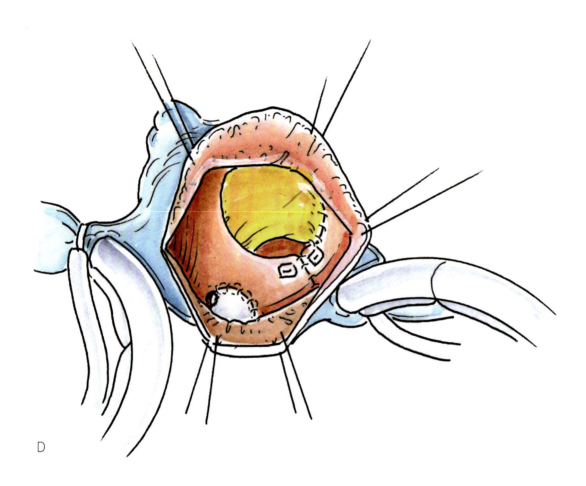

D

（2）Starnes 单心室修补手术：对于三尖瓣瓣叶发育很差的患者采用单心室矫治方法（图 16-4）。

(2) Starnes procedure: Single ventricle repair is adopted in patients with poorly developed tricuspid leaflets (Figure 16-4).

图 16-4　Starnes 单心室修补手术
A. 用一块固定好的自体心包直接将三尖瓣瓣口关闭。
B. 在补片上开口 4mm，以减小右心室压力。

Figure 16-4　Starnes procedure
A. The tricuspid valve orifice is closed directly with a fixed piece of the native pericardium.
B. An opening of 4 mm is placed on the patch to reduce the pressure of the right ventricle.

Continued

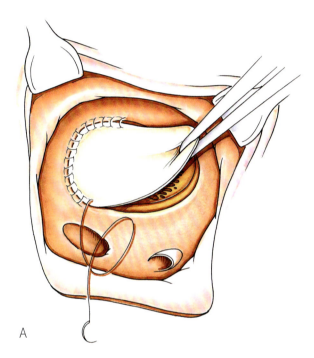

A

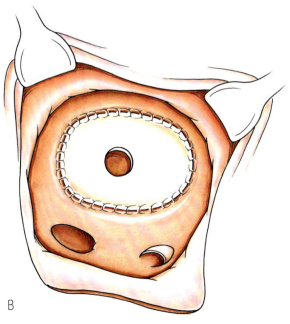

B

图 16-4（续）

C. 房间隔切除扩大。肺动脉横断，分别
连续缝合关闭。取 3.5~4mm ePTFE 管
道做 B-T 分流。

Figure 16-4 cont'd

C. The atrial septal defeat is enlarged. The pulmonary artery is transected and closed with separate running sutures. Take a 3. 5-4 mm ePTFE conduit for B-T shunt.

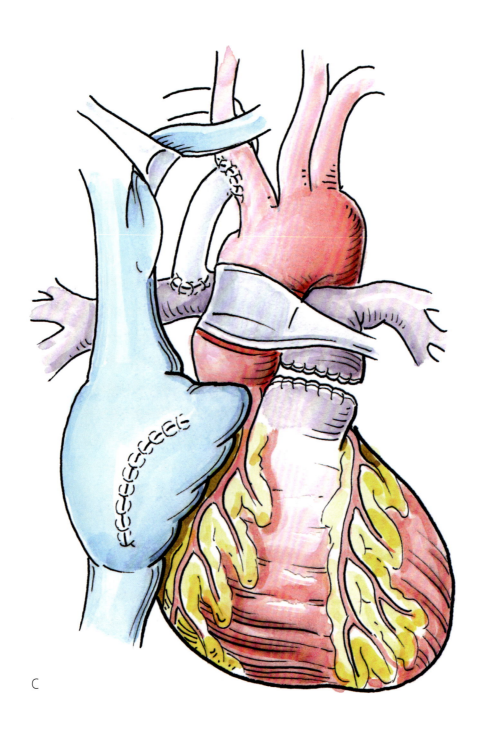

C

2. 传统的三尖瓣重建手术 Danielson 医生早在 1972 年提出了一种重建方法,即通过三尖瓣前瓣与室间隔对合在一起,来获得瓣膜的关闭性能。这种修补还包括三尖瓣瓣环后缘的瓣环成形术。以后又有一些改良,将部分三尖瓣沿根部切开游离,将瓣叶缝合在正常的三尖瓣瓣环位置。同时做部分心房化心室的横向折叠和瓣环缩小。Hetzer 医生介绍了双孔方法,即将三尖瓣前瓣和隔瓣用 5-0 Prolene 缝线做对合缝合,也取得了较好的效果(图 16-5)。

2. Conventional tricuspid valve reconstruction In 1972, Dr. Danielson proposed the reconstruction of a deformed tricuspid valve in which the anterior leaflet of the tricuspid valve was coapted with the ventricular septum to obtain the closing competence of the valve. This repair also includes annuloplasty of the posterior edge of the tricuspid annulus. Later, there were some improvements. Part of the tricuspid valve was cut away along the root, and the leaflets were sutured to the normal tricuspid annulus. Simultaneously, part of the atrialized ventricle was plicated horizontally, and the annulus was reduced. Dr. Hetzer described a two-hole approach with satisfactory results, in which the anterior tricuspid leaflet and septal leaflet were sutured using a 5-0 Prolene suture (Figure 16-5).

A、B. 通过三尖瓣前瓣与室间隔对合在一起,来获得瓣膜的关闭性能。

A, B. The anterior leaflet of the tricuspid valve was coapted with the ventricular septum to obtain the closing competence of the valve.

Continued

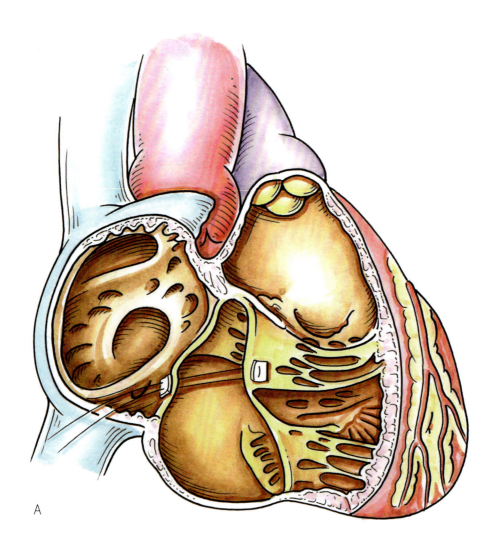

A

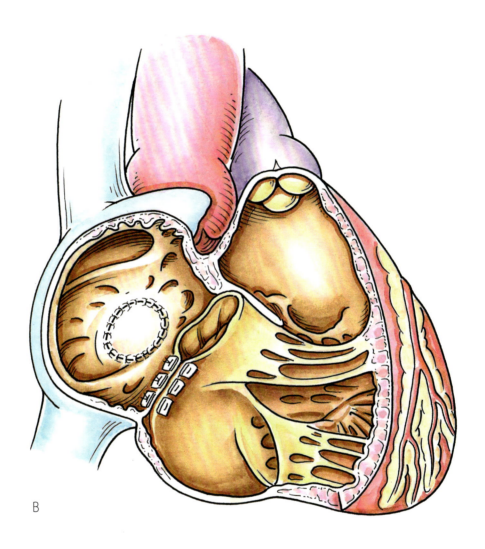

B

图 16-5（续）

C. 三尖瓣瓣环后缘的瓣环成形术。

D. 将部分三尖瓣沿根部切开游离。

Figure 16-5 **cont'd**

C. Annuloplasty of the posterior edge of the tricuspid annulus.

D. Part of the tricuspid valve was cut away along the root.

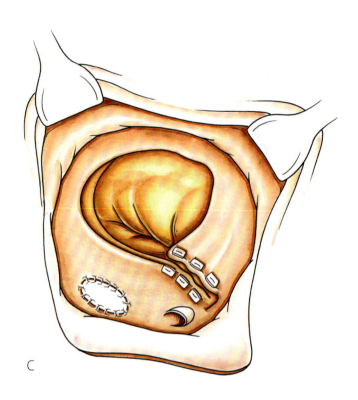

C

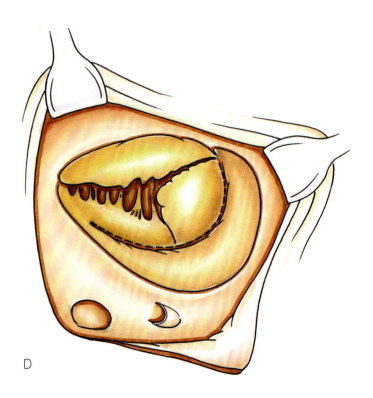

D

图 16-5（续）

Figure 16-5 cont'd

E、F. 将瓣叶缝合在正常的三尖瓣瓣环位置，同时做部分心房化心室的横向折叠和瓣环缩小。

E, F. The leaflets were sutured to the normal tricuspid annulus. Simultaneously, part of the atrialized ventricle was plicated horizontally, and the annulus was reduced.

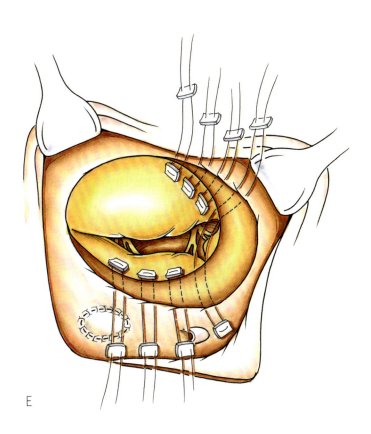

E

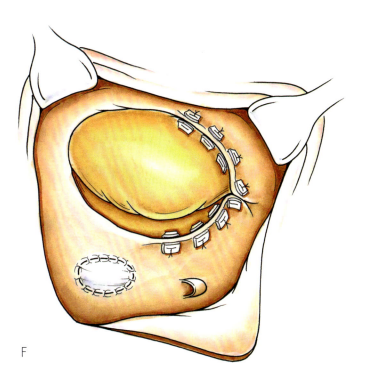

F

图 16-5（续）

G、H. 双孔法：将三尖瓣前瓣和隔瓣用 5-0 Prolene 缝线做对合缝合。

Figure 16-5 cont'd

G, H. The two-hole approach: the anterior tricuspid leaflet and septal leaflet were sutured using a 5-0 Prolene suture.

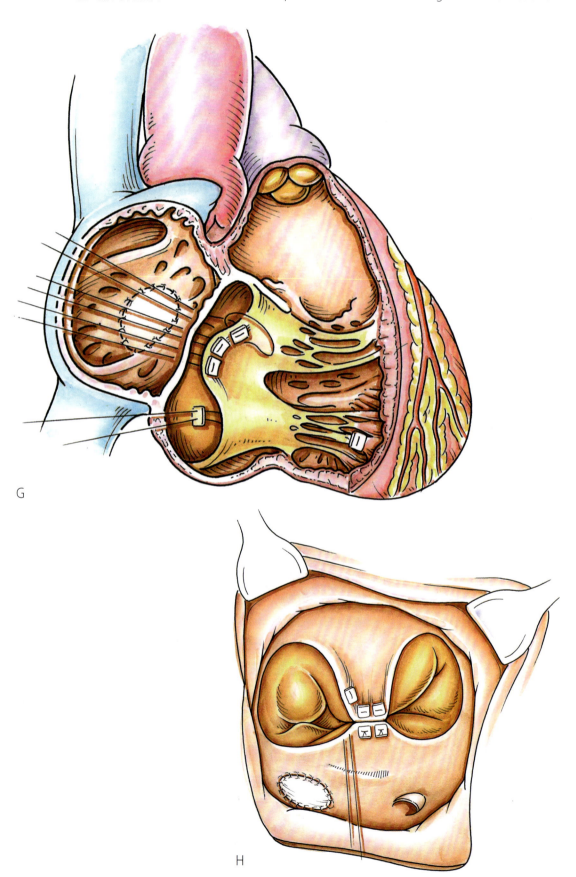

G

H

3. 三尖瓣锥形重建手术（图 16-6）

3. Tricuspid valve cone reconstruction (Figure 16-6)

图 16-6　三尖瓣锥形重建手术

A. 常规行心肺转流术，右心房纵行切口。

B. 采用四根心房牵引线暴露瓣膜，注水测试瓣膜反流情况。

Figure 16-6　Tricuspid valve cone reconstruction

A. Cardiopulmonary bypass is performed routinely, and a longitudinal incision is performed to the right atrium.

B. The valve is exposed with four atrial traction lines, and the valve regurgitation is tested with cold saline injection.

Continued

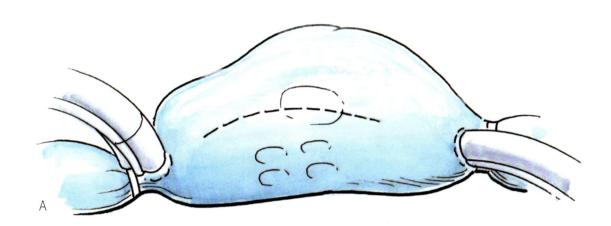

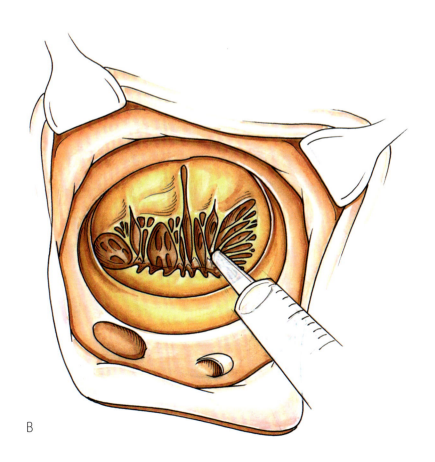

图 16-6(续)

C. 在三尖瓣前瓣距瓣环 2~3mm 处将
瓣叶切下，并充分游离瓣下组织，使瓣
叶能充分抬起并旋转。

Figure 16-6 cont'd

C. Cut the valve leaflets off the anterior tricuspid valve at 2-3 mm
from the annulus, and fully free the subvalvular tissues so that
the leaflets can be fully lifted and rotated.

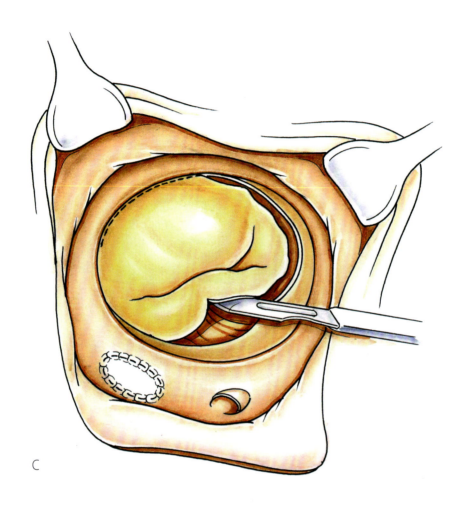

C

图 16-6（续）

D. 如隔后瓣处仍有部分瓣叶组织也一同给予游离。将前瓣顺时针方向旋转与松解的部分隔瓣组织缘对缘缝合。一般采用 5-0 Prolene 缝线间断缝合。

Figure 16-6 cont'd

D. If there is still part of the valve leaflet tissue at the posterior septal leaflet, it will be freed together. The anterior leaflet is rotated clockwise and sutured, in an edge-to-edge way, to the mobilized part of the septal leaflet. The interrupted sutures are made with 5-0 Prolene suture.

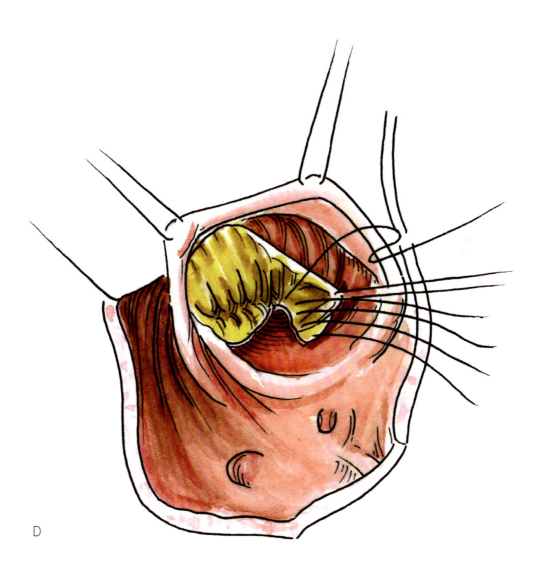

D

图 16-6（续）

E. 将房化心室部分切除或直接纵向折叠缝合,将三尖瓣瓣叶重新固定在三尖瓣环处。

Figure 16-6 cont'd

E. Part of the atrialized ventricle is excised or longitudinally plicated and sutured. The tricuspid valve leaflets are refixed at the tricuspid valve annulus.

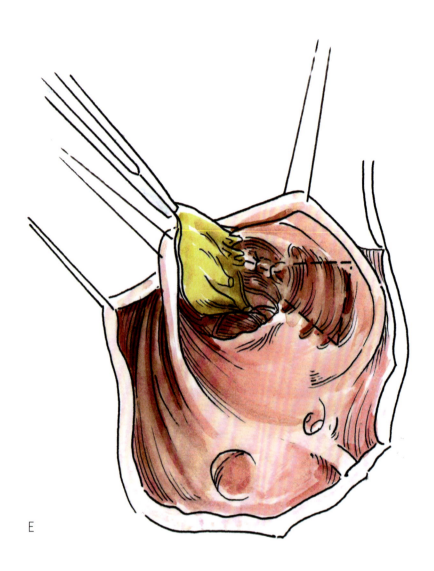

E

图 16-6（续）

F. 靠隔瓣处带垫 U 形间断缝合，其余部分可连续缝合。三尖瓣瓣环做部分环缩。

Figure 16-6 cont'd

F. U-shaped interrupted sutures with pledget are applied near the septal leaflet, and running sutures may be applied for the rest part. The tricuspid annulus is partially reduced in size.

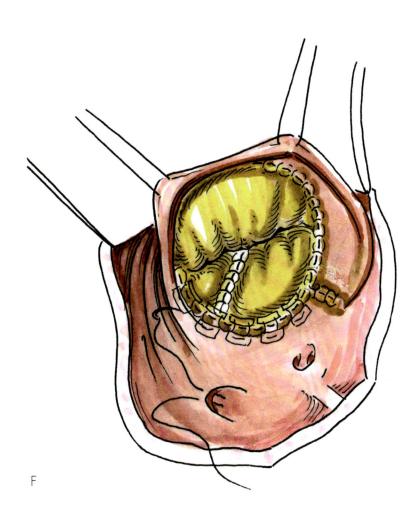

F

图 16-6(续)

Figure 16-6 cont'd

G、H. 重建后的三尖瓣形成一个"锥形"。

G, H. The reconstructed tricuspid valve forms a cone shape.

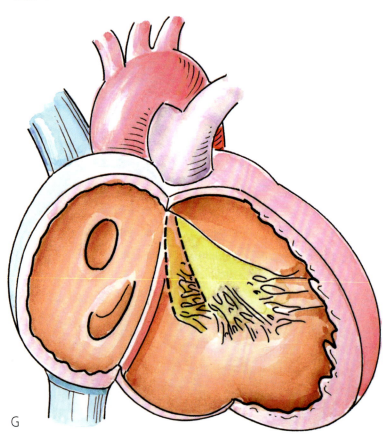

G

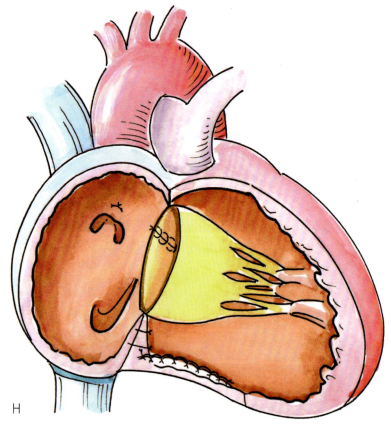

H

4. 三尖瓣置换术　对于三尖瓣发育很差或整形手术后效果仍不满意的患儿需考虑瓣膜置换手术。与成人不同的是，因兼顾到儿童的体格生长和瓣膜使用的耐久性，儿童三尖瓣置换大多选用机械瓣。缝合方法与二尖瓣置换相同。但重要的是带垫U形缝合时要注意避免损伤传导组织。垫片一般放在右房面（图16-7）。

4. Tricuspid valve replacement　Tricuspid valve replacement should be considered in infants with poor tricuspid valve development or after tricuspid valvuloplasty with unsatisfactory outcomes. Different from adults, mechanical valves are the most common choice in tricuspid valve replacement for children, as the physical growth of children calls for a durable valve. The same suturing method as that in mitral valve replacement is applied. It is important to avoid damaging conductive tissue when using a pledget-supported U-shape suture. The pledget is typically placed on the right atrial surface (Figure 16-7).

图 16-7　瓣膜置换术
A. 如果冠状窦与瓣环之间有足够空间可将垫片放在二者之间，冠状窦开口右心房。

Figure 16-7　Tricuspid valve replacement
A. If there is enough space, the pledget can be placed between the coronary sinus and the annulus, and the coronary sinus can open at the right atrium.

Continued

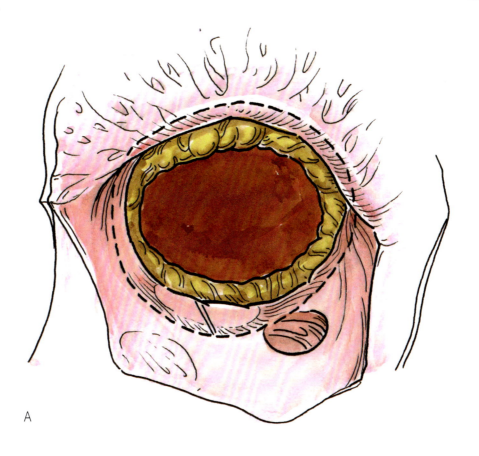

A

图 16-7（续）

B. 如果间距太小可将垫片放在冠状窦外缘，冠状窦开口在右心室。

Figure 16-7 cont'd

B. If there is not enough space between the coronary sinus and the annulus, the pledget may be placed on the outer edge of the coronary sinus, and the coronary sinus can open in the right ventricle.

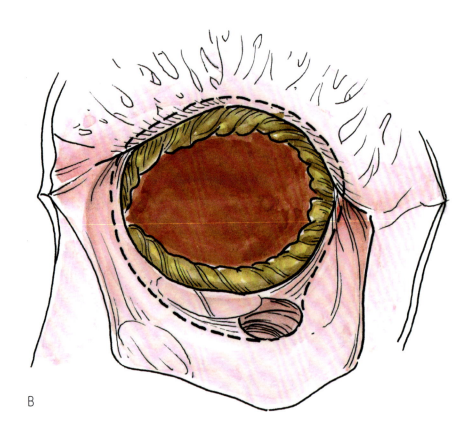

B

图 16-7(续)

C. 如三尖瓣瓣环过大，可在缝合时同时缩小瓣环。

Figure 16-7 cont'd

C. If the tricuspid annulus is too large, the annulus may be reduced when suturing.

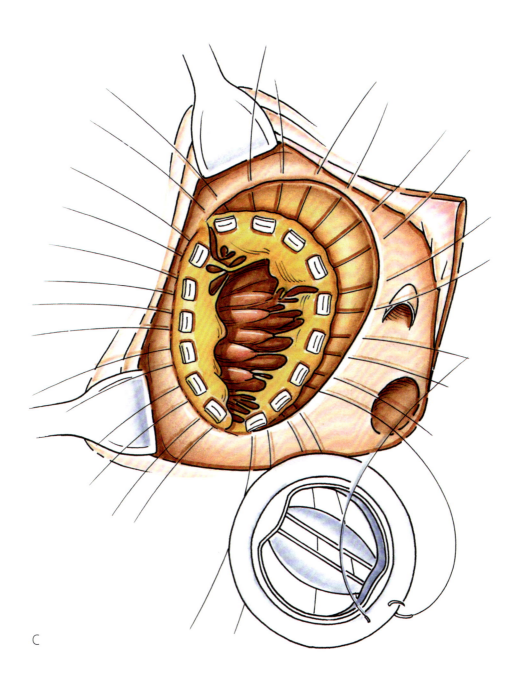

C

图 16-7(续)

D. 注意打结时均匀受力，每个垫片必须
紧贴右心房。

Figure 16-7 cont'd

D. Note that the force is evenly applied when knotting the
suture, and each pledget must be close to the right atrium.

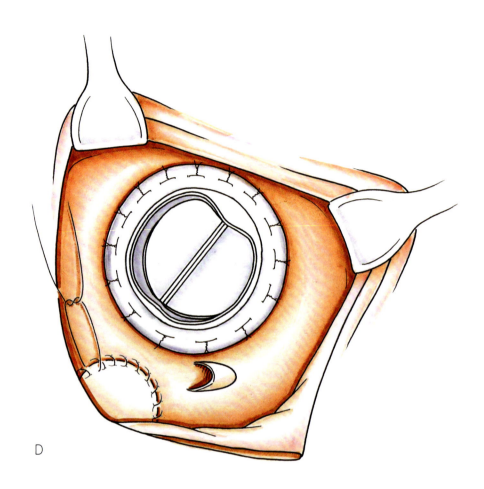

D

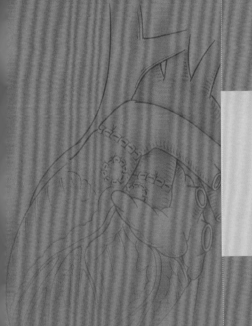

17 房间隔缺损

17 Atrial Septal Defect

一、解剖分型

房间隔缺损（atrial septal defect, ASD）主要有三类：继发孔型房间隔缺损（80%）、静脉窦型房间隔缺损（10%）和原发孔型房间隔缺损（10%）。原发孔型通常合并有房室瓣畸形，又称为部分型房室隔缺损，将在第二十一章叙述。此外，ASD 的其他类型还有卵圆孔未闭、冠状窦型房间隔缺损（无顶冠状窦）和共同心房（图 17-1）。

I. Anatomical Typing

Atrial septal defect (ASD) mainly includes three types: ostium secundum defect (80%), Sinus venosus atrial septal defect (10%), and ostium primum defect (10%). The ostium primum defect, usually associated with an atrioventricular valve malformation, is also called partial atrioventricular septal defect, which will be introduced in Chapter 21. In addition, other types of ASD include patent oval foramen, coronary sinus defect (unroofed coronary sinus), and common atrium (Figure 17-1).

图 17-1　房间隔缺损的解剖分型
A. 继发孔型房间隔缺损。

Figure 17-1　Anatomical typing of atrial septal defect
A. Ostium secundum defect.

Continued

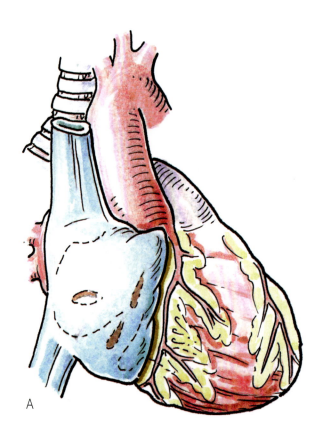

图 17-1（续）

Figure 17-1 cont'd

B. 静脉窦型房间隔缺损。C. 原发孔型
房间隔缺损。

B. Sinus venosus atrial septal defect. C. Ostium primum
defect.

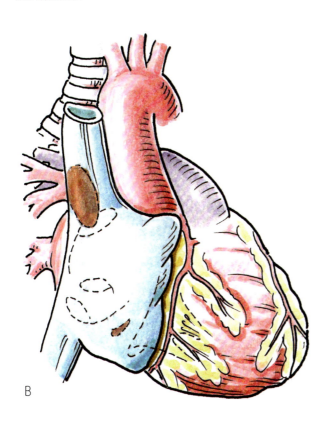

B

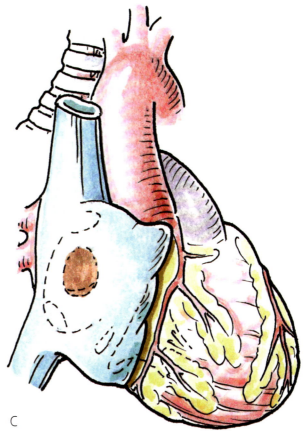

C

图 17-1（续）

Figure 17-1 cont'd

D. 卵圆孔未闭。E. 冠状窦型房间隔缺损。

D. Patent oval foramen. E. Coronary sinus defect.

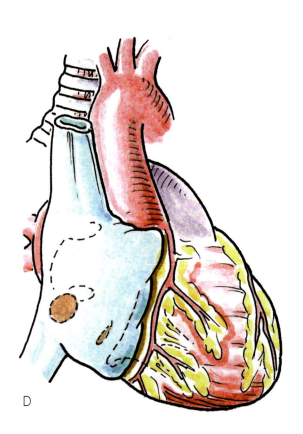

D

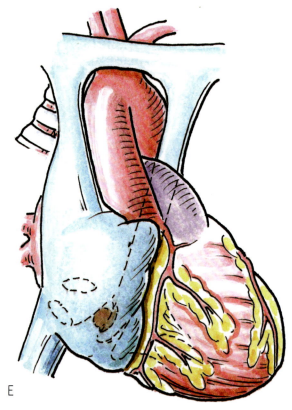

E

图 17-1（续）
F. 共同心房。

Figure 17-1 cont'd
F. Common atrium.

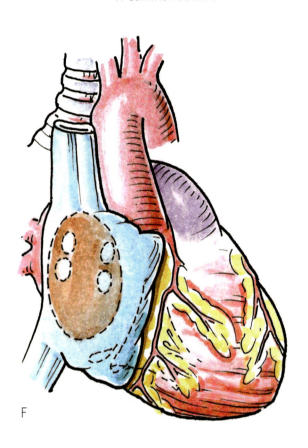

F

二、手术方法

II. Surgical Methods

1. 卵圆孔未闭导管介入治疗 位于第二房间隔（继发隔）和第一房间隔（原发隔）之间的小型心房间交通，现大多采用心导管介入治疗，采用封堵伞将其关闭。若合并其他心内畸形，则在手术时同时关闭（图 17-2）。

1. Interventional therapy for patent oval foramen Generally, patent oval foramen, a small interatrial communication between the septum primum and septum secundum, is treated with cardiac catheterization and closed with an occlusion umbrella. For patent oval foramen complicated with other intracardiac malformations, the closures will be performed at the same time during operation (Figure 17-2).

图 17-2　卵圆孔未闭导管介入
　　　　治疗

Figure 17-2　Interventional therapy for patent oval
foramen

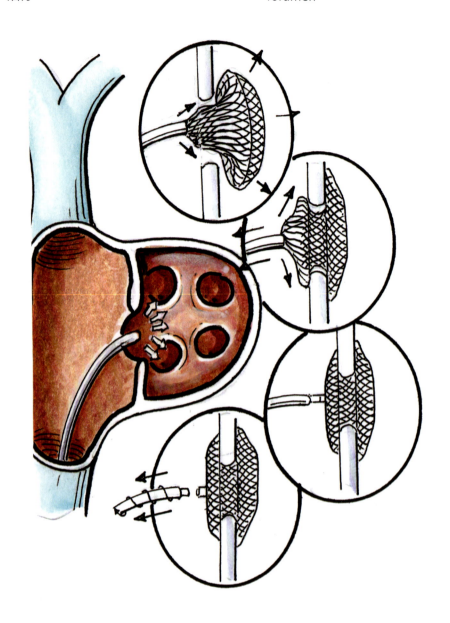

2. 中央型或下腔型房间隔缺损（图 17-3）

2. Central or inferior vena cava atrial septal defect (Figure 17-3)

图 17-3　中央型或下腔型房间隔缺损

A、B. 中央型房间隔缺损若直径小于 1cm，通常可直接缝合。

Figure 17-3　Central or inferior vena cava atrial septal defect

A, B. If the diameter of the central atrial septal defect is less than 1 cm, it can usually be sutured directly.

Continued

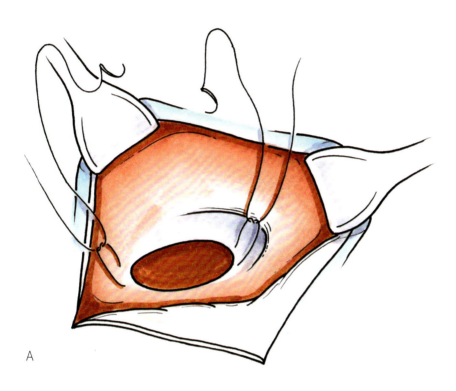

A

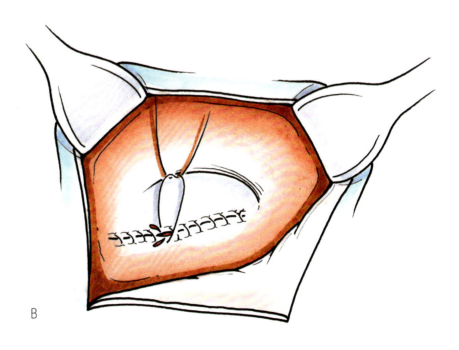

B

图 17-3（续）

Figure 17-3 cont'd

C、D. 如 ASD 大于 1cm 或为下腔型，则多采用心包补片缝合修补。

C, D. If the ASD is larger than 1 cm or the inferior vena cava type, a pericardial patch is often used.

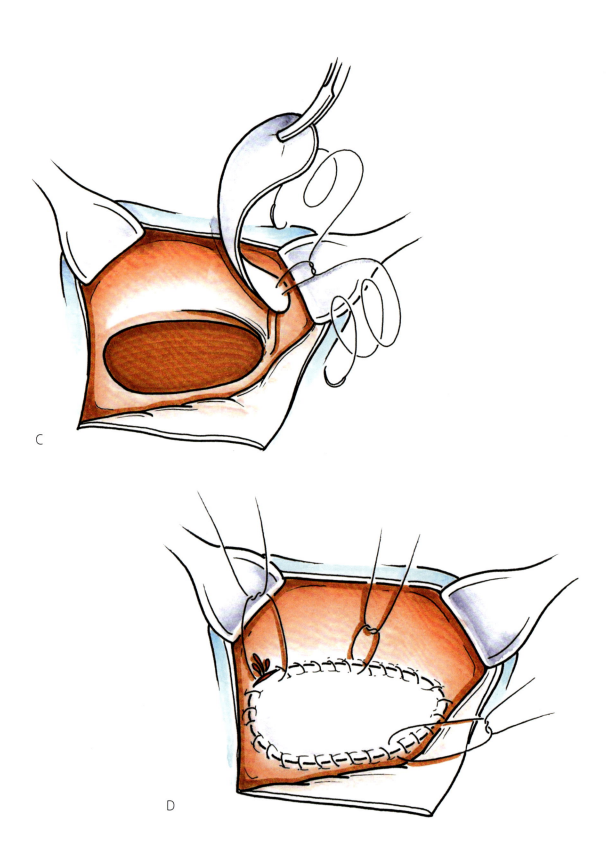

C

D

3. 静脉窦型房间隔缺损 多发生在上腔静脉和右心房连接处，故又称为上腔型 ASD（图 17-4）。对缺损位置较高，加之有部分肺静脉开口异常，直接补片修补易导致上腔静脉回流受阻，可采用 Warden 手术（图 17-5）。

3. Sinus venosus atrial septal defect (SVASD) Most SVASD occur at the junction between the superior vena cava (SVC) and the right atrium, so they are also called superior vena cava ASD (Figure 17-4). For SVASD at the superior aspect of the atrial septum complicated with abnormalities of partial pulmonary vein drainage, one patch repair easily obstructs the SVC reflux, so the Warden procedure can be used to repair the defects (Figure 17-5).

图 17-4　**静脉窦型房间隔缺损**
A. ASD 位于上腔静脉开口和上嵴束之间，有时可合并右上肺静脉开口在 ASD 边缘。

Figure 17-4　Sinus venosus atrial septal defect
A. ASD locates between the SVC ostium and the superior limbic band and sometimes associates with the ostium of the right superior pulmonary vein adjacent to the edge of the ASD.

Continued

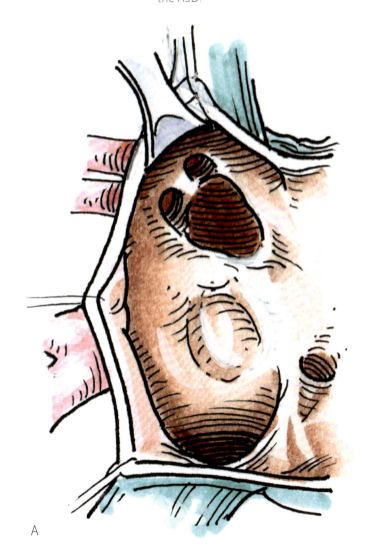

A

图 17-4（续）

B. 先将房间隔切开,扩大 ASD,取心包补片关闭 ASD,确保上腔静脉和肺静脉回流畅通。

Figure 17-4 cont'd

B. Incise the atrial septum, enlarge ASD, and close the ASD with pericardial patches to ensure unobstructed flow of the SVC and pulmonary vein.

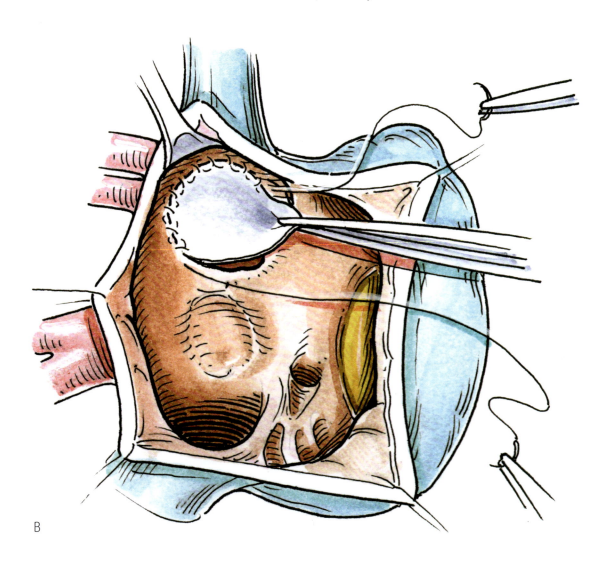

B

图 17-5　Warden 手术
A. 上腔静脉使用直角插管，位置要高。

Figure 17-5　Warden procedure
A. High cannulation of the SVC is performed with a right-angle cannula.

Continued

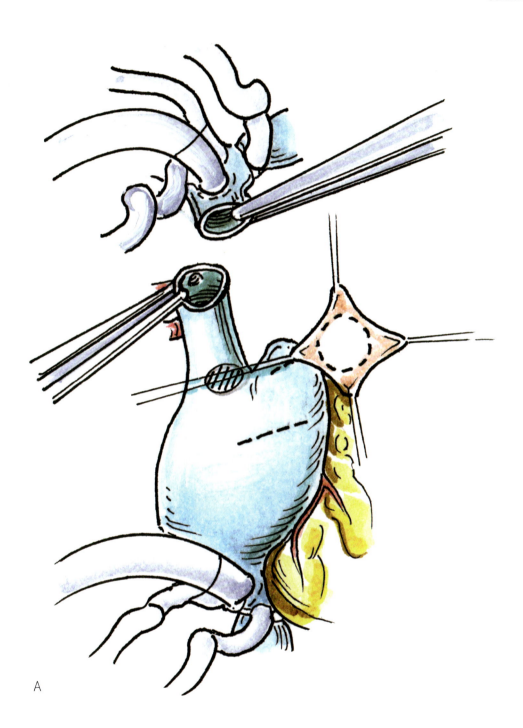

A

图 17-5（续）

B. 上腔静脉离断，近心端缝闭。右心耳做一切口，并将内面的肌小梁切除。

Figure 17-5 cont'd

B. Dissect SVC and close the cardiac orifice of the SVC. Make an incision in the right atrial appendage and then excise the trabeculations in the inner wall.

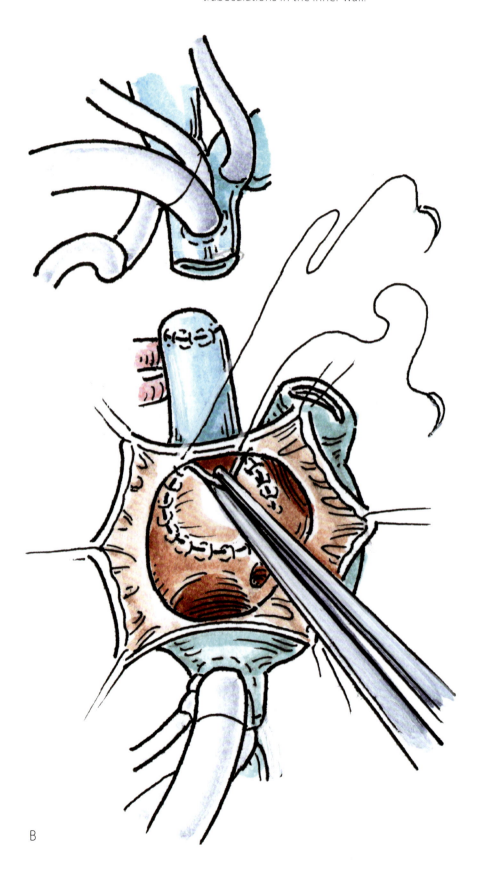

B

图 17-5（续）

Figure 17-5 cont'd

C. 用心包补片修补 ASD，同时将上腔静脉心内开口一并隔入左心房。

C. Repair the ASD with a pericardial patch and at the same time, the SVC is baffled to the left atrium.

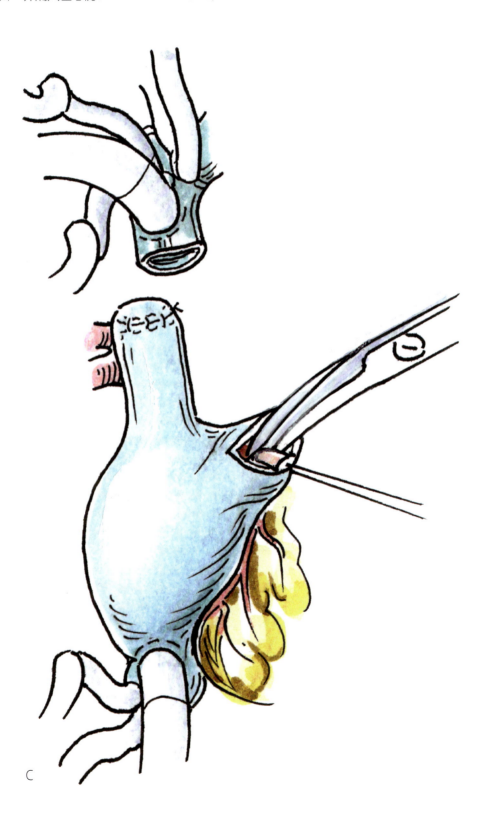

C

图 17-5（续）

Figure 17-5 cont'd

D. 将上腔静脉远心端与右心耳开口做端侧吻合。

D. The distal end of the SVC is anastomosed end-to-side with the right atrial appendage.

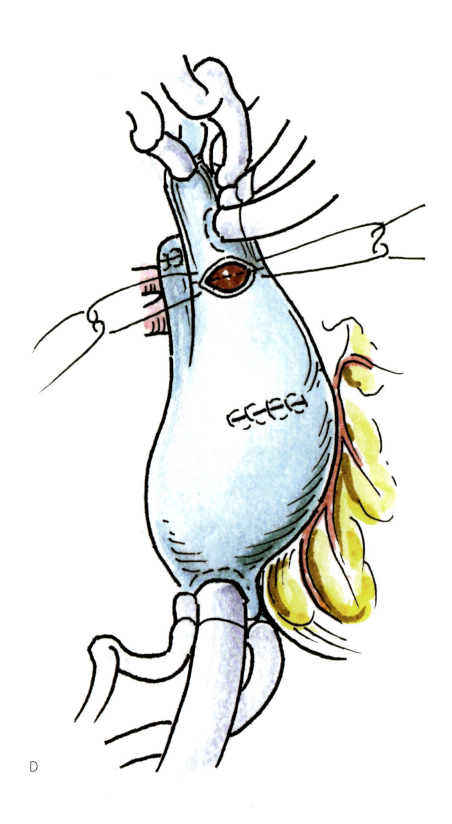

D

4. 冠状窦型（无顶冠状窦）房间隔缺损　在冠状窦的管状结构和左心房之间存在直接交通，造成左心房血液经冠状窦缺损进入右心房（图 17-6）。

4. Coronary sinus septal defect (Unroofed Coronary Sinus)　Direct communication between the tubular structure of the coronary sinus and the left atrium results in blood inflow from the left atrium through the coronary sinus defect into the right atrium (Figure 17-6).

图 17-6　冠状窦型（无顶冠状窦）房间隔缺损

A. 将 ASD 与冠状窦开口之间的部分房间隔打开，并将其扩大。

Figure 17-6　Coronary sinus septal defect (unroofed coronary sinus)

A. Open and expand partial interatrial septa between the ASDs and the coronary sinus ostium.

Continued

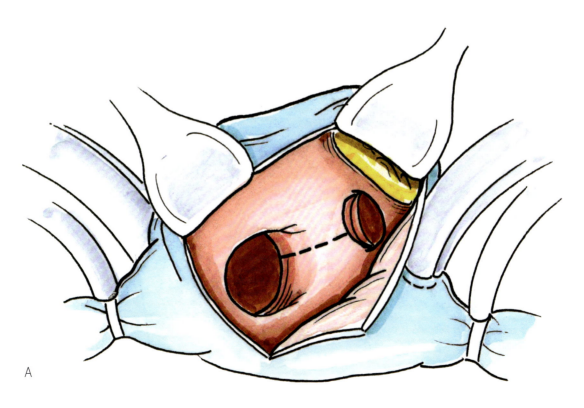

A

图 17-6(续)

Figure 17-6 cont'd

B、C. 取自身心包补片修补扩大的房间隔缺损。

B. C. Repair the enlarged atrial septum with pericardial patches.

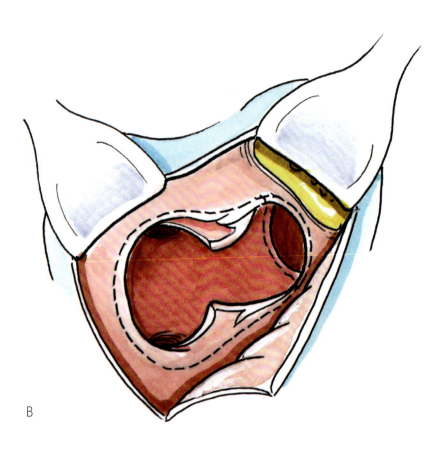

B

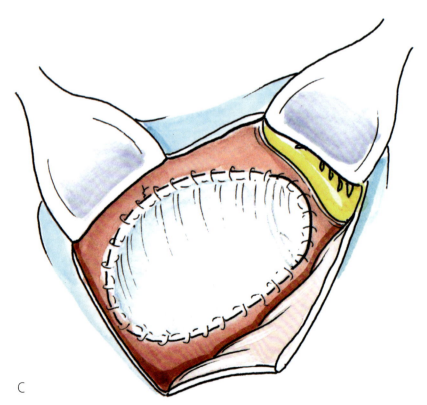

C

图 17-6(续)

Figure 17-6 cont'd

D. 术后冠状窦血液进入左心房,造成轻微的右向左分流。这些患者通常会存在左上腔静脉残存部分,术中需将左上腔静脉直接连接在右心房。

D. After the operation, the coronary sinus blood enters the left atrium, resulting in a slight right-to-left shunt. These patients usually have left SVC remnants, and hence, the left SVC is to be connected directly to the right atrium during the procedure.

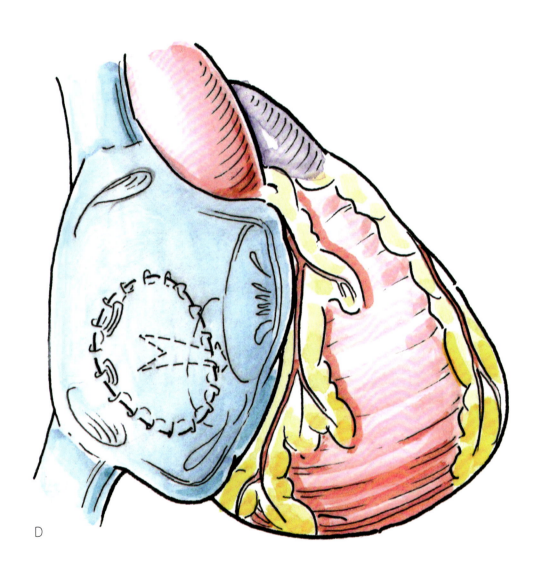

D

5. 共同心房（图 17-7）

5. Common atrium (Figure 17-7)

图 17-7　共同心房

A. 房间隔完全缺损,经右心房顶便可看到左侧的二尖瓣和肺静脉开口。

Figure 17-7　Common atrium

A. Complete atrial septal defect with left mitral and pulmonary vein ostia visible through the roof of the right atrium.

Continued

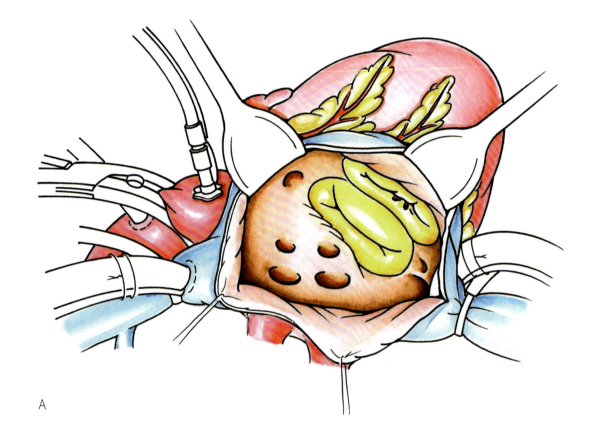

A

图 17-7（续）

B. 取一块大的补片，先从二尖瓣和三尖瓣交界处开始缝合。缝针不宜太深，避免损伤传导组织。

Figure 17-7 cont'd

B. Take a large patch and start suturing at the commissure of the mitral and tricuspid valves. Care must be taken not to take deep bites to avoid injury to conductive tissue.

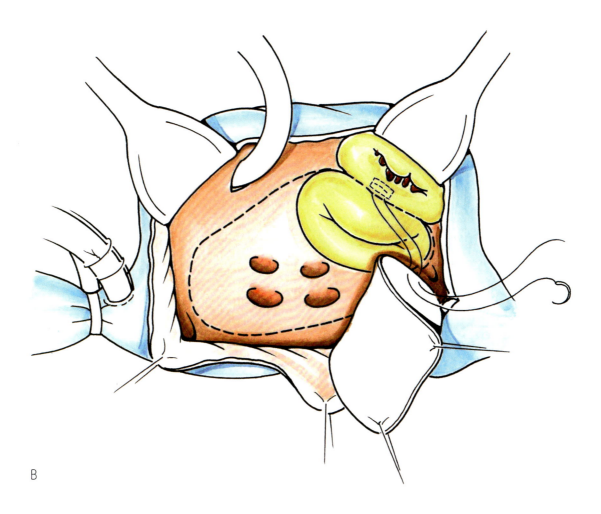

B

图 17-7（续）

Figure 17-7 cont'd

C. 从两侧将残留的部分房间隔缝合
完成。

C. Suture the residual partial septum from both sides.

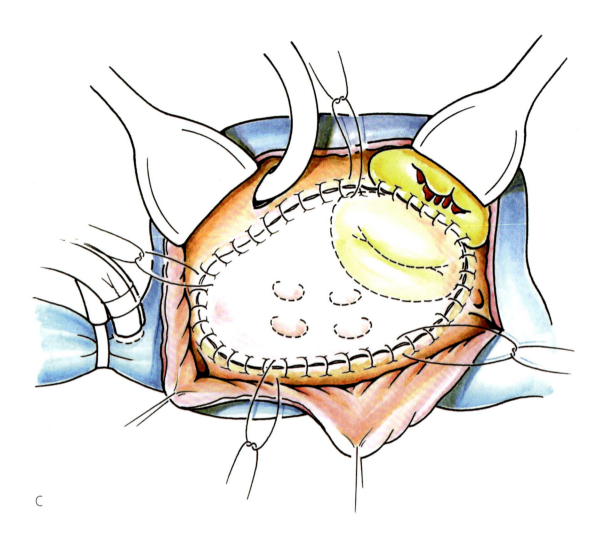

C

6. 部分型肺静脉异位连接 部分型肺静脉异位连接最多见于右上或右中肺静脉进入上腔静脉与右心房交接处,大多会合并静脉窦型ASD(图 17-8)。

6. Partial anomalous pulmonary venous connection (PAPVC) In most PAPVCs, the right superior or right middle pulmonary vein abnormally drains into the junction of the SVC and right atrium. PAPVCs are usually associated with sinus venous ASD (Figure 17-8).

图 17-8 **部分型肺静脉异位连接**
A. 右房平行切口。

Figure 17-8 Partial anomalous pulmonary venous connection

A. A parallel incision is made to the right atrium.

Continued

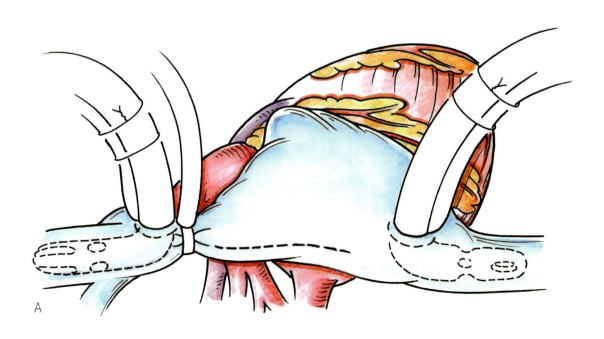

A

图 17-8 (续)

Figure 17-8 cont'd

B. 如果需要扩大房间隔缺损,沿缺损下缘朝卵圆窝方向剪开。

C. 切除部分房间隔组织,确保肺静脉回流至左心房畅通。

B. If it is necessary to enlarge the ASD, the incision is made along the inferior margin of the defect toward the fossa ovalis.

C. Part of the atrial septal tissue is excised to ensure unobstructed reflow of the pulmonary veins to the left atrium.

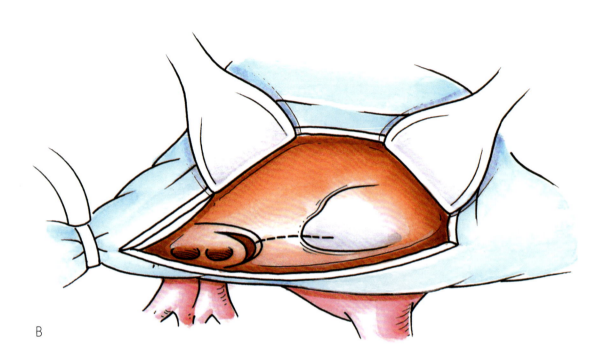

B

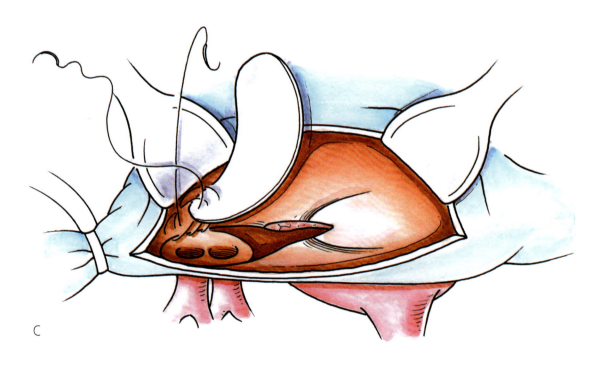

C

图 17-8（续）

D. 取自体或牛心包补片修补 ASD，将肺静脉开口隔入左心房内。

E. 直接缝合或用另一块心包补片扩大右心房切口。

Figure 17-8 cont'd

D. The ASD is repaired with an autologous or bovine pericardial patch and the pulmonary ostium is baffled in the left atrium.

E. The patch is directly sutured, or the right atrial incision is enlarged with another pericardial patch.

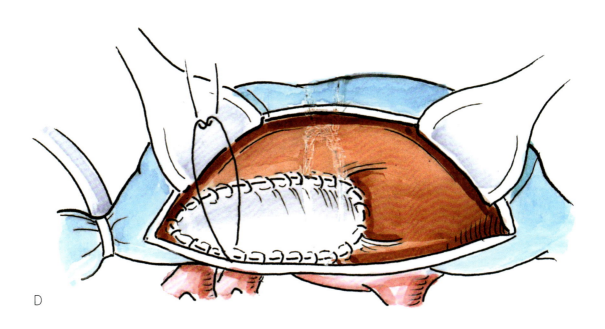

D

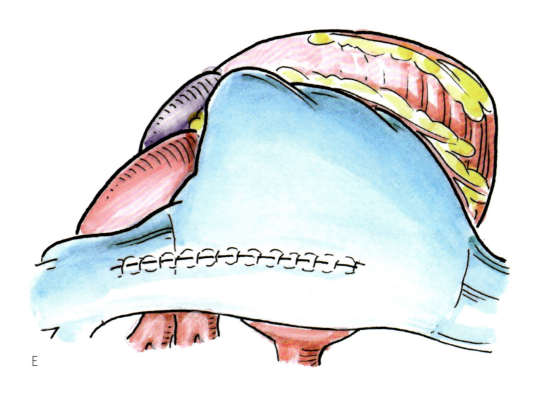

E

7. 弯刀综合征 部分型肺静脉异位连接的一种类型,即右肺的所有或部分肺静脉形成一根垂直静脉连接至下腔静脉,常伴有右肺发育不良,以及从腹主动脉发出的异常体动脉穿过横膈进入右肺,术中需要将体动脉分支予以离断(图 17-9)。

7. Scimitar syndrome Scimitar syndrome is a variant of PAPVC, which comprises of entire or partial pulmonary veins of the right lung join to form a single vertical trunk that connects to the inferior vena cava (IVC). This syndrome is usually associated with right lung dysplasia and an anomalous systemic artery arising into the right lung from the abdominal aorta penetrating the septum. The branches of the systemic artery are to be transected during the operation (Figure 17-9).

图 17-9 弯刀综合征
A. 右肺的所有或部分肺静脉形成一根垂直静脉连接至下腔静脉。

Figure 17-9　Scimitar syndrome
A. Entire or partial pulmonary veins of the right lung join to form a single vertical trunk that connects to the IVC.

Continued

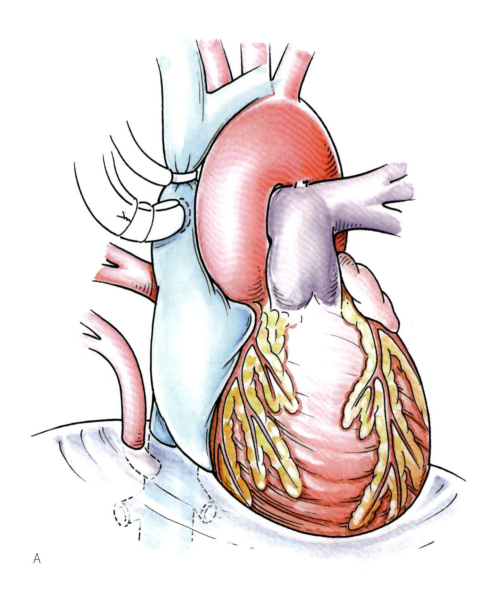

A

图 17-9（续）

B. 可将该异常走行静脉直接吻合到左心房。

Figure 17-9 cont'd

B. The anomalous vein can be directly anastomosed to the left atrium.

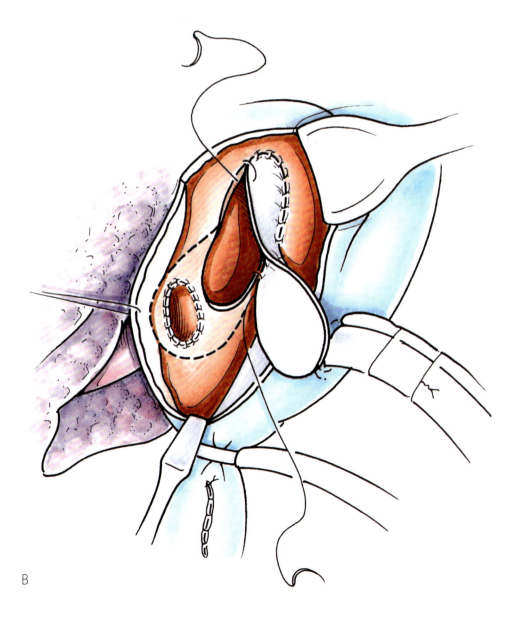

B

图 17-9（续）

C~F. 也可使用心包补片作为板障,将房间隔扩大,同时将右下肺静脉血流导入左心房。

Figure 17-9 cont'd

C-F. Or a pericardial patch is used as a baffle to augment the atrial septum. Meanwhile, the right inferior pulmonary vein flow is introduced into the left atrium.

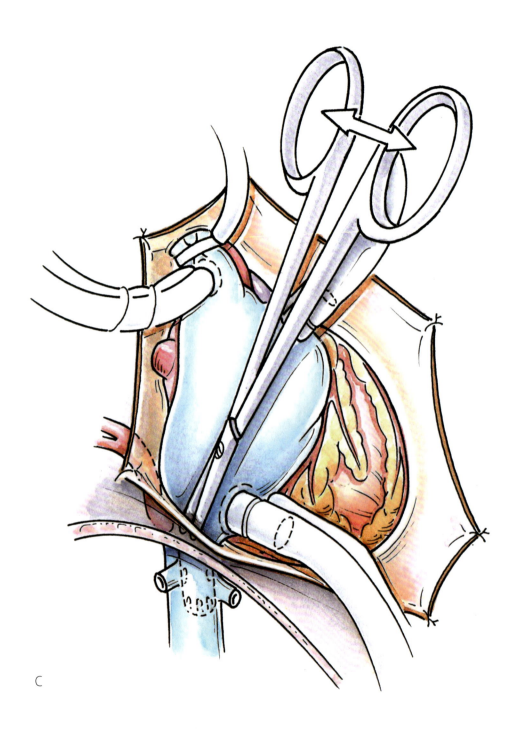

C

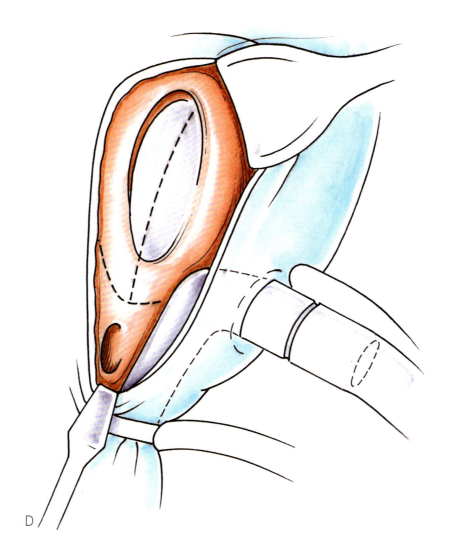

D

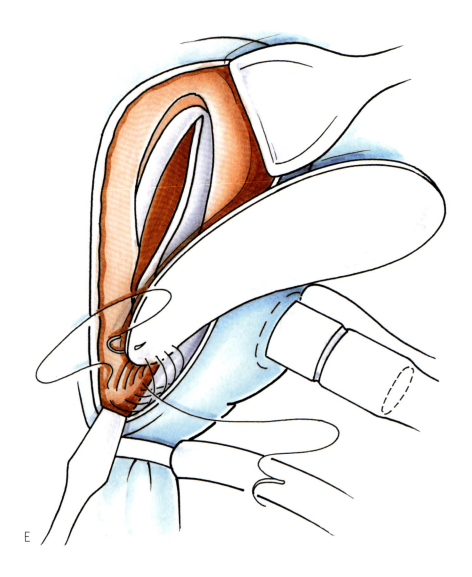

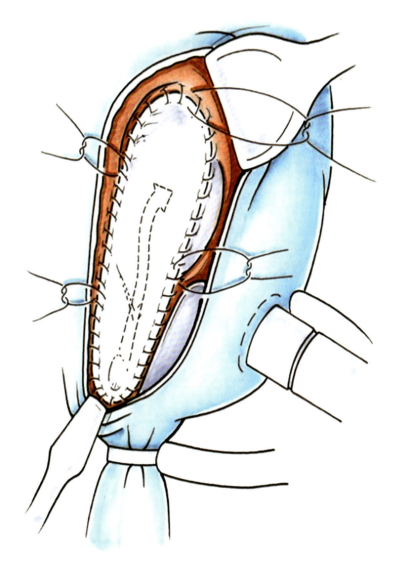

F

图 17-9（续）

G. 右心房切口可用心包补片扩大。

Figure 17-9 cont'd

G. The right atrial incision can be augmented with a pericardial patch.

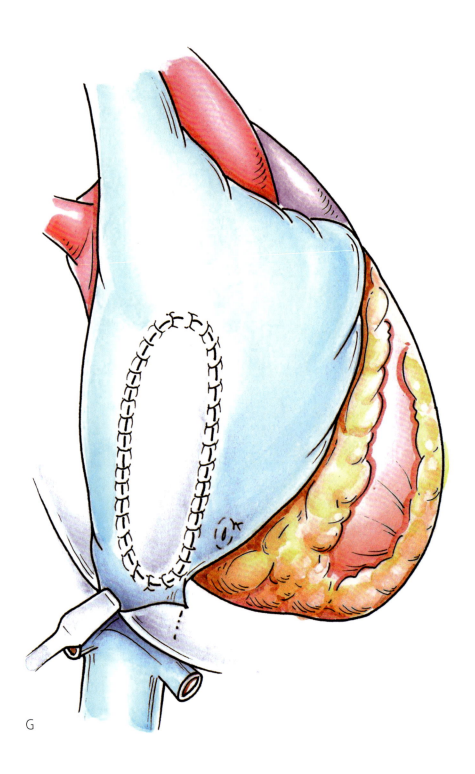

G

18 三房心和肺静脉狭窄

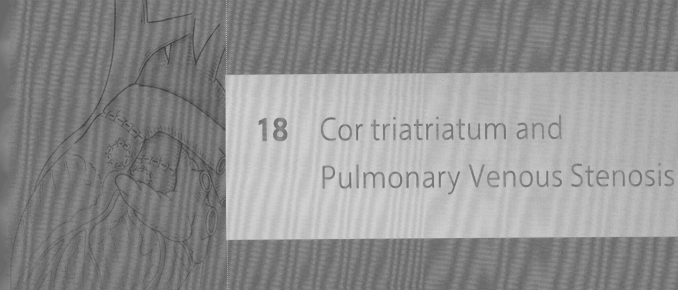

18 Cor triatriatum and
Pulmonary Venous Stenosis

三房心又可分为左侧三房心和右侧三房心,后者极为少见。通常说三房心畸形指的是左侧三房心。

Cor triatriatum consists of cor triatriatum sinister and cor triatriatum dexter, and the latter is rare. Therefore, cor triatriatum is usually used to refer to cor triatriatum sinister.

一、解剖分型

I. Anatomic Typing

按照 Lucas-Schmidt 分型,三房心包括以下几种类型(图 18-1)。

According to the Lucas-Schmidt classification, cor triatriatum includes the following types (Figure 18-1).

1. 副心房接受所有肺静脉,并与左心房有交通。

1. The accessory atrium receives all pulmonary veins and communicates with the left atrium.

(1)没有其他连接(经典三房心)。

(1) No other connections (classic cor triatriatum).

(2)有其他异位连接:①直接连接到右心房;②合并完全型肺静脉异位引流。

(2) With other anomalous connections: ① Direct connection to right atrium; ② Combined with total anomalous drainage of the pulmonary vein.

2. 副心房接受所有肺静脉,但与左心房无交通。

2. The accessory atrium receives all pulmonary veins but does not communicate with the left atrium.

(1)直接连接到右心房。

(1) Direct connection to the right atrium.

(2)合并完全型肺静脉异位引流。

(2) Combined with total anomalous drainage of the pulmonary vein.

3. 不完全型三房心

(1)副心房接受部分肺静脉,并连接到左心房:①其余肺静脉连接正常;②其余肺静脉连接异常。

3. Subtotal cor triatriatum

(1) The accessory atrium receives a portion of the pulmonary veins and connects to left atrium: ① Normal connection of remaining pulmonary veins; ② Anomalous connection of remaining pulmonary veins.

（2）副心房接受部分肺静脉并连接到右心房，其余肺静脉连接正常。

(2) The accessory atrium receives part of the pulmonary veins and connects to the right atrium, and the remaining pulmonary veins connect normally.

图 18-1　Lucas-Schmidt 分型
A. 肺静脉回流至副心房，三房心隔膜开口是肺静脉唯一出口。
B. 除隔膜开口外，副心房和右心房之间存在交通。

Figure 18-1　Lucas-Schmidt classification
A. The pulmonary vein returns to the accessory atrium, and the only egress for the pulmonary vein is through the opening in the cor triatriatum membrane.
B. There is communication between the accessory atrium and right atrium in addition to the opening in the cor triatriatum membrane.

Continued

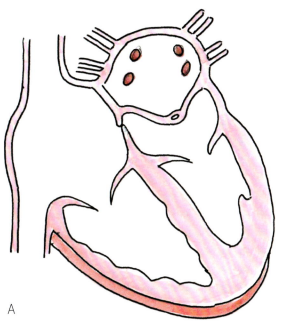

A

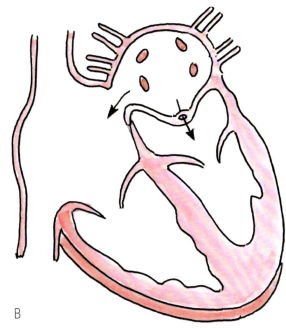

B

图 18-1（续）

C. 除隔膜开口外，副心房与无名静脉存在连接。肺静脉回流血通过垂直静脉、无名静脉再入上腔静脉和右心房。

D. 肺静脉回流经副心房和右心房之间的交通至右心房，再经房间隔缺损入左心房。

Figure 18-1 cont'd

C. Except for the opening in the cor triatriatum membrane, there is an anomalous connection between the accessory atrium and the innominate vein. The pulmonary venous return reaches the superior vena cava and the right atrium through the vertical vein and the innominate veins.

D. Pulmonary venous return reaches the right atrium through a communication between the accessory atrium and the right atrium, and blood reaches the left atrium via the atrial septal defect.

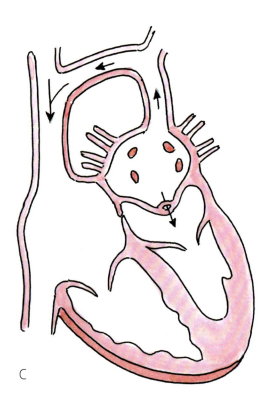

C

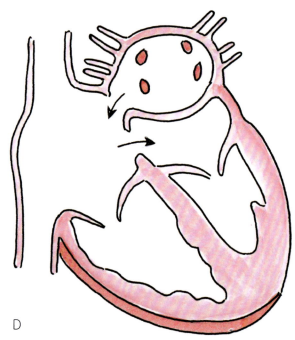

D

图 18-1（续）

E. 副心房经垂直静脉引流至门静脉和下腔静脉。

F. 右肺静脉经一狭窄的开口与左心房交通，左侧肺静脉直接开口在左心房。

Figure 18-1 cont'd

E. Accessory atrium decompresses via a vertical vein to the portal vein and inferior vena cava.

F. The right pulmonary vein communicates with the left atrium through a stenotic orifice, and the left pulmonary vein opens directly to the left atrium.

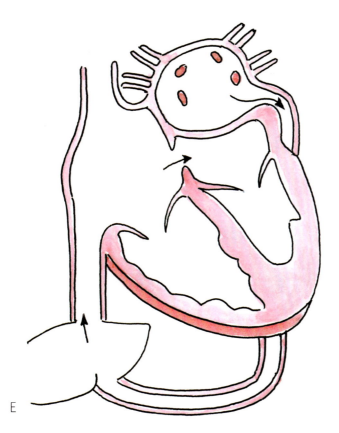

E

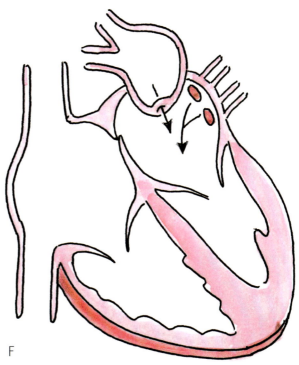

F

图 18-1（续）

G. 右肺静脉经狭窄开口与左心房交通，左肺静脉与无名静脉相连。

H. 右肺静脉经狭窄开口与右心房交通，左肺静脉开口正常。

Figure 18-1 cont'd

G. The right pulmonary vein communicates with the left atrium through a stenotic orifice, and there is connection of the left pulmonary vein to the left innominate vein.

H. The right pulmonary vein communicates with the right atrium via a stenotic orifice, and the left pulmonary vein connects normally.

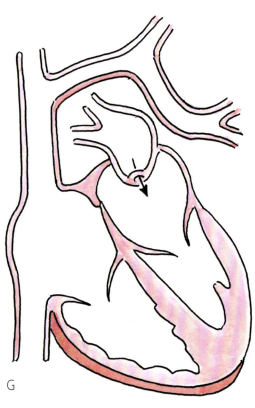

G

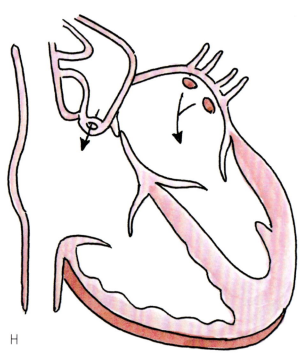

H

二、手术方法

1. 隔膜切除 术前明确诊断后，应用常规心肺转流术，经右心房通过房间隔或左心房切口暴露心内解剖结构。外科手术原则包括完整切除隔膜，术中需注意识别四个肺静脉的开口位置。年龄较小的婴幼儿切除隔膜时需特别小心，注意避免损伤二尖瓣和左心房壁（图18-2）。对同时合并部分型或完全型肺静脉异位连接的患者，则需要在切除心内隔膜的同时做肺静脉异位引流矫治手术（参考《完全性肺静脉异位连接》一章）。

II. Surgical Methods

1. The resection of the membrane After the preoperative diagnosis is confirmed, the left atrium anatomy is exposed via the right atrial, trans-septal approach, or the left atrial approach under a routine cardiopulmonary bypass. The surgical principles include complete resection of the obstructing membrane, and careful identification of the four ostia of the pulmonary vein (PV). When resecting the membrane in younger infants, care should be taken to avoid injuries to the mitral valve and left atrial wall (Figure 18-2). In patients present with partial or total anomalous pulmonary venous connection, corrective procedures of anomalous pulmonary venous connection should be performed at the same time when resecting the membrane (refer to the chapter dealing with total anomalous pulmonary venous connection).

图 18-2　隔膜切除

A、B. 在常规心肺转流术时经右心房通过房间隔或左心房切口暴露心内解剖结构。

Figure 18-2　The resection of the membrane

A, B. The intra-LA anatomy is exposed via the right atrial, trans-septal approach, or the left atrial approach under a routine cardiopulmonary bypass.

Continued

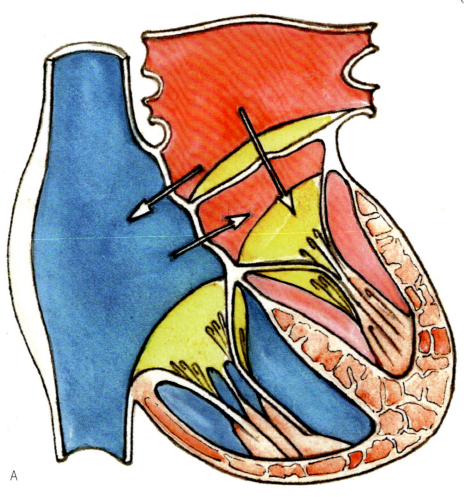

A

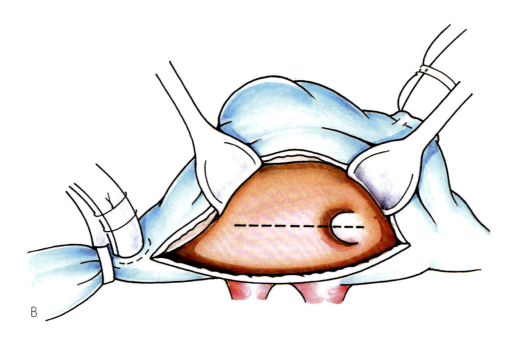

B

图 18-2（续）

Figure 18-2 cont'd
C~E. 完整切除隔膜。

C-E. Complete resection of the obstructing membrane.

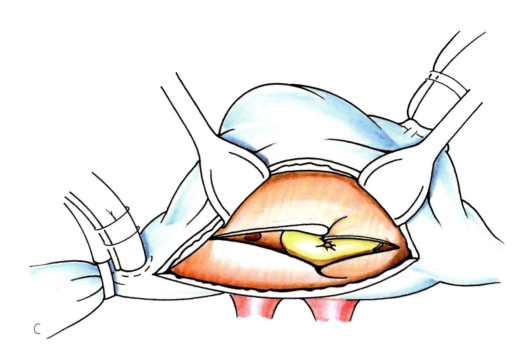

C

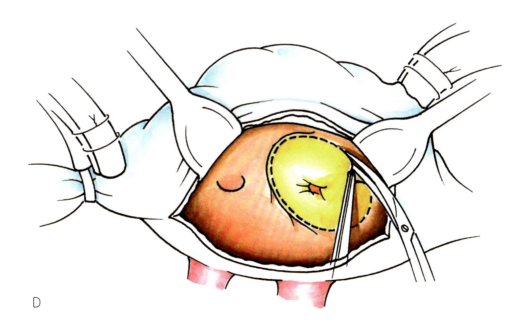

D

图 18-2（续）

C~E. 完整切除隔膜。

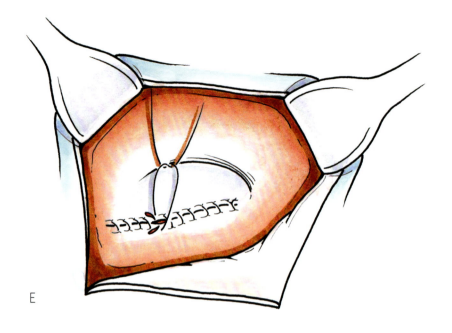

E

图 18-2（续）

F. 年龄较小的婴幼儿切除隔膜时需注意避免损伤二尖瓣和左心房壁。

Figure 18-2 cont'd

F. When resecting the membrane in younger infants, care should be taken to avoid injuries to the mitral valve and left atrial wall.

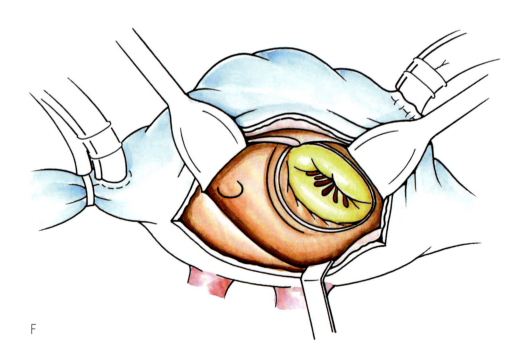

F

2. 肺静脉狭窄处理 肺静脉狭窄患者临床表现取决于受累肺静脉的数量和梗阻的严重程度。根据狭窄程度可分为长段发育不良、局限性隔膜、局限性内膜纤维化。对局限性隔膜型狭窄，通常行狭窄环切开、内嵴切除，并用自身心包补片扩大。可以先用两片小的心包扩大肺静脉开口，再用一片大的心包扩大左心房，也可直接用一块大的心包补片扩大肺静脉和左心房，但再狭窄的发生率较高（图18-3）。

2. Management of pulmonary vein stenosis The clinical presentation of patients with PV stenosis depends on the number of affected PVs and the severity of the obstruction. Depending on the degree of stenosis, it can be divided into long-segment dysplasia, discrete diaphragm, and focal intimal fibrosis. For discrete diaphragm stenosis, the stenosis ring is usually dissected, the internal ridge is resected, and the incision is augmented with an autologous pericardial patch. The PV ostium may be enlarged firstly with two small pericardium pieces, and the left atrium with a large pericardium piece later. As an alternative, the PV ostium and the left atrium may also be directly enlarged with a large pericardial patch. However, above pericardial patch angioplasties are associated with a very high rate of pulmonary vein stenosis recurrence (Figure 18-3).

图 18-3　**肺静脉狭窄处理**
A. 肺静脉狭窄的三种不同类型。

Figure 18-3　Management of pulmonary vein stenosis
A. Three types of pulmonary vein stenosis.

Continued

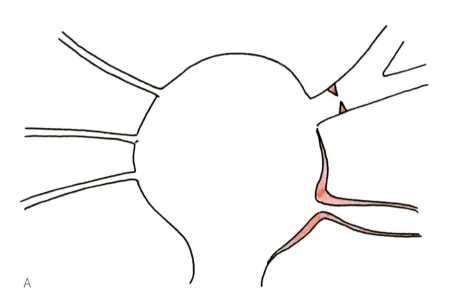

A

图 18-3（续）

Figure 18-3 cont'd

B. 局限性隔膜型狭窄。

C. 狭窄环切开。

B. Discrete diaphragm stenosis.

C. The stenosis ring is usually dissected.

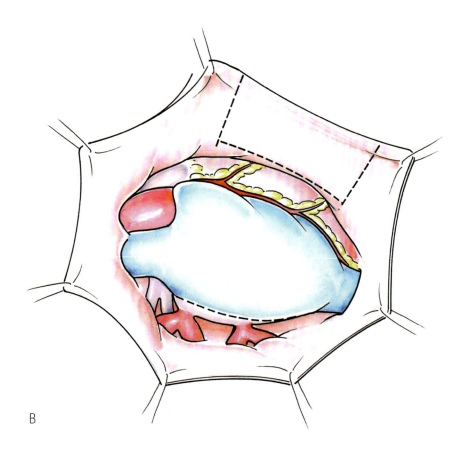

B

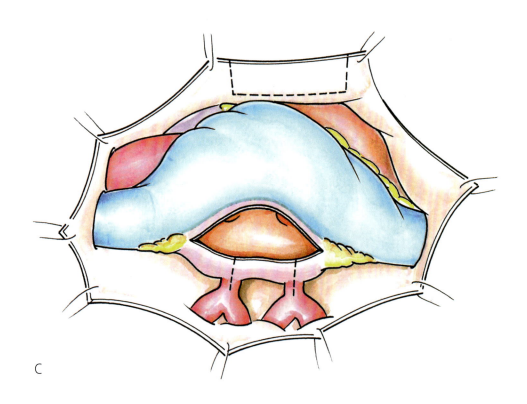

C

图 18-3（续）

D. 内嵴切除，用自身心包补片扩大。

E. 先用两片小的心包扩大肺静脉开口。

Figure 18-3 cont'd

D. The internal ridge is resected, and the incision is augmented with an autologous pericardial patch.

E. The PV ostium may be enlarged firstly with two small pericardium pieces.

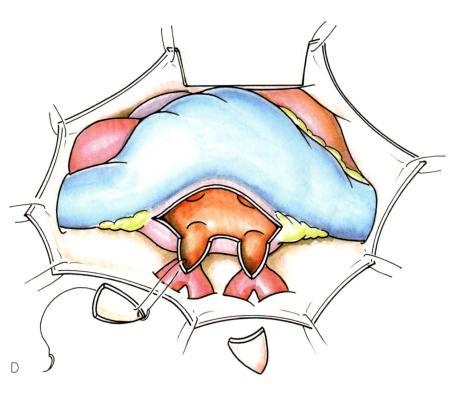

D

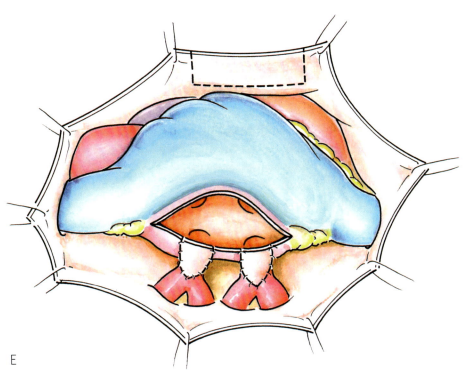

E

图 18-3 (续)

F. 再用一片大的心包扩大左心房。

G. 也可直接用一块大的心包补片扩大
肺静脉和左心房。

Figure 18-3 cont'd

F. The left atrium with a large pericardium piece later.

G. The PV ostium and the left atrium may also be directly enlarged with a large pericardial patch.

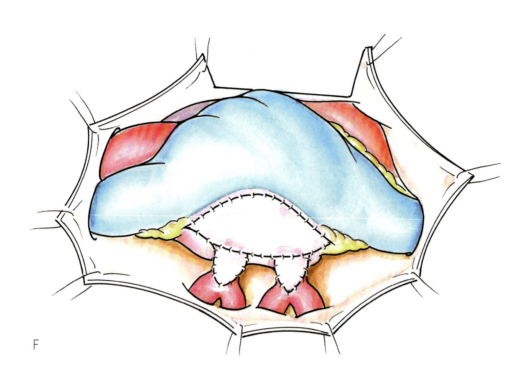

F

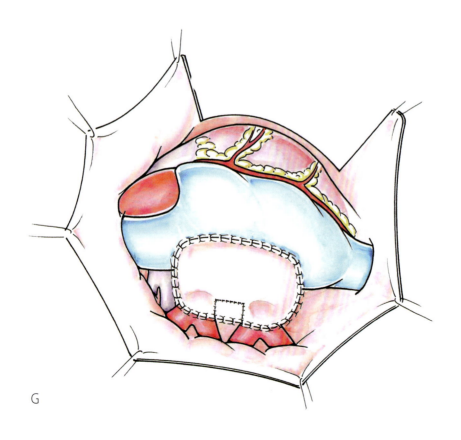

G

图 18-3（续）

H. 对左侧肺静脉开口狭窄可采用左心耳和肺静脉联合切口，再采用心包补片扩大。

Figure 18-3 cont'd

H. For the stenosis of the left pulmonary vein openings, the left atrial appendage and pulmonary vein combined incision can be used, and then the pericardial patch can be used.

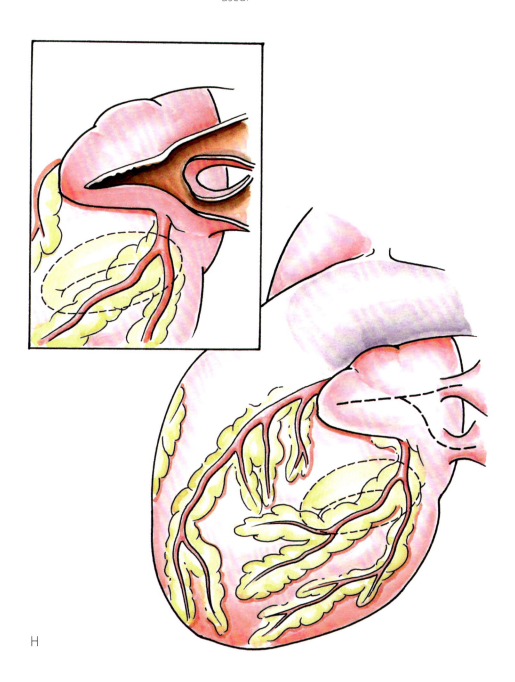

H

3. Sutureless 技术 目前对肺静脉狭窄大多采用 Sutureless 技术，即在狭窄的肺静脉和与之相邻的左心房做一个切口，在这些切口的上方构建一个心包囊袋，避免对于肺静脉的直接缝合（图 18-4）。

3. Sutureless technique At present, the sutureless technique is adopted for pulmonary vein stenosis. that is, an incision is made in the narrow pulmonary vein and adjacent left atrium, and a pericardial pouch is constructed over these incisions to avoid direct sutures of the pulmonary veins (Figure 18-4).

图 18-4　Sutureless 技术

A. 在左心房做一个切口（虚线所示），切口分别延伸至右上和右下肺静脉开口。

Figure 18-4　Sutureless technique

A. An incision (dotted line) is made into the left atrium and extended to both right superior and right inferior PV ostia, respectively.

Continued

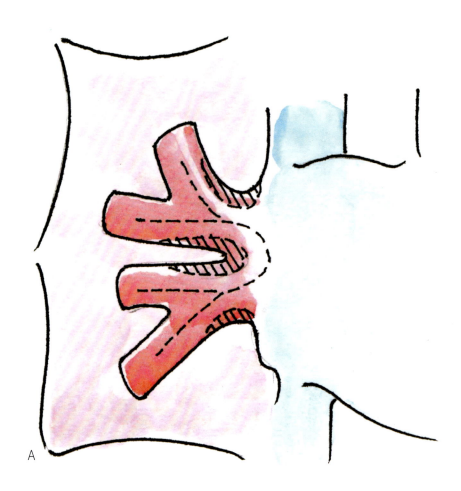

A

图 18-4（续）

B. 剪开邻近的心包组织，从紧靠右上肺静脉和左心房交界处开始缝合。

Figure 18-4 cont'd

B. The adjacent pericardial tissue is cut open, and suturing is begun in the pericardium just above the junction of the right superior pulmonary vein and left atrium.

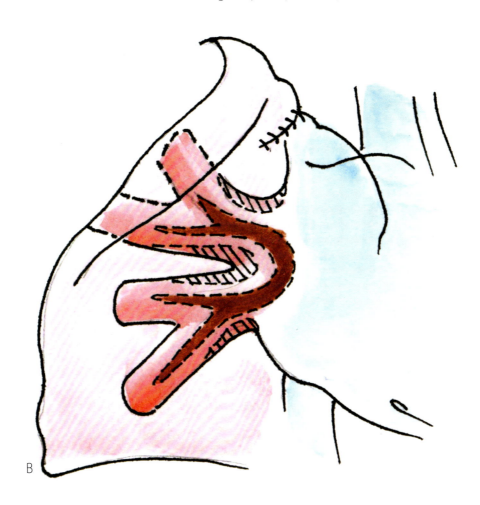

B

图 18-4（续）

Figure 18-4 cont'd

C. 另一侧的心包补片用另一根缝线从右下肺和左心房交界处开始缝合，与上端的缝线汇合打结。

C. The pericardial patch on the other side is sutured with a second inferior suture, which starts from the junction of the right lower lung and the left atrial to join the superior suture line, and knot is made there.

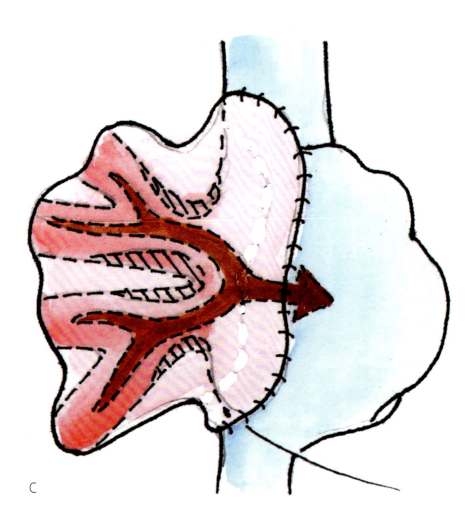

C

19 完全性肺静脉异位连接

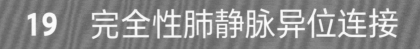

19 Total Anomalous Pulmonary Venous Connection

一、解剖分型

正常肺静脉是在心脏的背面左右上下共四个开口直接汇入左心房。通常将完全性肺静脉异位连接（total anomalous pulmonary venous connection，TAPVC）分成四型。Ⅰ型（心上型）：肺总静脉与心脏以上的结构相连，即右上腔静脉、奇静脉、左上腔静脉或无名静脉；Ⅱ型（心内型）：肺总静脉与心内结构相连，即右心房或冠状窦；Ⅲ型（心下型）：肺静脉汇总后向横膈下方走行，与下腔静脉、门静脉系统相连；Ⅳ型（混合型）：上述情况混搭出现（图19-1）。

I. Anatomical Typing

The normal pulmonary veins return directly into the left atrium from the left, right, upper, and lower openings on the back of the heart. Total anomalous pulmonary venous connections (TAPVC) are usually classified into four types. Type Ⅰ (supracardiac TAPVC): Common pulmonary vein is connected to structures above the heart, i. e., the right superior vena cava, azygos vein, left superior vena cava, or innominate vein; Type Ⅱ (intracardiac TAPVC): Common pulmonary vein is connected to intracardiac structures, namely the right atrium or coronary venous sinus; Type Ⅲ (infracardiac TAPVC): Pulmonary veins confluence courses below the diaphragm and are connected to the inferior vena cava or portal venous system; Type Ⅳ (mixed TAPVC): It is a mix of the above three conditions (Figure 19-1).

图 19-1　完全性肺静脉异位连接的解剖分型

A. 正常肺静脉。

Figure 19-1　Anatomical typing of total anomalous pulmonary venous connections

A. The normal pulmonary veins.

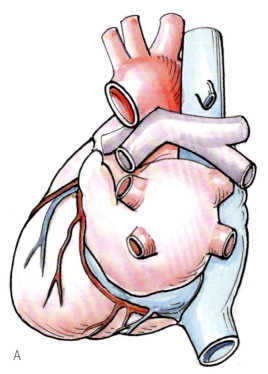

A

Continued

图 19-1（续）

B. 心上型：肺总静脉与心脏以上的结构
相连。

C. 心内型：肺总静脉与右心房连接。

Figure 19-1 cont'd

B. Supracardiac TAPVC: Common pulmonary vein is
connected to structures above the heart.

C. Intracardiac TAPVC: Common pulmonary vein is
connected to the right atrium.

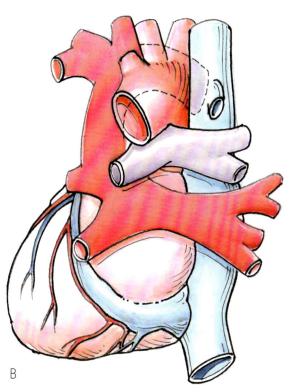

B

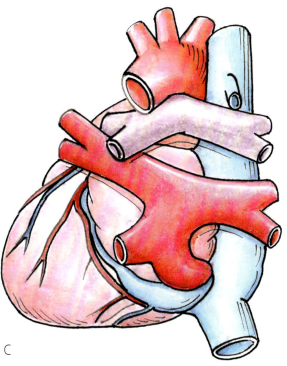

C

图 19-1（续）

D. 心内型：肺总静脉与冠状窦连接。

E. 心下型：肺静脉汇总后向横膈下方走行，与下腔静脉、门静脉系统相连。

Figure 19-1 cont'd

D. Intracardiac TAPVC: Common pulmonary vein is connected to the coronary venous sinus.

E. Infracardiac TAPVC: Pulmonary veins confluence courses below the diaphragm and are connected to the inferior vena cava or portal venous system.

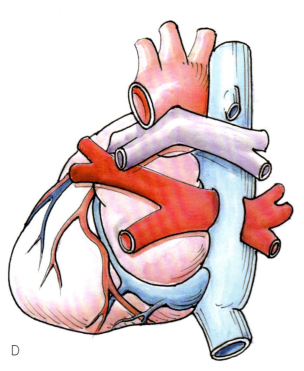

D

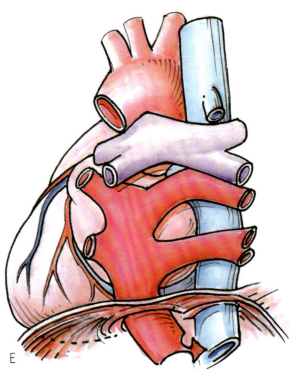

E

二、手术方法

II. Surgical Methods

1. 心上型手术（图 19-2）

1. Surgery of supracardiac TAPVC (Figure 19-2)

图 19-2　心上型手术
A. 传统的方法是在右心房做一横切口，并在卵圆孔水平剪开房间隔进入左心房，并延伸至左心耳根部。

Figure 19-2　Surgery of supracardiac TAPVC
A. Traditionally, make a transversal incision in the right atrium and horizontally cut the atrial septum at the foramen ovale to enter the left atrium and extend to the root of the left atrial appendage.

Continued

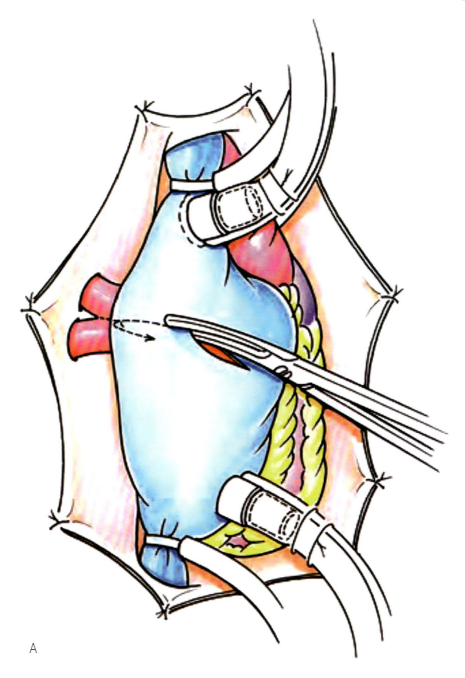

A

图 19-2 (续)

B. 在下方的肺静脉汇合处做一个与左心房切口平行的切口，用 6-0 Prolene 缝线直接做侧侧吻合。

C. 吻合从最左端开始，若左心房偏小，可缝合一部分右心房组织，确保吻合口足够宽。

Figure 19-2 cont'd

B. Make an incision parallel to the left atrium incision at the lower pulmonary vein confluence and make a direct side-to-side anastomosis with 6-0 Prolene suture.

C. The anastomosis starts from the far-left end. If the left atrium is too small, part of the right atrium tissue may be sutured to ensure that the anastomosis is wide enough.

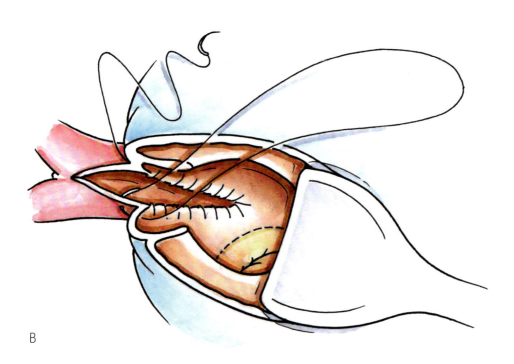

B

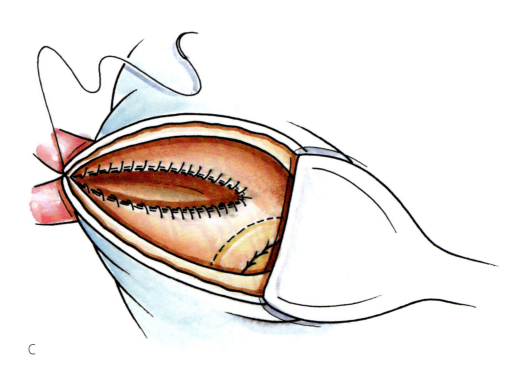

C

图 19-2（续）

Figure 19-2 cont'd

D、E. 取心包补片扩大缝合剪开之房间隔，同时也扩大发育较小的左心房。

D. E. The pericardial patch is taken to enlarge and suture the incised atrial septum, and the smaller left atrium is enlarged at the same time.

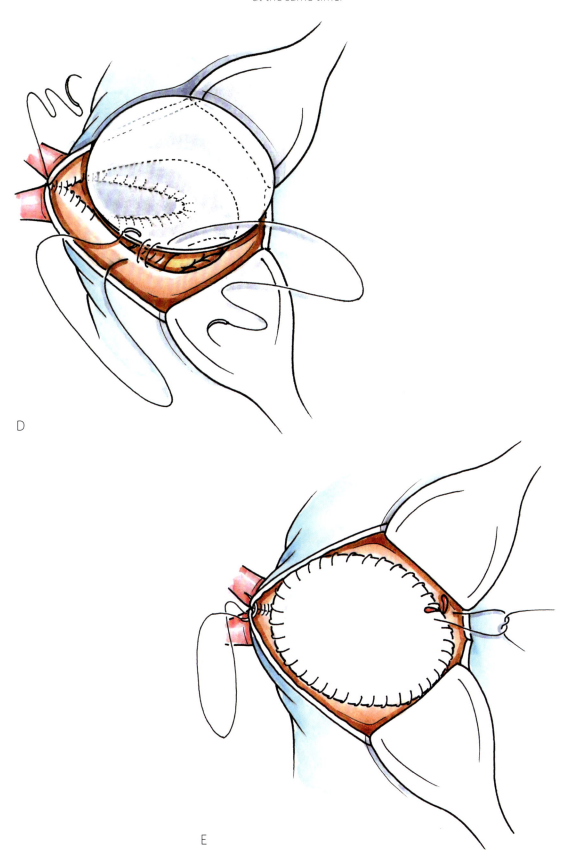

D

E

图 19-2（续）

Figure 19-2 cont'd

F. 直接缝合右心房切口。

F. The right atrium incision is directly sutured.

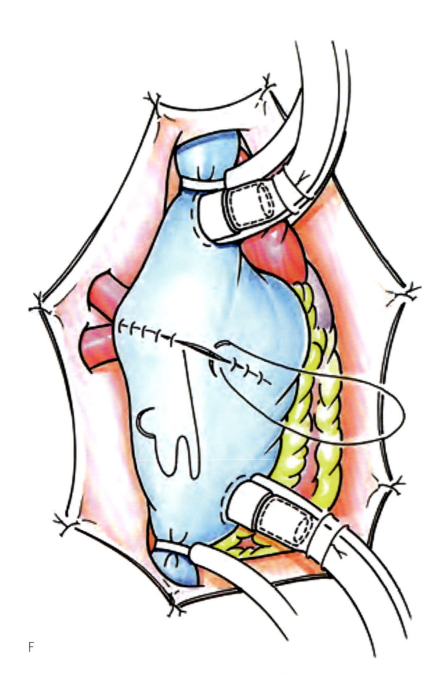

F

图 19-2（续）

G. 另一种手术方法是从主动脉和上腔静脉之间的上方径路,即在左心房顶部进行操作。该技术更适用于年龄稍大的患儿。

Figure 19-2 cont'd

G. An upper approach between the aorta and the superior vena cava could be taken. That is, the operation is performed on the roof of the left atrium. This technique is more suitable for elder children.

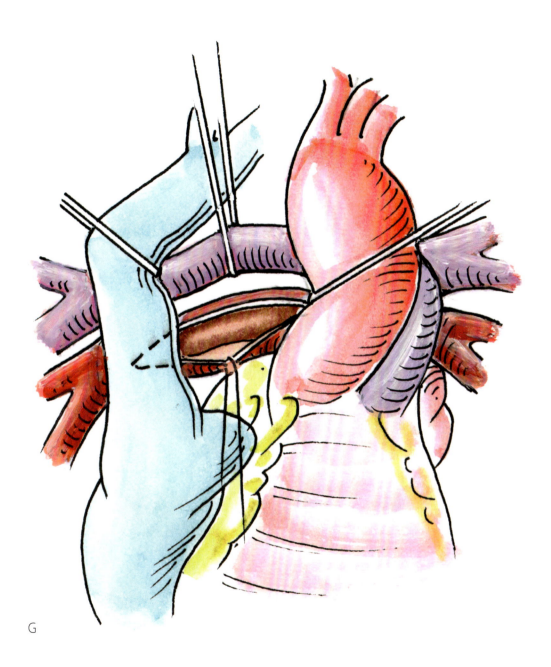

G

2. 心内型手术（图 19-3）

2. Surgery of intracardiac TAPVC (Figure 19-3)

图 19-3　心内型手术

A. 切开右心房暴露扩大的冠状窦和房间隔缺损或未闭的卵圆孔。切开两者之间的房间隔组织（虚线所示）。

B. 将冠状窦顶部组织切开，并向心房后壁延伸。确认清楚所有肺静脉开口和左侧房室瓣开口，确保两者之间无任何梗阻。

C. 取一块大的心包组织修补冠状窦去顶产生的房间隔缺损，冠状窦直接开口在左心房。

Figure 19-3　Surgery of intracardiac TAPVC

A. Cut the right atrium to expose the enlarged coronary sinus and atrial septal defect or open foramen ovale. Incise the septal tissue between the two (shown by the dotted line).

B. The roof of the coronary sinus is dissected toward the posterior wall of the atrium. Identify all pulmonary ostia and the left atrioventricular valve ostium to confirm there is no obstruction between the two.

C. A large piece of pericardial tissue is taken to repair the atrial septal defect caused by the unroofed coronary sinus. The coronary sinus opens directly to the left atrium.

Continued

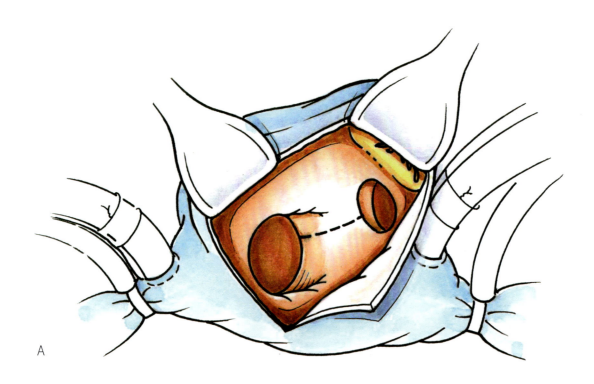

A

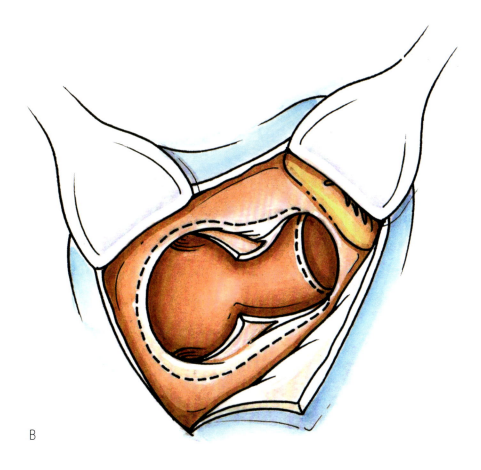

B

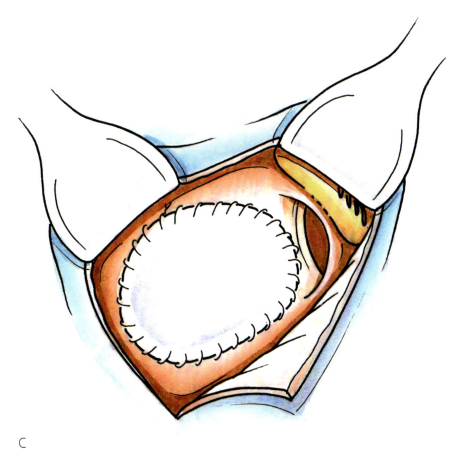

C

图 19-3（续）

D. 术毕肺静脉血流直接经二尖瓣进入左心室。

Figure 19-3 cont'd

D. After the operation, the pulmonary vein blood returns directly into the left ventricle through the mitral valve.

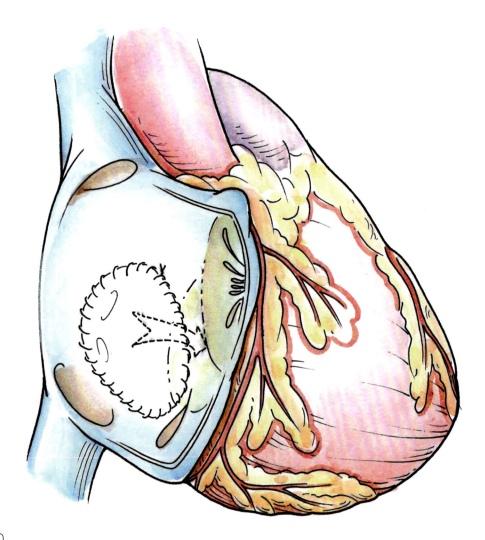

D

3. 心下型手术（图 19-4）

3. Surgery of infracardiac TAPVC (Figure 19-4)

图 19-4　心下型手术

A. 首先将垂直静脉在最靠横膈处缝扎切断。在左心耳和左房与相应汇总静脉做纵向切开（见虚线处）。若汇总静脉较短，可以利用一部分近端垂直静脉。

Figure 19-4　Surgery of infracardiac type

A. First, the vertical vein is ligated at the point closest to the diaphragm. Make a longitudinal incision in the left atrial appendage and the left atrium, corresponding to the confluence vein (see the dotted line). If the PV confluence is short, a part of the proximal vertical vein may be used.

Continued

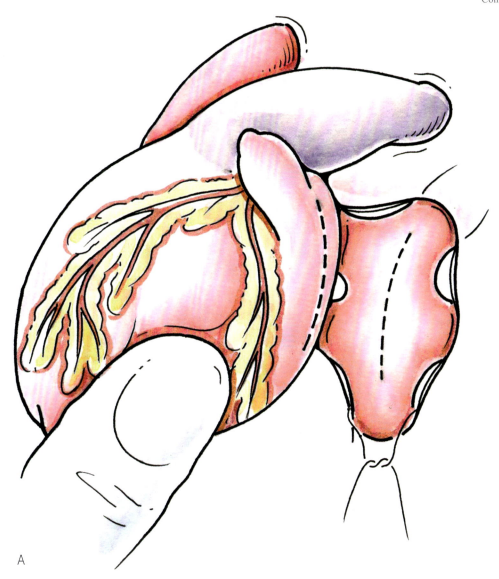

A

图 19-4（续）

Figure 19-4 cont'd

B. 用 6-0 或 7-0 Prolene 缝线做左心房与肺静脉侧侧吻合。吻合时需注意两者之间的位置不可有过度牵拉或扭曲，避免肺静脉回流受阻。

B. Make a side-to-side anastomosis between the left atrium and pulmonary vein with 6-0 or 7-0 Prolene sutures. It is necessary to ensure there is no excessive stretching or twisting between the left atrium and the PV during anastomosis to avoid obstruction of pulmonary venous return.

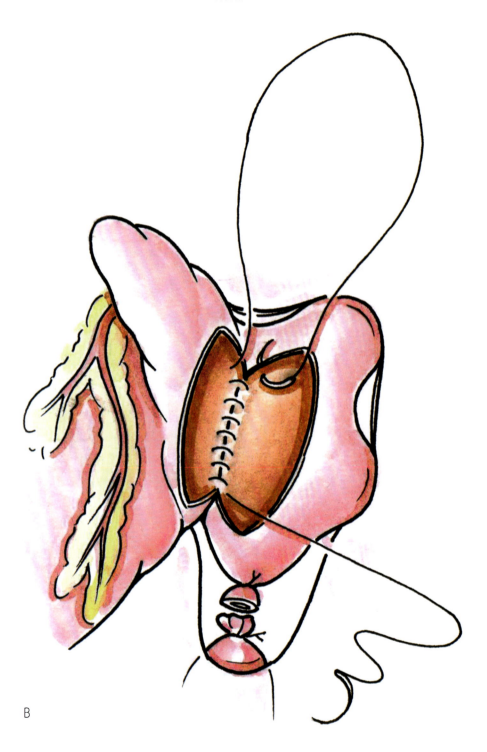

B

图 19-4（续）

Figure 19-4 cont'd

C. 术毕从心脏背面看肺静脉与左心房之间连接情况。

C. The connection between the pulmonary vein and the left atrium is seen from the back of the heart postoperatively.

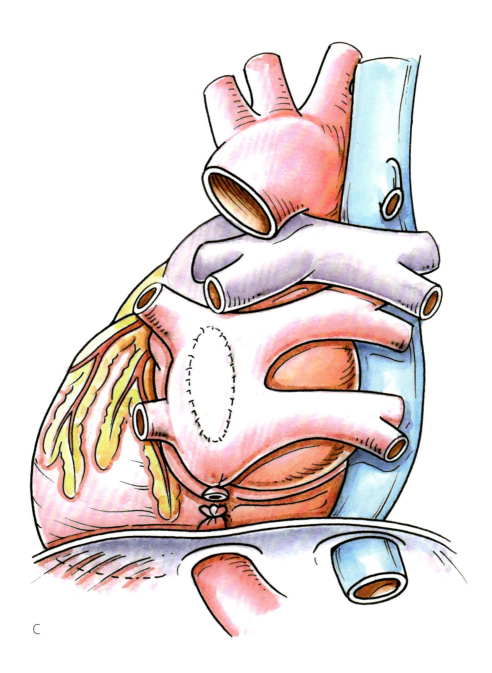

C

4. Sutureless 技术 该技术多用于心下型肺静脉异位连接和术后肺静脉再狭窄的患者（在三房心与肺静脉狭窄中已有描述）。本部分重点介绍心下型 TAPVC 缝合方法（图 19-5）。

4. Sutureless technique This technique is commonly used in patients with infracardiac anomalous pulmonary venous connection and postoperative pulmonary vein restenosis (described in the chapter on pulmonary vein stenosis). This section focuses on the infracardiac TAPVC suturing methods (Figure19-5).

图 19-5　Sutureless 技术
A. 心下型 TAPVC，将位于心脏后方的汇总肺静脉切开，将左心房切开并延伸至左心耳，形成一个尽量宽的开口（虚线所示）。

Figure19-5　Sutureless technique
A. In the infracardiac TAPVC, the pulmonary vein confluence located behind the heart is incised, and the left atrium is incised and extended to the left atrial appendage to form an opening as wide as possible (see the dotted line).

Continued

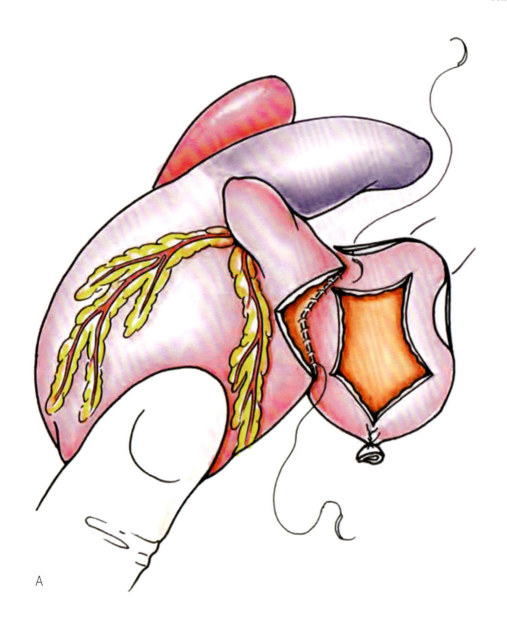

A

图 19-5（续）

B. 沿着如图所示的虚线位置，用 6-0 Prolene 缝线连续缝合，将左心房切口和边缘缝合至肺静脉外周的心包上，尽可能利用周边的心包组织，确保吻合口足够宽和没有牵拉（见虚线图示）。

Figure19-5 cont'd

B. Follow the dotted line as shown in the figure, and suture the left atrial incision and edge to the peripheral pericardium of the pulmonary vein with a running suture of 6-0 Prolene. Use the surrounding pericardial tissue as much as possible to ensure that the anastomosis is wide enough and free of traction (see dotted line).

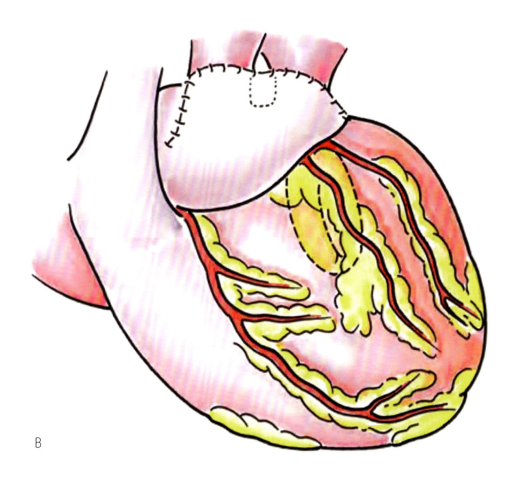

B

图 19-5（续）

C. 缝合后从心脏背面看肺静脉与左心房之间的连接情况。

Figure19-5 cont'd

C. The connection between the pulmonary vein and the left atrium was observed from the back of the heart after suturing.

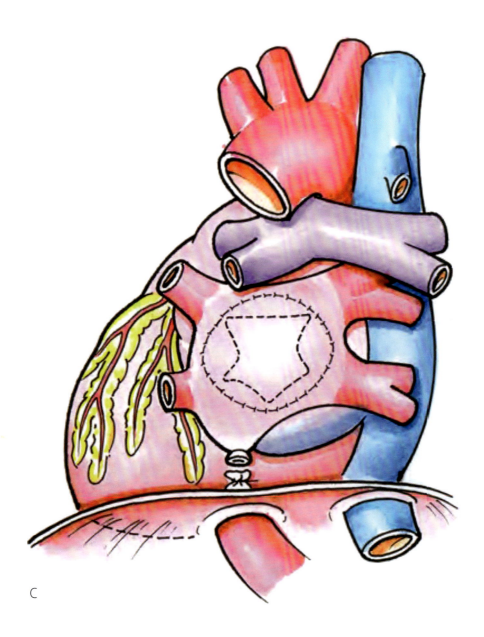

C

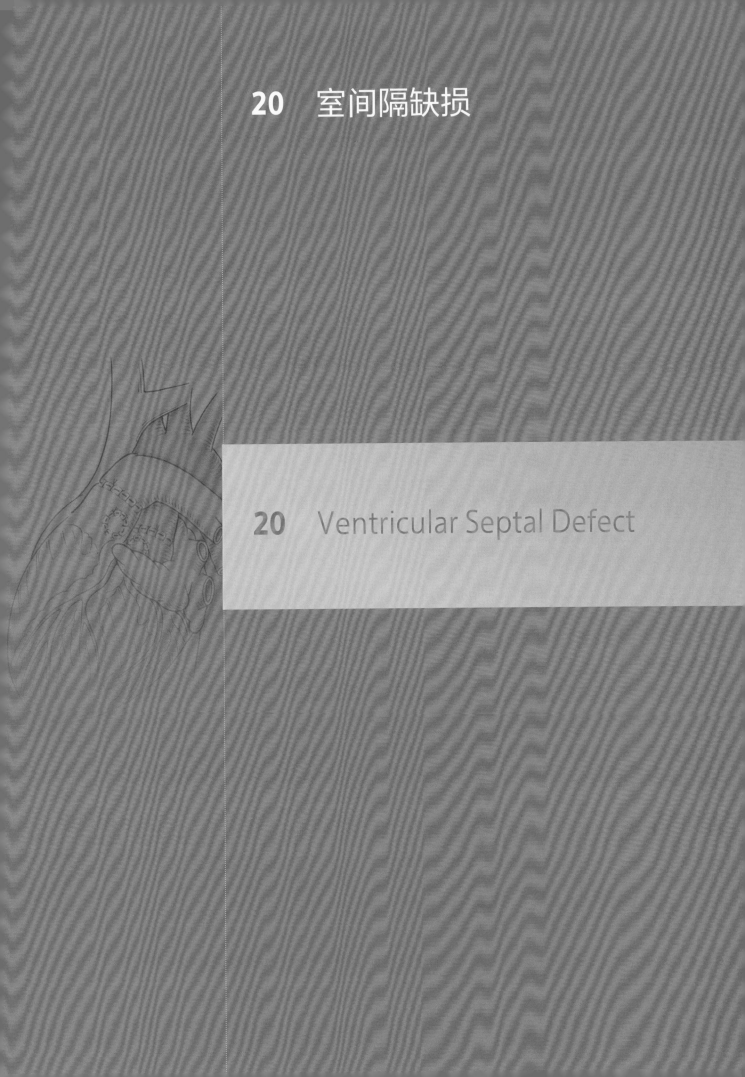

20 室间隔缺损

20 Ventricular Septal Defect

一、解剖分型

I. Anatomical Typing

室间隔缺损（ventricular septal defect，VSD）在先天性心脏病外科手术中占比最高，其解剖变异较多，为便于手术通常将缺损分为四个类型（图 20-1）。

Ventricular septal defect (VSD) is the most common malformation in congenital heart disease (CHD) surgeries, with many anatomic variations. To facilitate the operation, VSD is usually classified into four types (Figure 20-1).

Ⅰ型：VSD 与双动脉相关且位于动脉圆锥隔、室上嵴漏斗部和肺动脉瓣下。有时伴有主动脉瓣叶脱垂嵌入 VSD，引起主动脉瓣关闭不全。在著名病理学家 Van Praagh 医生的分类中，为圆锥隔缺损型。

Type I: A ventricular septal defect is associated with both great arteries and is usually a conal, supracrital, subpulmonary defect. It is sometimes associated with the prolapsed aortic leaflets embedded in the VSD, resulting in aortic insufficiency. In the classification of Dr. Van Praagh, a famous pathologist, this type of VSD belongs to a conal septal defect.

图 20-1　室间隔缺损的解剖分型
A. 圆锥隔缺损型 VSD。

Figure 20-1　Anatomical typing of ventricular septal defect
A. Conal VSD.

Continued

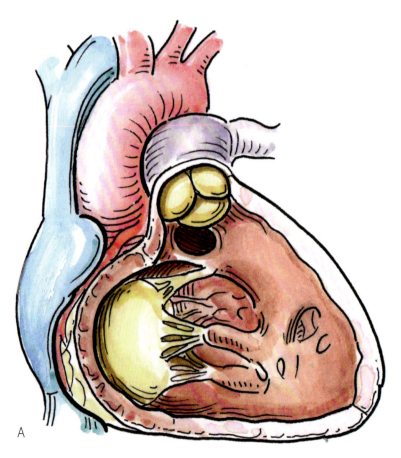

A

Ⅱ型：通常称为膜周型 VSD。术中碰到最多就是这类 VSD，缺损的表现特征是主动脉瓣叶和三尖瓣在缺损的后下缘存在纤维连续，这个区域包括膜部室间隔的房室部分。

Type Ⅱ: Perimembranous VSD. This type of VSD is the most frequently encountered in surgery, and the defect is characterized by fibrous continuity between the aortic valve leaflets and a tricuspid valve at the posteroinferior margin, and the area of the defect incorporates the atrioventricular portion of the membranous septum.

图 20-1（续）
B. 膜周型 VSD。

Figure 20-1 cont'd
B. Perimembranous VSD.

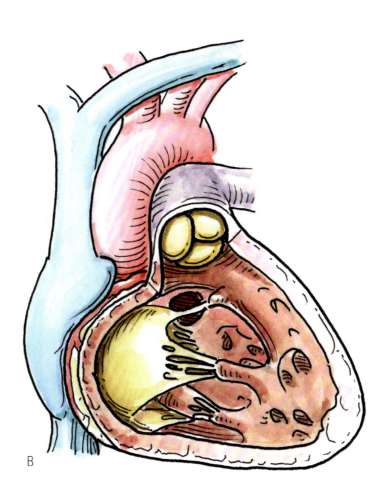

B

Ⅲ型：又称房室管型或流入道VSD。这类缺损通常较大，位于三尖瓣隔后瓣下。也有些缺损合并有三尖瓣瓣叶骑跨。缺损的下缘离房室结发出的传导束很近，术中需特别注意。在 Van Praagh 分类中，也被称为房室管型缺损。

Type Ⅲ : Inlet defect, also known as atrioventricular canal type (AV canal type). This type of defect is usually large and located below the septal and posterior leaflets of the tricuspid valve septa. There are also some defects associated with straddling tricuspid valve leaflets. The inferior margin of the defect is close to the conduction bundle from the atrioventricular node, and special attention should be paid during the operation. This type is also referred to as an atrioventricular canal defect in the Van Praagh classification.

图 20-1（续）
C. 房室管型 VSD。

Figure 20-1 cont'd
C. Atrioventricular canal type.

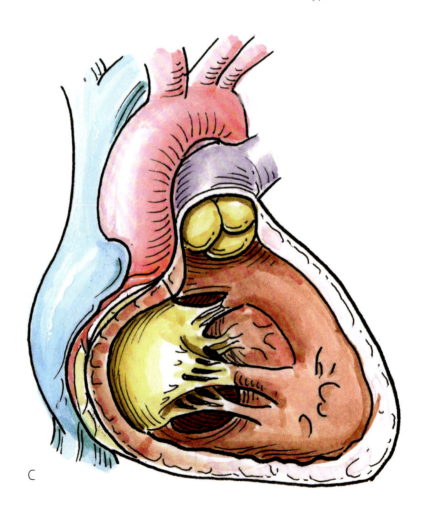

IV型：也称为肌部缺损。其缺损位置可以位于肌部室间隔的任意部位，可单一或多发。特别是位于心尖部的肌部缺损，可呈多个蜂窝状缺损，故又被称为"瑞士干酪"样缺损，很难直接修补，目前临床治疗大多采用介入封堵的方法。

Type IV : Muscular defect. The defect can be located anywhere in the interventricular septum, presenting as single or multiple deformities. Muscular defects, especially those located in the apical part, such as "Swiss cheese", which is presented as multiple honeycomb shape, are difficult to be repaired directly. At present, interventional closure is the primary choice for muscular VSDs.

图 20-1（续）
D. 肌部缺损。

Figure 20-1 cont'd
D. Muscular VSD.

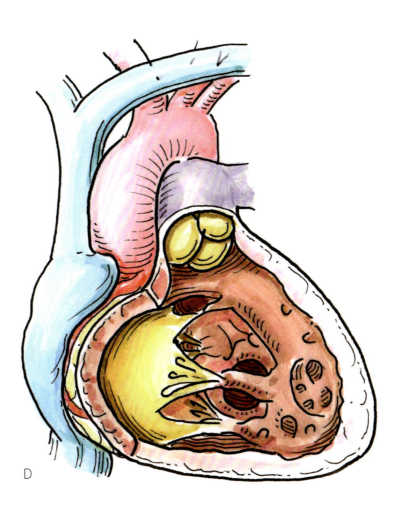

D

除此之外,还有一些特殊类型的室间隔缺损,如左心室右心房分流,较少见。

In addition, other special types of VSDs, such as a shunt from the left ventricular to the right atrium, are rare.

二、手术方法

II. Surgical Methods

术前判定 VSD 的位置,决定选择不同心脏切口做修补。尽量做到暴露清晰,避免导致室间隔缺损周边组织的损伤。通常有 5 个手术径路:右心房切口径路、肺动脉切口径路、主动脉切口径路、右心室切口径路和左心室切口径路。

Choose a cardiac incision for repair by the VSD location determined before surgery. Try to make a clear exposure and avoid damaging the surrounding tissues of VSDs. There are usually five surgical approaches: the right atrial approach, the transpulmonary arterial approach, the transaortic approach, the right ventricular approach, and the left ventricular approach.

1. 右心房切口径路　绝大多数 VSD 手术都可采用此径路,尤其是膜周型 VSD(图 20-2)。

1. Right atrial approach　Right atrial approach is appropriate for the majority of VSD procedures, especially those for perimembranous VSD (Figure 20-2).

A. 膜周型 VSD 右心房径路，切开右心
房，牵开三尖瓣组织暴露 VSD。

A. Right atrial approach for perimembranous VSD: incise the right atrium, distract tricuspid valve tissue to expose the VSD.

Continued

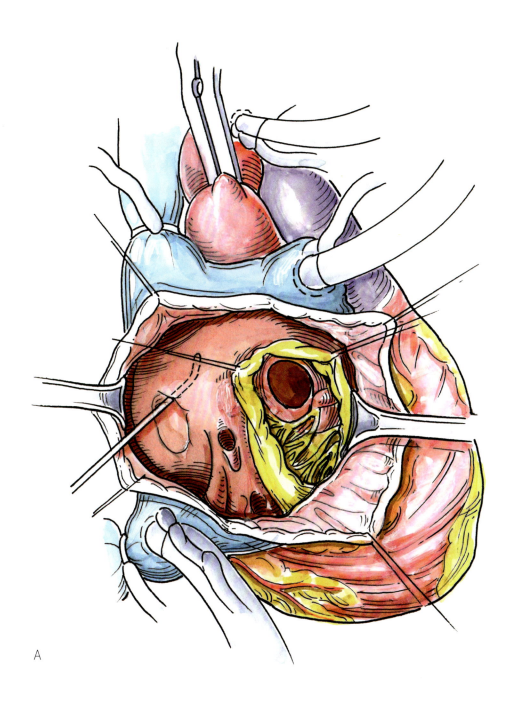

A

图 20-2（续）

B、C. 为了清楚暴露缺损的边缘,可将室隔瘤或部分三尖瓣隔瓣组织切开。

Figure 20-2 cont'd

B, C. In order to expose the surrounding structures of the defect clearly, dissect the false aneurysm of membrance septum or part of the tricuspid septal tissues.

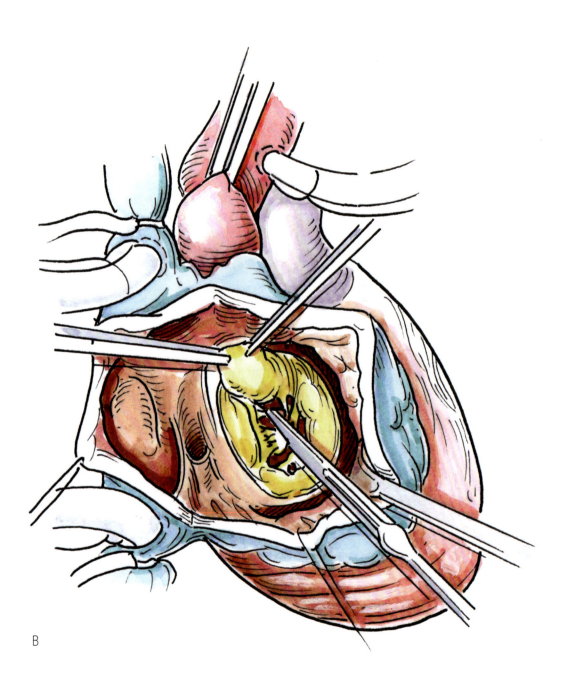

B

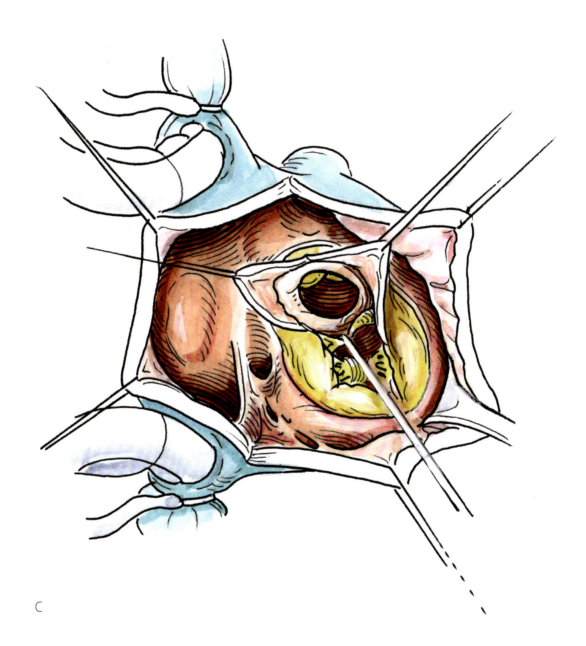

C

图 20-2（续）

D. 可采用多针带垫的双头针间断褥式缝合。也可采用一针带垫双头针连续缝合。

Figure 20-2 cont'd

D. The defect is usually closed using interrupted pledgetted mattress sutures with multiple double-armed needles or single pledget-supported running sutures with a double-armed needle.

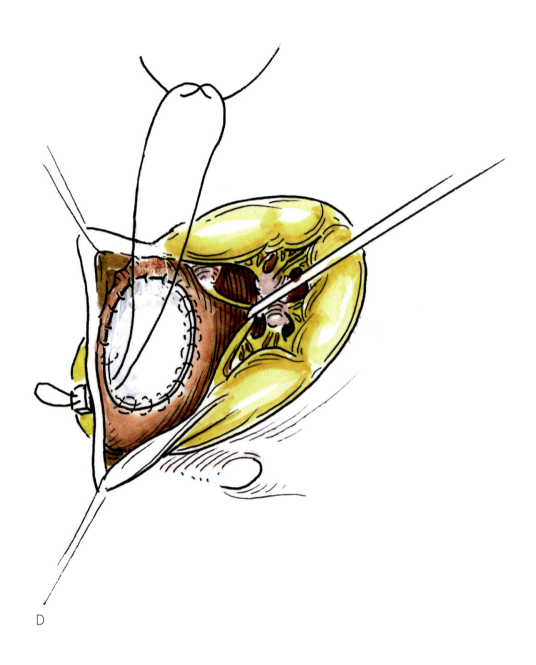

D

图 20-2（续）

E. 将切开之三尖瓣组织缝合修补。注水测试三尖瓣反流情况。膜周偏流出道的 VSD 缝合时需注意沿缺损后下缘从圆锥乳头肌处开始，一直到靠近 Koch 三角顶端区域的三尖瓣瓣环，缝线不能太深，避免损伤传导系统。

Figure 20-2 cont'd

E. The incised tricuspid valve is repaired through sutures. Tricuspid regurgitation is examined by the cold saline injection test. When closing perimembranous VSD extending slightly to the outlet, the sutures shall be placed superficially and carefully along the posterior and inferior edge of the defeat, beginning from the muscle of Lancisi and continuing to the tricuspid annulus near the apex region of Koch's triangle, to avoid damaging to the conduction system.

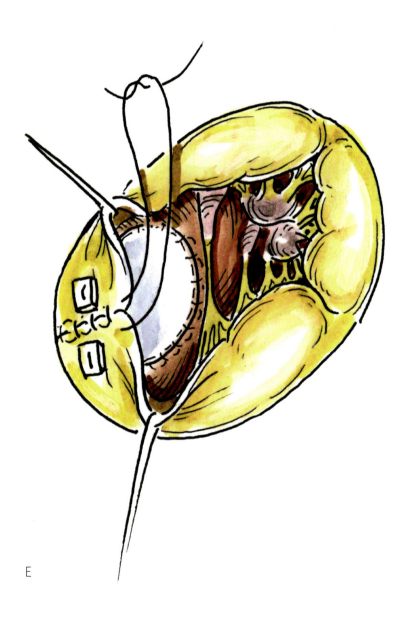

E

图 20-2（续）

F. 当室间隔缺损偏向主动脉瓣下，并有三尖瓣腱索横跨遮挡时，为清晰暴露，可将三尖瓣隔前瓣根部切开暴露。在三尖瓣隔、前瓣处距瓣环 1~2mm 作一横向切口（见虚线）。

Figure 20-2 cont'd

F. When VSD lie inferior to the aortic valve and are shielded by the tricuspid chordae tendineae, the root of the septal and anterior leaflets of the tricuspid valve can be dissected for a clear exposure. A transverse incision is made at the tricuspid septum and the anterior leaflet, keeping 1-2mm away from the annulus (dotted liney).

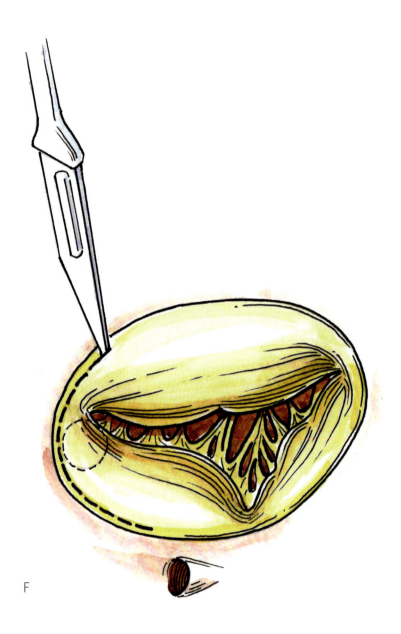

F

图 20-2（续）

G、H. 将三尖瓣牵开，暴露室间隔缺损边缘。可采用间断或连续缝合。

Figure 20-2 cont'd

G, H. The tricuspid valve is retracted to expose the rim of the VSD, and it can be closed by interrupted or running sutures;

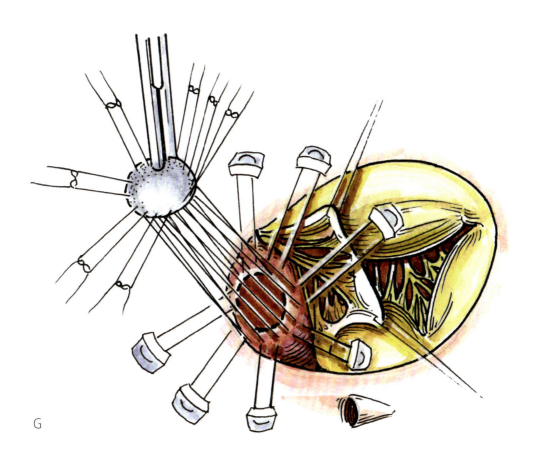

G

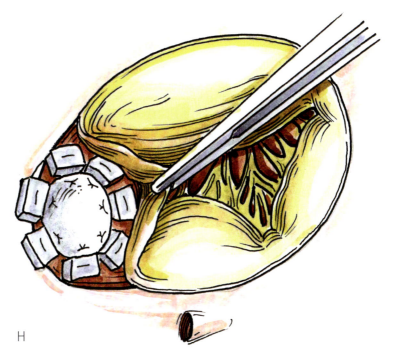

H

图 20-2（续）

I. 将剪开之三尖瓣瓣叶重新缝合固定到原来位置。

Figure 20-2 cont'd

I. The incised tricuspid valve leaflets are resuspended to the original position.

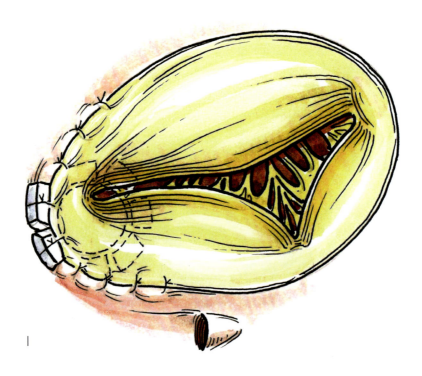

I

2. 肺动脉切口径路（图 20-3）

2. Transpulmonary arterial approach (Figure 20-3)

图 20-3　肺动脉切口径路修补室间隔缺损

A. 肺动脉瓣环上 5~10mm 做一纵行或横行切口，牵开肺动脉瓣暴露间隔缺损部位及周边关系。

Figure 20-3　Transpulmonary arterial approach for VSD repair

A. A longitudinal or transverse incision is made 5-10mm above the pulmonary annulus, and the pulmonary valve is distracted to reveal the location of the septal defect and the relationship of the atrial septal defect (ASD) to the surrounding structures.

Continued

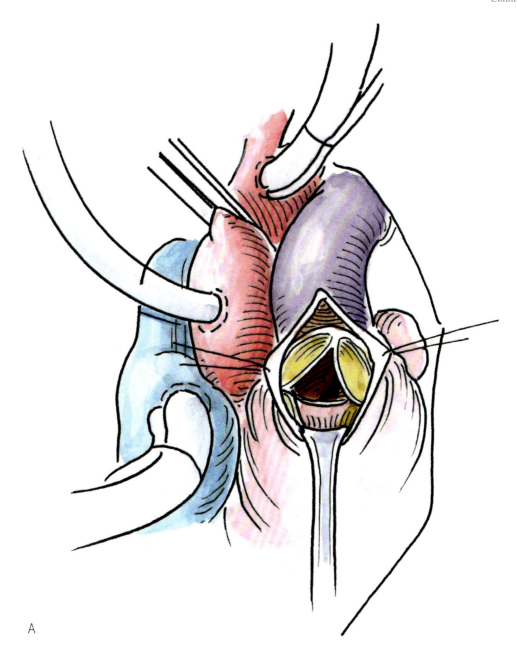

A

图 20-3（续）

Figure 20-3 cont'd

B. 可用带垫 U 形间断缝合或连续缝合。

B. The defect can be closed with U-shaped interrupted or running sutures with pledgets.

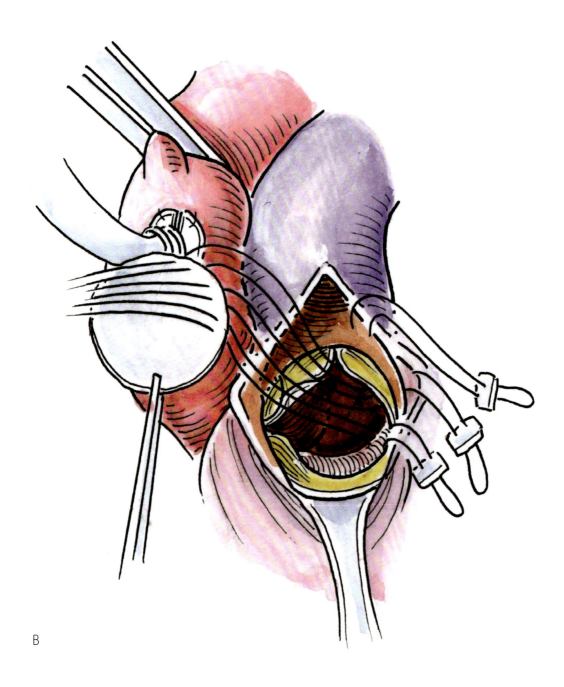

B

图 20-3（续）

Figure 20-3 cont'd

C. 在缝合缺损上缘同主、肺动脉瓣之间没有肌性室间隔，故将部分缝线经肺动脉瓣根部穿入缝合。

C. At the superior portion of the defect, since there is no muscular septum between the leaflets of the aortic and pulmonary valves, part of the sutures should be placed through the root of the pulmonary valve.

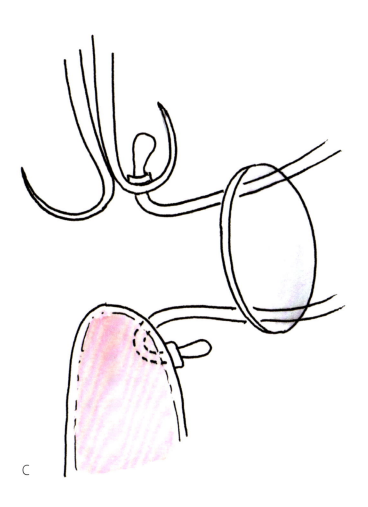

C

图 20-3（续）

Figure 20-3 cont'd

D. 从侧面看缝线与主动脉瓣、肺动脉瓣之间关系。尤其是缺损上缘不能缝合太深,注意避免损伤主动脉瓣。

D. Lateral view shows the relationship of the sutures to the aortic and pulmonary valves. In particular, the superior margin of the defect cannot be sutured too deeply to avoid damaging the aortic valve.

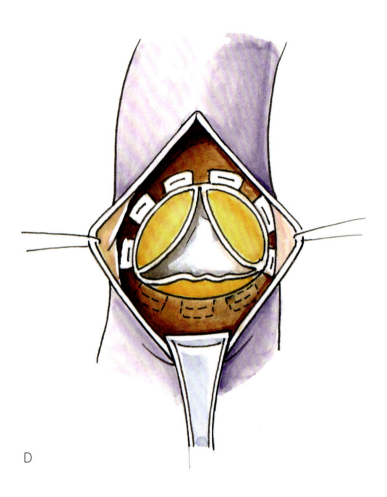

D

3. 主动脉切口径路 这种切口通常对室间隔缺损合并主动脉瓣脱垂,需要对瓣膜做整形或悬吊,或在修补室间隔缺损的同时处理瓣膜狭窄或瓣下狭窄时选用(图 20-4)。

3. Transaortic approach This approach applies to the VSDs complicated with aortic valve prolapse when there is a need to perform the valvoplasty or suspension for prolapsed leaflets or a need for treatment of valve stenosis or subvalvular stenosis apart from VSD closure (Figure 20-4).

图 20-4 **主动脉切口径路修补室间隔缺损**

A. 在升主动脉前部瓣环上 2cm 做一斜行切口,直视下将切口向右下,朝着主动脉无冠窦中央延伸。

Figure 20-4 Transaortic approach for VSD repair

A. An oblique incision is started 2 cm above the aortic annulus in the anterior aspect of the ascending aorta, carried inferiorly and to the right under direct vision toward the center of the noncoronary sinus of the aorta.

Continued

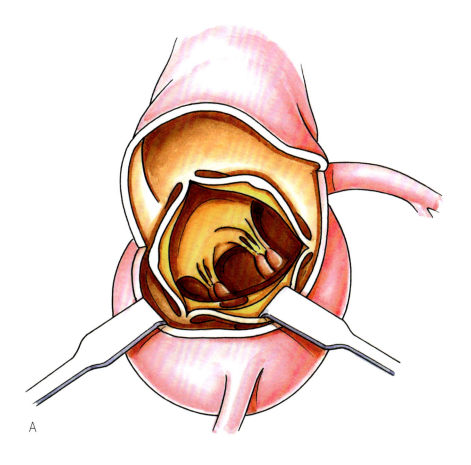

A

图 20-4（续）

B. 小心牵开主动脉瓣叶，充分暴露 VSD 边缘。用 5-0 Prolene 带垫缝线连续或间断缝合补片修补。

Figure 20-4 cont'd

B. Carefully distract the aortic valve leaflets for enough exposure of the edge of the VSD and then close the defect using running or interrupted sutures with pledget-supported Prolene 5-0 suture.

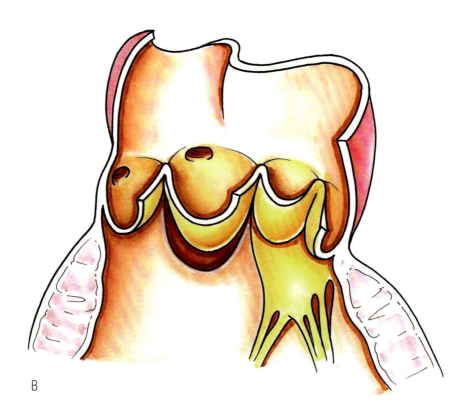

B

图 20-4（续）

C、D. 若缺损较小可用带垫褥式间断直接缝合。

Figure 20-4 cont'd

C, D. Smaller defect can be directly closed with interrupted mattress sutures buttressed with pledgets.

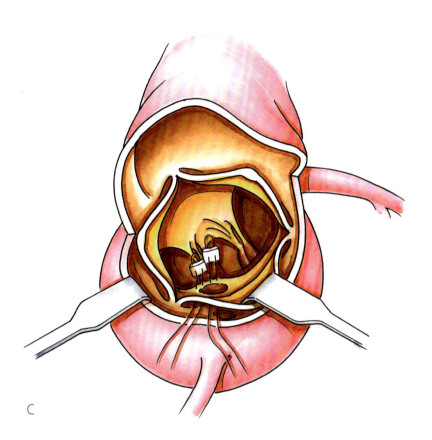

C

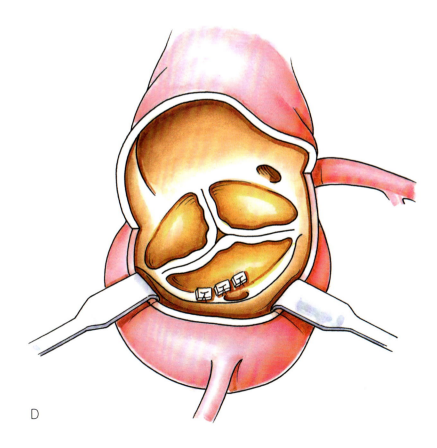

D

图 20-4（续）

E. 大多室间隔缺损都需要用补片修补。可采用带垫间断 U 形缝合。有时室间隔缺损上缘没有肌性或纤维组织，可采用带垫片褥式缝线从主动脉窦内部穿过主动脉壁缝合。

Figure 20-4 cont'd

E. In most cases, patches are needed, and interrupted, pledget-supported U-shaped sutures can be applied. Occasionally, as there are no muscular or fibrous tissues at the superior edge of the VSD, pledget-supported mattress sutures may be placed through the aortic wall from the inside of the aortic valvar sinus.

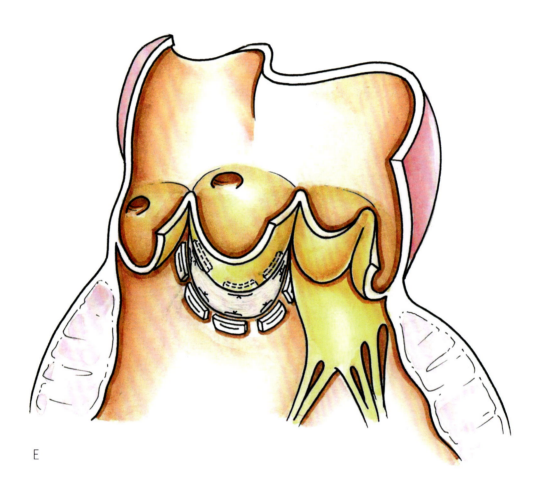

E

4. 右心室切口径路 单纯VSD 很少应用这类切口。通常合并有右室双腔,同时需做右心室流出道梗阻解除的患者可采用这种径路(图 20-5)。

4. Right ventricular approach This approach is rarely applied in isolated VSD but is mainly used for patients with VSD complicated with double-chambered right ventricle who also need the treatment of a right ventricular outflow tract obstruction (RVOTO)(Figure 20-5).

图 20-5 **右心室切口径路修补室间隔缺损**
A. 切口可选择横切口或纵行切口,但要仔细辨认在右心室流出道附近的冠状动脉分支,避免损伤冠状动脉。

Figure 20-5 Right ventricular approach for VSD repair
A. Either a transverse incision or a longitudinal incision can be made after careful identification of the coronary branches near the right ventricular outflow tract, and care is taken to avoid injuries to the coronary arteries.

Continued

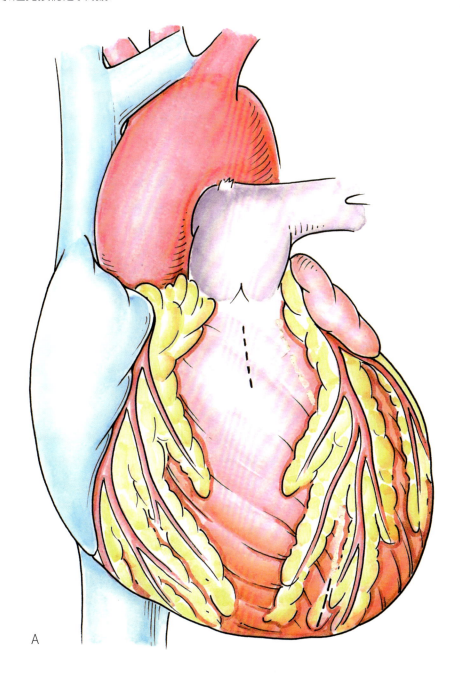

A

图 20-5（续）

B. 牵开后暴露室间隔缺损，如室间隔缺损周边有异常肌束，可切断以暴露得更清楚。

Figure 20-5 cont'd

B. Retract the incision to expose VSD. If there are abnormal muscle bundles around the defect, they can be excised to optimize the exposure of VSD.

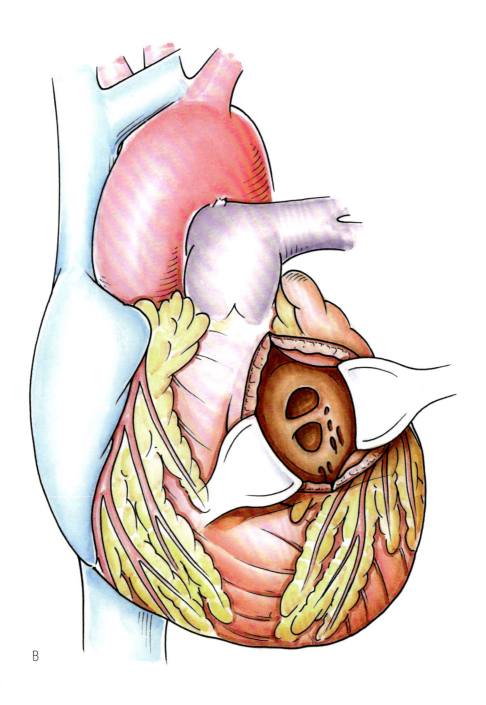

B

图 20-5 (续)

Figure 20-5 cont'd

C. 室间隔缺损可采用带垫 U 形间断缝合，也可采用连续缝合，一般都需补片修补。

C. The VSD can be closed with U-shaped interrupted sutures or running sutures with pledgets, and usually, the patches are needed.

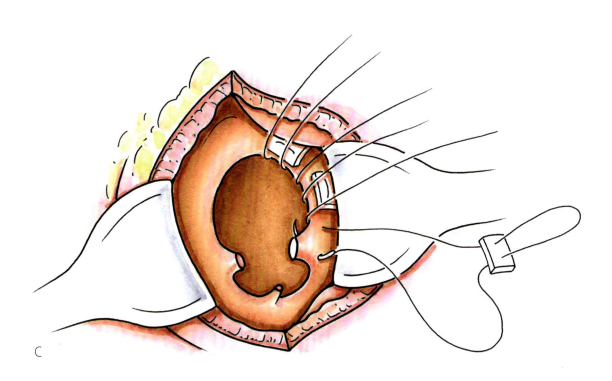

C

图 20-5（续）

Figure 20-5 cont'd

D. 对靠近心尖部的肌部缺损也可采用右心室切口径路修补，取右心室近心尖处小切口，避开冠状血管。仔细探查室间隔缺损位置。

D. For the apical muscular VSD, the right ventricular incision can also be used to repair. A small incision was made near the apex of the right ventricle, avoiding the coronary vessels. Carefully explore the location of the ventricular defect.

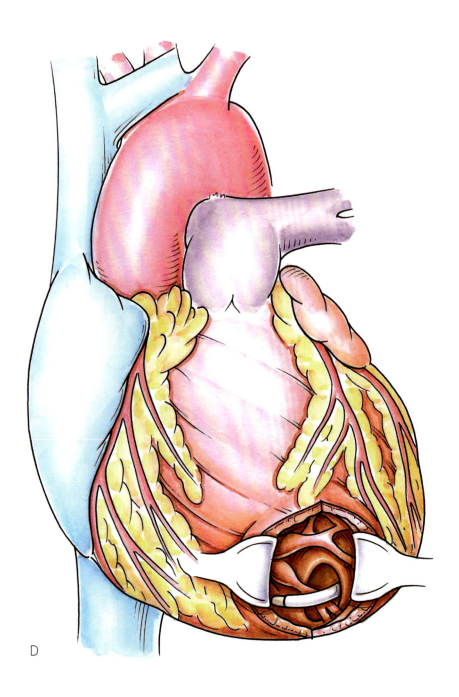

D

图 20-5（续）

E. 必要时可切断部分小肌束，带垫片双头针 U 形缝合，置补片修补。

F. VSD 边缘非常靠近心尖部的，可将部分垫片放置在右心室表面。

Figure 20-5 cont'd

E. If necessary, part of the small muscle bundles can be cut off, a pledget-supported double-ended needle was used to suture in a U shape, and repair the VSD with a patch.

F. If the edge of VSD is very close to the apex, some pledgets can be placed on the surface of the right ventricle.

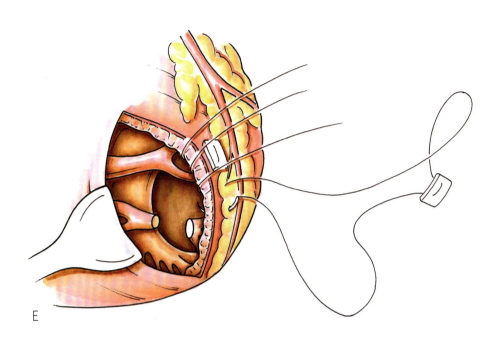

E

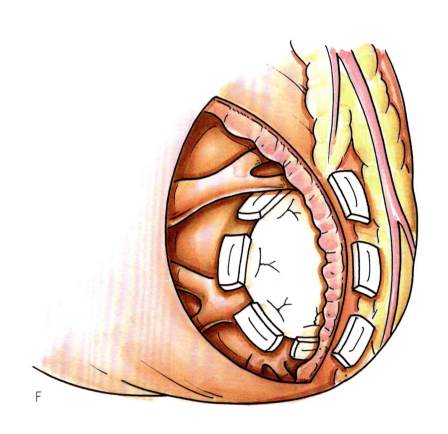

F

5. 经左心室切口径路 这种径路极少使用,以前主要用于心尖肌部 VSD。因这类缺损在右室面较难获得清晰的暴露,常常是多孔状,而左室面则单一开口。但目前这类室间隔缺损大多已选择经皮或经胸封堵治疗(图 20-6)。

5. Trans-left ventricular approach This rare approach was previously limited to the apical muscular VSD. Because there are multiple openings on the right side and a single opening on the left side of the septum, the defect cannot be exposed clearly from the right side. However, at present, most patients of this kind of VSD have been treated with percutaneous or transthoracic closure (Figure 20-6).

图 20-6 **经左心室切口径路修补室间隔缺损**

A. 将左心尖轻轻抬起,切口选择在左心尖无血管裸区,切口不宜太大,避免损伤周边冠状血管和保护心功能。

Figure 20-6 Trans-left ventricular approach for VSD repair

A. Gently lift the left heart apex and make a small incision in the bare avascular area near the left heart apex to avoid injuries to the peripheral coronary vessels and protect heart function.

Continued

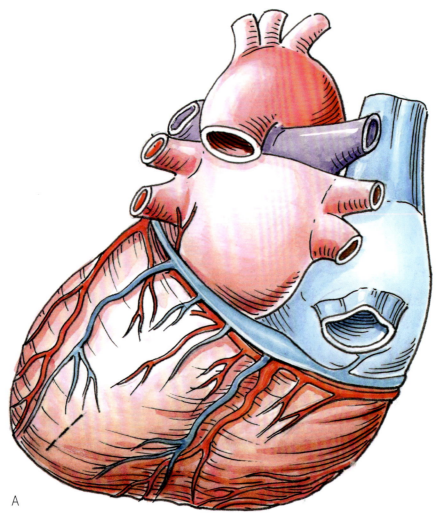

A

图 20-6（续）

B. 暴露 VSD 后用带垫缝线间断缝合或
补片修补。

Figure 20-6 cont'd

B. Closed with pledget-supported interrupted sutures or
with patches after the exposure of the defect.

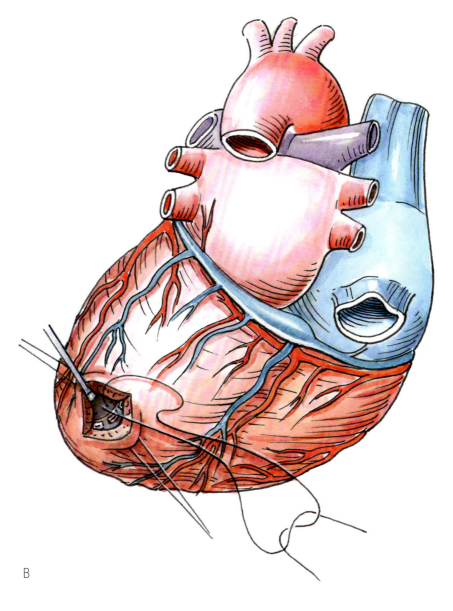

B

图 20-6（续）

C. 左心尖切口须带垫褥式缝合，必要时可采用带毡垫补片加固。

Figure 20-6 cont'd

C. The left apical incision requires pledget-supported mattress stitches and can be reinforced with a felt patch if necessary.

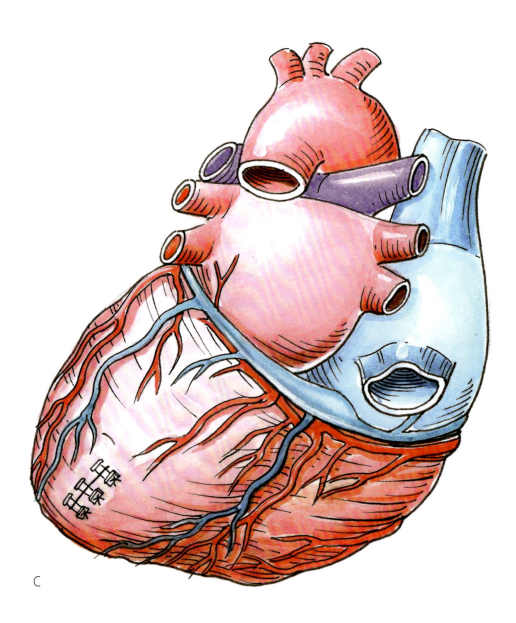

C

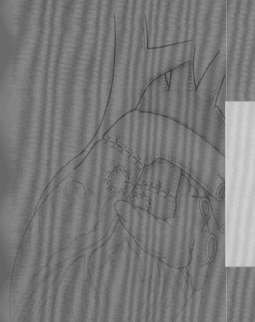

21　房室隔缺损

21　Atrioventricular Septal Defect

一、解剖分型

房室隔缺损（atrioventricular septal defect，AVSD）可分为部分型、过渡型和完全型。而完全型房室隔缺损依据 Rastelli 医生提出的分类方法，又可分为 A、B、C 三型。

1. 部分型房室隔缺损 典型特征是一个较大的原发孔型房间隔缺损伴有二尖瓣前瓣根部的裂缺。由于二尖瓣和三尖瓣的共同连接平面向心尖方向移位，使左心室流出道的长度延长，在影像学上表现为"鹅颈样改变"。

2. 过渡型房室隔缺损 其特征是除了有上述部分型房室隔缺损的表现，还伴有一个限制性 VSD。室间隔缺损大多局限于二尖瓣前瓣和三尖瓣隔瓣交界处。有时可形成室隔瘤，仅有少量分流。

3. 完全型房室隔缺损 A 型：最常见。室间隔嵴上方的共同瓣完全分割，瓣叶腱索分别附着在室间隔两侧。B 型：相对少见。常伴有左、右心室发育不平衡。这类患者腱索可有骑跨，即二尖瓣腱索跨越入右心室或三尖瓣腱索跨入左心室。C 型：位于室间隔嵴上方的共

I. Anatomical Typing

Atrioventricular septal defect (AVSD) can be divided into partial AVSD, transitional AVSD, and complete AVSD. The complete atrioventricular septal defect can be subdivided into three types: A, B, and C according to the classification method proposed by Dr. Giancarlo Rastelli.

1. Partial AVSD Its typical feature is a large ostium primum defect associated with a cleft at the root of the anterior mitral valve. Due to the displacement of the connection plane of the mitral and tricuspid valves towards the apex, the left ventricular outflow tract is lengthened and radiographically visualized as a "gooseneck change".

2. Transitional AVSD It is characterized by a restrictive ventricular septal defect (VSD) in addition to the defect described above in the partial AVSD. VSDs are mostly confined to the commissure between the anterior leaflet of the mitral valve and the septal leaflet of the tricuspid valve. Occasionally, a ventricular septal aneurysm can be formed with only a small amount of shunt.

3. Complete AVSD Type A: The most common one in which the common superior bridging leaflet above the septal ridge is split in two, and the two leaflet chordae are entirely over two sides of the interventricular septum. Type B: Relatively uncommon. It is usually associated with an unbalanced development of the left and right ventriculars. In such patients, the chordae

同瓣未分割或部分分割,通常没有腱索从瓣叶中央部位附着到室间隔嵴上(图 21-1)。

tendineae may have an straddling, i. e., the chordae tendineae of the mitral valve is attached to the right ventricle, or the chordae tendineae of the tricuspid valve is attached to the left ventricle. Type C: The common superior bridging leaflets above the ventricular septal ridge are unsplit or partially split. There is usually no chordae tendineae attached to the interventricular septum from the central portion of the leaflet (Figure 21-1).

图 21-1　**完全型房室隔缺损的解剖分型**

A. A 型:室间隔嵴上方的共同瓣完全分割,瓣叶腱索分别附着在室间隔两侧。

Figure 21-1　**Anatomical typing of complete AVSD**

A. Type A: The common superior bridging leaflet above the septal ridge is split in two, and the two leaflet chordae are entirely over two sides of the interventricular septum.

Continued

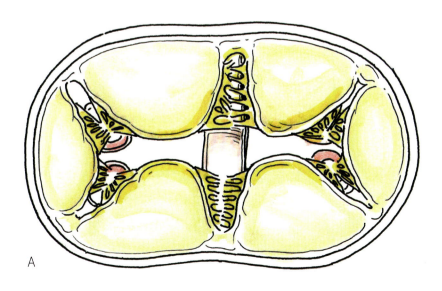

A

图 21-1（续）

B. B 型：常伴有左、右心室发育不平衡。

C. C 型：位于室间隔嵴上方的共同瓣未分割或部分分割。

Figure 21-1 cont'd

B. Type B: It is usually associated with an unbalanced development of the left and right ventricular.

C. Type C: The common superior bridging leaflets above the ventricular septal ridge are unsplit or partially split.

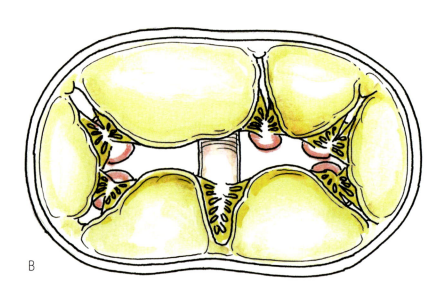

B

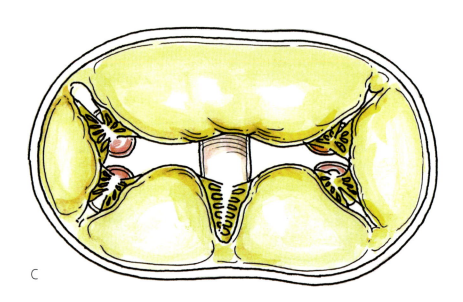

C

二、手术方法　Ⅱ. Surgical Methods

1. 部分型房室隔缺损(图 21-2)

1. Partial AVSD (Figure 21-2)

图 21-2　部分型房室隔缺损
A. 行常规心肺转流术,切开右心房,注水探查二尖瓣和三尖瓣关闭状况。
B. 5-0 或 6-0 Prolene 带心包小垫片间断缝合二尖瓣前瓣裂缺。

Figure 21-2　Partial AVSD
A. Routine cardiopulmonary bypass is established, the right atrium is incised, and the cold saline injection is employed to investigate the mitral and tricuspid valves closure.
B. The anterior mitral valve cleft can be closed using interrupted sutures of 5-0 or 6-0 Prolene suture with pericardial patches.

Continued

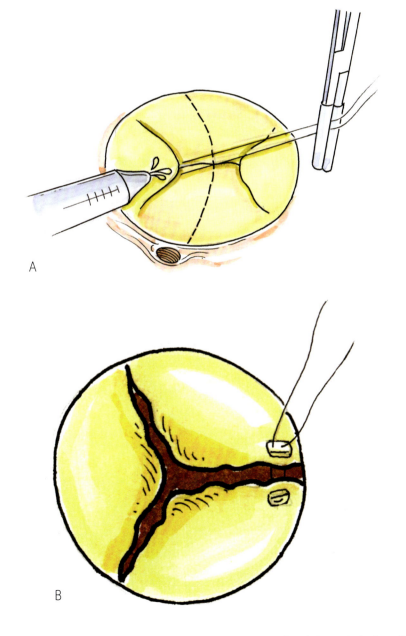

A

B

图 21-2（续）

C. 若瓣环扩大,可用带垫缝线折叠缝合前、后瓣交界处,达到瓣环成形减轻反流的目的,若同时合并有继发孔型房间隔缺损,可将原发孔与继发孔之间房间隔剪开。

Figure 21-2 cont'd

C. If the annulus is enlarged, pledget-supported sutures are used to the plicated anterior and posterior valve commissure to achieve the purpose of annuloplasty to reduce regurgitation. If an ostium secundum defect is present at the same time, the septum between the ostium primum and the ostium secundum defect can be cut open.

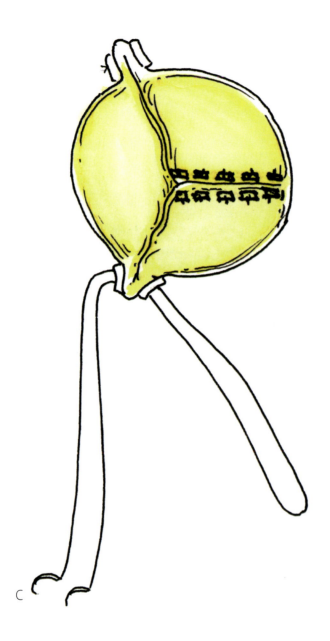

图 21-2（续）

D. 取一块自身心包补片关闭缝合房间隔缺损。根据房间隔缺损与冠状窦的位置,可将冠状窦置于右心房侧或左心房侧。

Figure 21-2 cont'd

D. An autologous pericardial patch is used to close the atrial septal defect. Depending on the location of the atrial septal defect and the coronary sinus, the coronary sinus can be placed either on the right atrial side or the left atrial side.

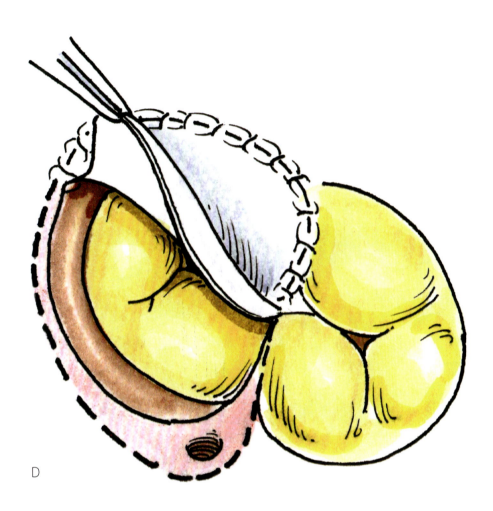

D

2. 过渡型房室隔缺损(图 21-3)

2. Transitional AVSD (Figure 21-3)

图 21-3 过渡型房室隔缺损

A. 经右心房切口暴露二尖瓣前瓣、三尖瓣裂缺并测试反流情况,用一把小的直角钳仔细探查心室水平是否还有交通。

Figure 21-3 Transitional AVSD

A. The right atrial incision is used to expose the clefts of the anterior mitral valve and tricuspid valves and test the regurgitation condition. A small right-angle clamp is used to carefully investigate whether there is communication at the ventricular level.

Continued

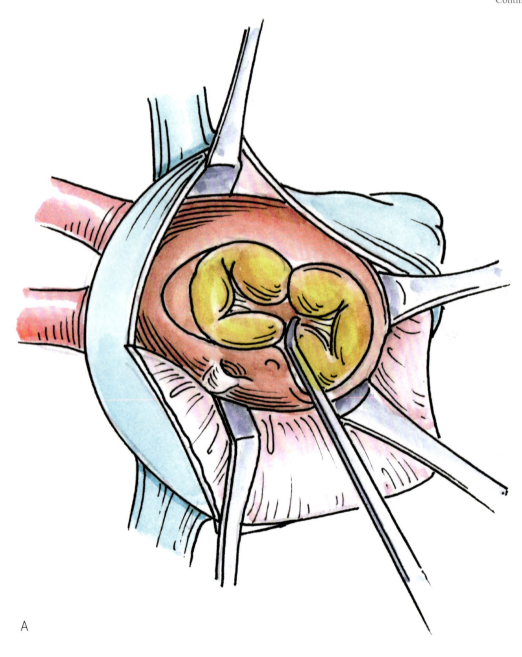

A

图 21-3（续）

B. 带心包小垫片间断缝合二尖瓣裂缺，心包补片缝合关闭原发孔缺损。

Figure 21-3 cont'd

B. Mitral valve cleft is closed with small pledget-supported interrupted sutures, and the ostium primum defect is closed by sutures with a pericardial patch.

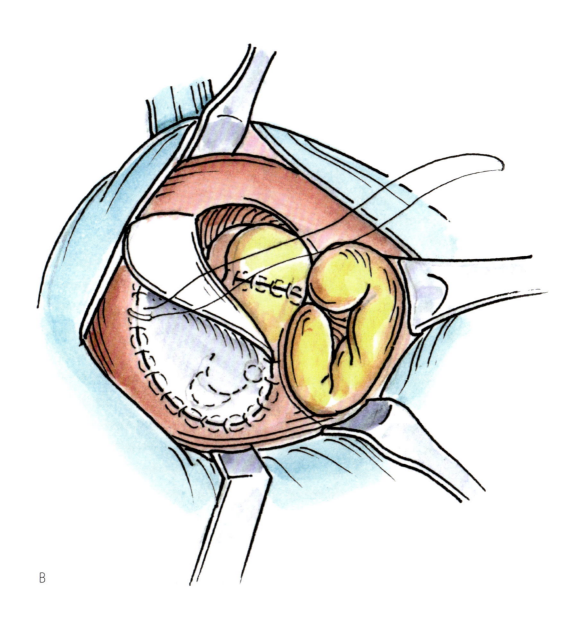

B

3. 完全型房室隔缺损

（1）单片法技术（图 21-4）

3. Complete AVSD (CAVSD)

(1) Single patch technique (Figure 21-4)

图 21-4　**单片法技术修补完全型房室隔缺损**

A. 右心房切开后用牵引线将右心房牵开，暴露原发孔缺损、房室瓣及瓣下缺损。用一针间断缝线将上、下桥瓣靠根部对合，注水测试瓣膜反流情况和空间隔缺损距瓣叶的高度。

Figure 21-4　Single patch technique for complete AVSD repair

A. The right atrium is dissected and retracted with a tether to expose the ostium primum defect, the atrioventricular valve, and the subvalvular defect. The upper and lower bridge valves are coapted against the roof with interrupted sutures, and the valve regurgitation and the height of the ventricular septal defect from the septal leaflet are measured with the cold saline injection.

Continued

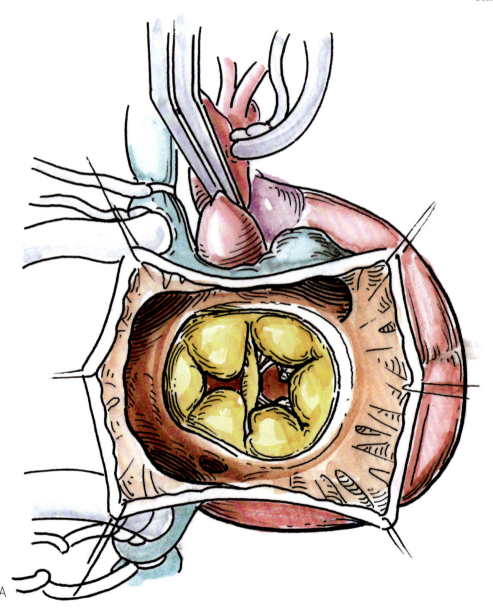

图 21-4（续）

B、C. 剪一块较大心包补片，带垫间断缝合或连续缝合室间隔缺损下缘。

Figure 21-4 cont'd

B. C. Cut a comparatively large pericardial patch to suture the inferior margin of the defect with pledget-supported interrupted sutures or running sutures.

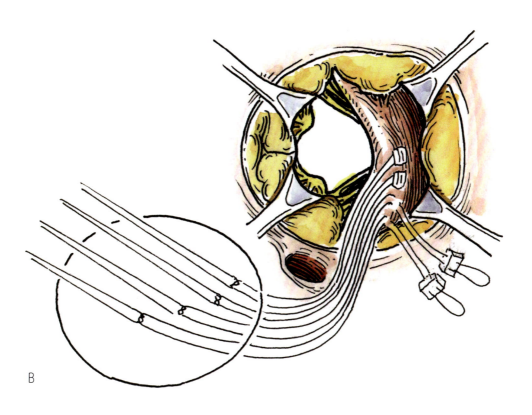

B

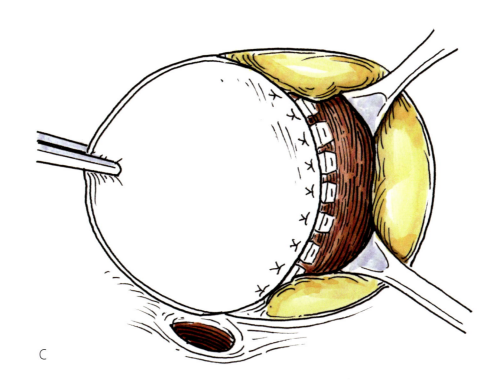

C

图 21-4(续)

D. 将心包补片提起,用一排褥式缝线将左右两侧房室瓣组织固定在心包补片的适当高度,打结固定。为了避免房室瓣撕裂,可在缝线两侧用心包条加固。间断缝合二尖瓣裂缺,测试瓣叶反流状况。

Figure 21-4 cont'd

D. Lift the pericardial patch, secure the right and left atrioventricular valve tissue to the appropriate height of the pericardial patch with a row of mattress sutures, and tie the knots to fix it. In order to avoid tearing the atrioventricular valve, reinforcement can be performed on both sides of the suture with pericardium strips. Interrupted sutures are applied to the mitral valves, and the leaflets' competency is tested.

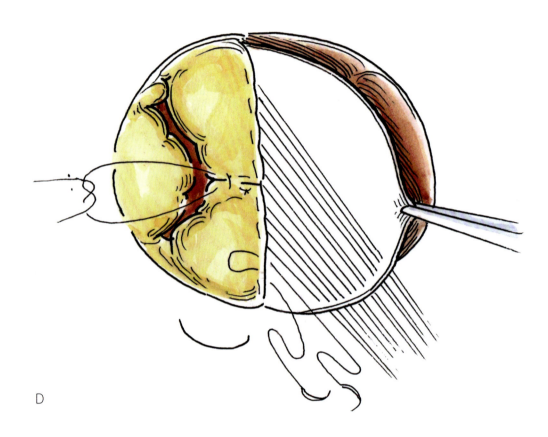

D

图 21-4(续)

E. 将剩余补片连续缝合关闭房间隔原发孔缺损。

Figure 21-4 cont'd

E. The remaining patch is used to close the ostium primum defect with running sutures.

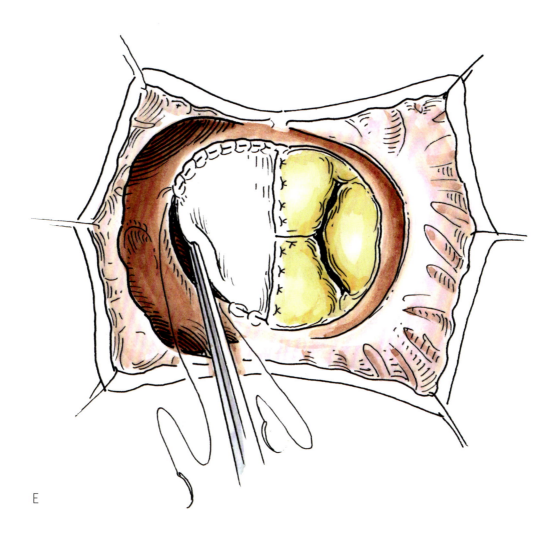

E

（2）双片法技术（图 21-5）

(2) Two-patch technique (Figure 21-5)

图 21-5 双片法技术修补完全型 房室隔缺损

A. 探查和测试瓣叶反流状况同前。确认室间隔缺损的大小，一般室间隔缺损较大的患者采取双片法。取心包补片或 ePTFE 补片剪成"月牙状"的补片。

Figure 21-5 Two-patch technique for complete AVSD repair

A. The exploration of AVSD and test of the valve leaflet regurgitation are the same as described above. The size of the VSD is confirmed, and the two-patch technique is generally adopted in patients with a large ventricular defect. Take a pericardial patch or ePTFF patch and cut it into a crescent-shape.

Continued

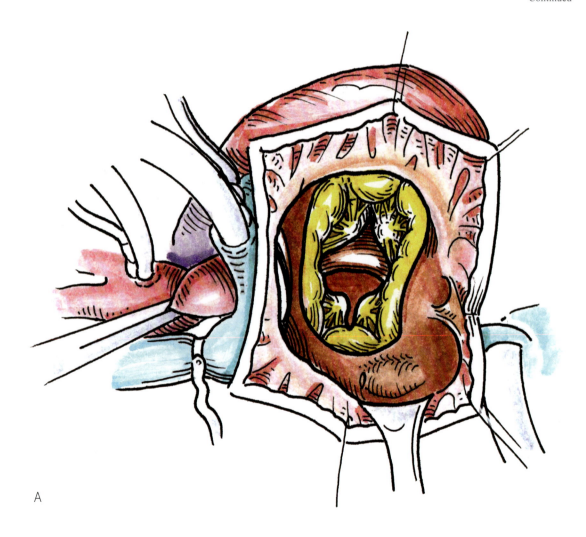

A

图 21-5（续）

B. 室间隔缺损下缘间断或连续缝合补片，打结固定。在补片两端将缝线穿出房室瓣进入右房面。

Figure 21-5 cont'd

B. Interrupted or running sutures are applied on the inferior margin of the defect with the patches, and the knots are made for fixation. The sutures are passed from the atrioventricular valve to the right atrial surface at both ends of the patch.

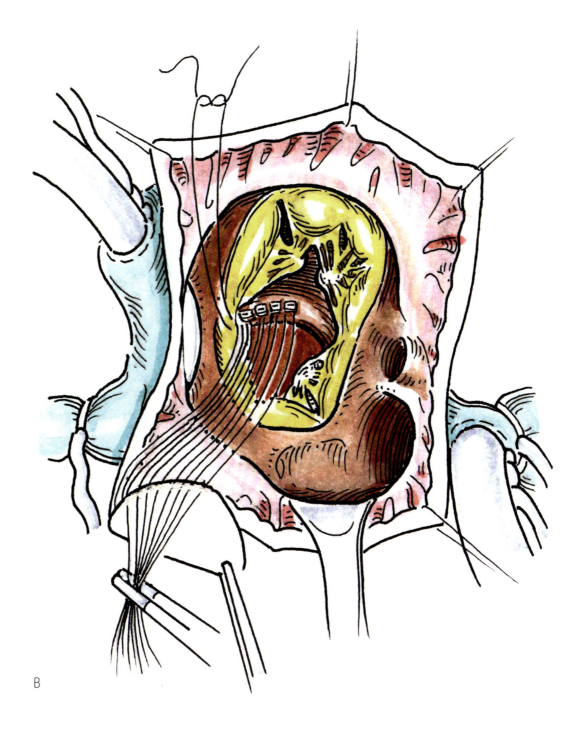

B

图 21-5（续）

C. 用一针牵引线对合二尖瓣裂缺，确定室间隔缺损补片的高度。

Figure 21-5 cont'd

C. A retracting suture is used to coapt with the mitral valve cleft, and the height of the patch for VSD is determined.

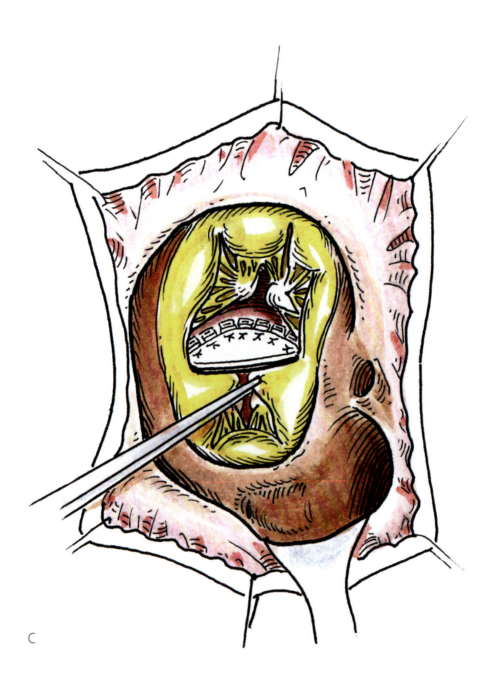

C

图 21-5（续）

D. 取自身心包补片关闭房间隔缺损，先用一组 5-0 Prolene 缝线将室间隔缺损上缘和二尖瓣缝合固定，具体缝法是先缝合室间隔缺损补片，再缝合二尖瓣和心包补片，这样二尖瓣瓣叶被夹在中间不易撕裂。

Figure 21-5 cont'd

D. An autologous pericardial patch is applied to close the atrial septal defect. A set of sutures of 5-0 Prolene is first used to secure the superior margin of the defect and mitral valve. The specific suture method is to suture the ventricular patch first, and then suture the mitral valve and pericardial patch. In this way, the mitral valve leaflets are sandwiched in the middle and are not easy to tear.

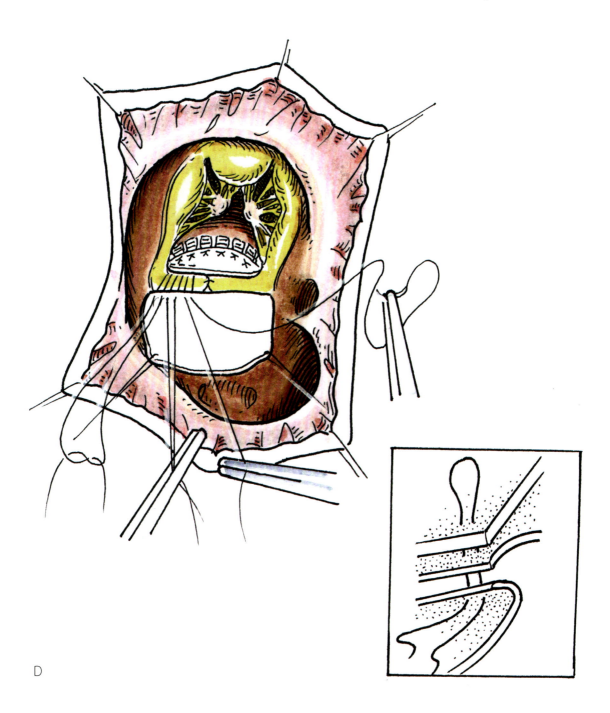

D

图 21-5（续）

E、F. 缝合二尖瓣裂缺，注水测试瓣叶反流情况。

Figure 21-5 cont'd

E, F. The mitral valve cleft is sutured, and the cold saline is injected to test the competency of valve leaflets.

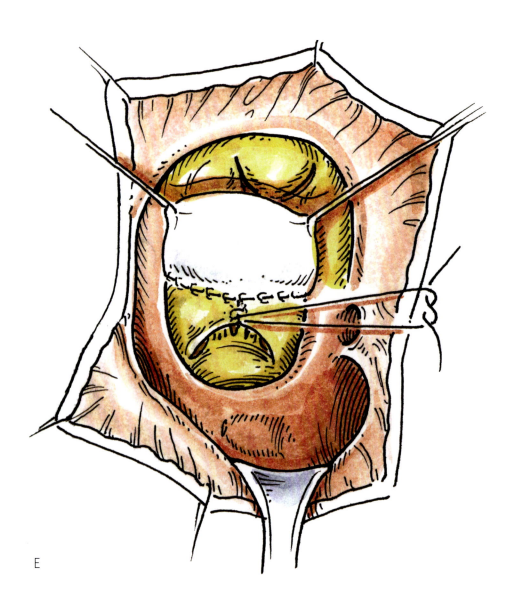

E

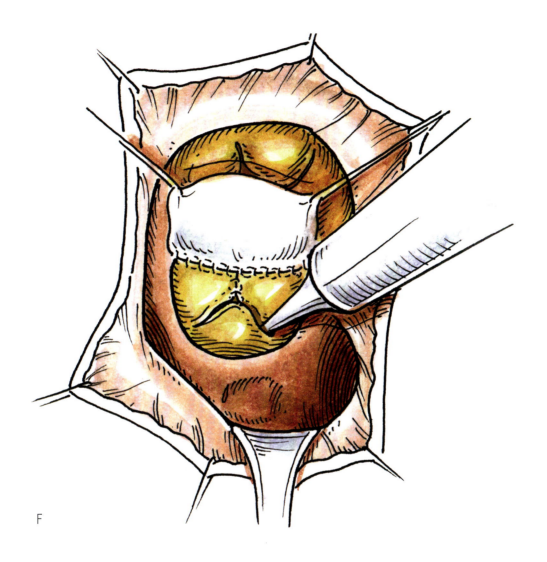

F

图 21-5（续）

G. 心包补片缝合房间隔缺损, 冠状窦置于右侧或左侧, 视房间隔缺损与冠状窦之间的距离而酌情处理。

Figure 21-5 cont'd

G. A pericardial patch is used to close the atrial septal defect, and depending on the distance between the atrial septal defect and the coronary sinus, the coronary sinus can be positioned on the right or left side of the patch.

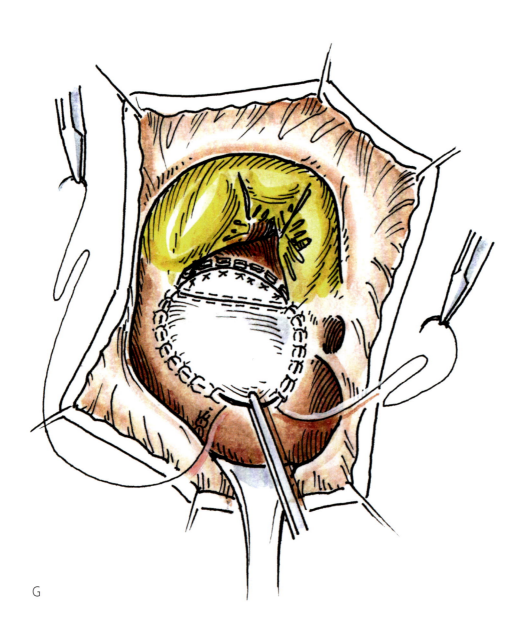

G

图 21-5（续）

Figure 21-5 cont'd

H. 再将右侧房室瓣缝合在房间隔缺损补片根部，注水测试三尖瓣反流情况，必要时间断缝合裂缺。

H. The right atrioventricular valve is sutured to the root of the atrial septal defect patch. The tricuspid valve is irrigated with the cold saline to see whether there is tricuspid regurgitation, which will determine the necessity of further interrupted sutures.

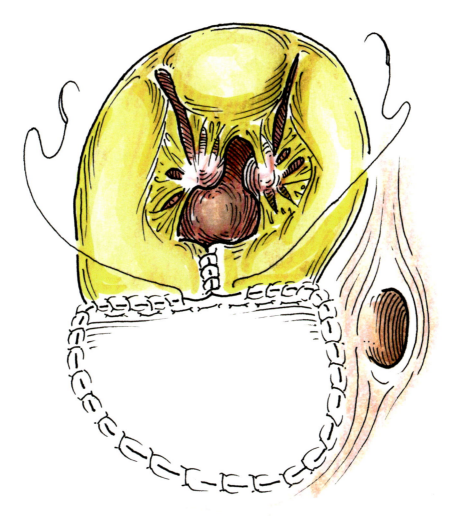

H

（3）改良单片法 该技术最早为澳大利亚墨尔本皇家儿童医院介绍，又称澳大利亚技术。该方法适宜应用在室间隔缺损不是太大的 A 型房室隔缺损患者（图 21-6）。

(3) Modified single patch technique The technique, also known as the "Australian" technique, was first introduced by the Royal Children's Hospital in Melbourne Australia. It is suitable for AVSD of type A without a too-large VSD (Figure 21-6).

图 21-6 改良单片法修补完全型房室隔缺损

A. 常规暴露原发孔型房间隔缺损、共同房室瓣和室间隔缺损。双头带垫 5-0 Prolene 缝线 8~10 针（视 VSD 大小）缝合在室间隔缺损下缘右侧面。

Figure 21-6 Modified single patch technique for Complete AVSD repair

A. After routine exposure of ostium primum defect, common atrioventricular valves, and VSD, 8-10 stitches (depending on the size of the VSD) are performed with double-ended pledget-supported sutures of Prolene 5-0 at the right side of the inferior margin of the VSD.

Continued

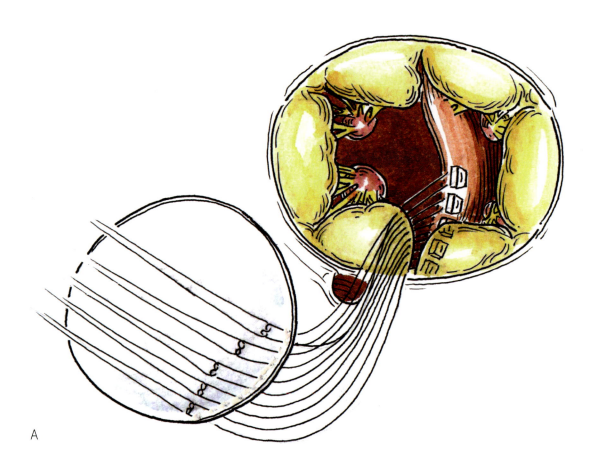

A

图 21-6（续）

B. 缝线先穿过共同瓣，然后再穿过心包补片，打结固定。

C. 将心包补片翻起，缝合左侧的房室瓣裂缺，注水测试瓣叶关闭情况。

Figure 21-6 cont'd

B. Theses sutures are first passed through the common leaflets, then penetrated through the pericardial patch, and finally tied for fixation.

C. Flip the pericardial patch over to close the atrioventricular valve cleft on the left side. Float the leaflets with injection of cold saline to test the leaflets' competency.

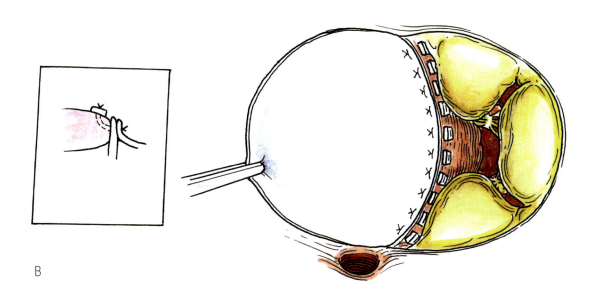

B

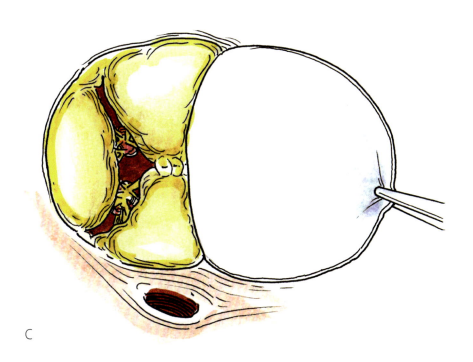

C

图 21-6（续）

D. 再将右侧房室瓣重建,固定在心包补片右侧面,用心包补片关闭房间隔缺损。

Figure 21-6 cont'd

D. The right atrioventricular valve is reconstructed and fixed to the right side of the pericardial patch, and the pericardial patch is used to close the atrial septal defect.

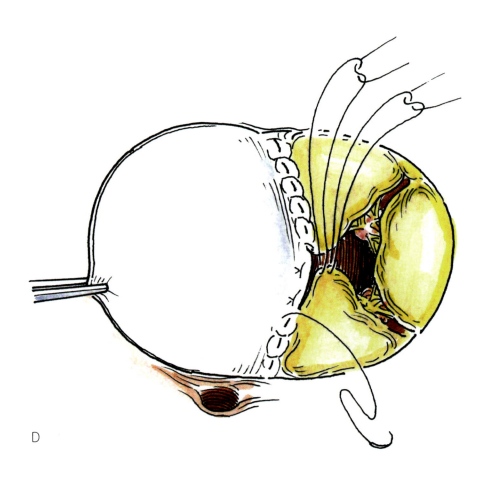

D

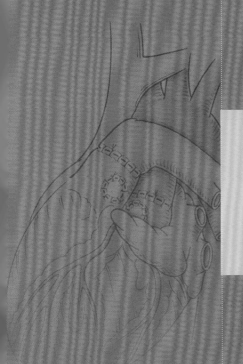

22 肺动脉狭窄

22 Pulmonary Stenosis

一、解剖分型

I. Anatomical Typing

单纯肺动脉狭窄通常仅限于肺动脉瓣水平的狭窄,也可继发漏斗部肥厚,造成右心室梗阻。

Isolated pulmonary stenosis usually refers to valvular pulmonary stenosis. There may also be secondary infundibular hypertrophy, resulting in right ventricular obstruction.

肺动脉狭窄通常分为新生儿危重型肺动脉狭窄和普通的婴幼儿肺动脉狭窄。前者的循环生理类似室间隔完整型的肺动脉闭锁患儿,出生后低氧严重,需急诊手术。而后者手术处理的原则是根据肺动脉瓣狭窄的程度,通常超声心动图测定肺动脉跨瓣压力阶差大于 50mmHg 就有手术指征。

It is usually divided into critical pulmonary artery stenosis in neonates and common pulmonary artery stenosis in infants. Neonates with severe pulmonary artery stenosis, whose circulatory physiology is like that in children with pulmonary atresia with an intact ventricular septum, are severely hypoxic after birth, and emergency surgery is required. For infants with common pulmonary artery stenosis, the principle of surgical treatment is based on the degree of pulmonary valve stenosis. Usually, the presence of the pulmonary artery transvalvular pressure gradient greater than 50mmHg measured by echocardiography is indicated for surgery.

二、手术方法

II. Surgical Methods

1. 新生儿危重型肺动脉狭窄 在新生儿期即出现症状的肺动脉狭窄一般都较危重。三个瓣叶融合形成一个鱼嘴样开口。有时会合并三尖瓣和右心室的发育不良,必须尽早治疗。

1. Critical pulmonary stenosis in neonates The presence of symptomatic pulmonary stenosis during the neonatal period is generally critical. The three leaflets fuse to form a fish-mouth-like opening. Sometimes, it is complicated with dysplasia of the tricuspid valve and right ventricle, which is indicated for prompt treatment.

(1)经胸球囊扩张术(图 22-1)

(1) Transthoracic balloon dilatation (Figure 22-1)

图 22-1　经胸闭塞球囊扩张术

A. 在右心室流出道无血管区用 5-0 Prolene 带垫缝线做褥式缝合。

Figure 22-1　Transthoracic balloon valvuloplasty

A. The pledget-supported mattress sutures are performed with a 5-0 Prolene suture in the avascular area near the right ventricular outflow tract.

Continued

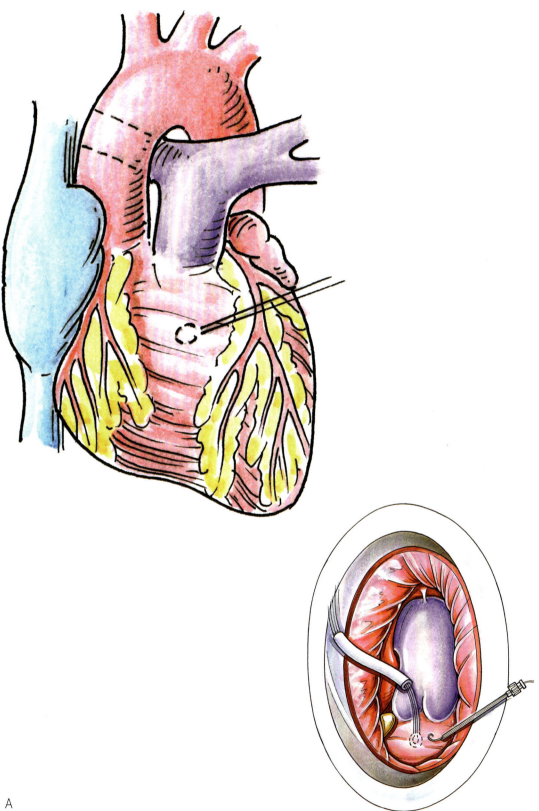

A

图 22-1（续）

B. 分别插入穿刺针和导引钢丝通过狭窄肺动脉瓣口，置入球囊导管做瓣叶扩张。

Figure 22-1 cont'd

B. A needle and a guide wire are inserted through the stenotic pulmonary valvular orifice, and a balloon catheter is placed for leaflet dilation.

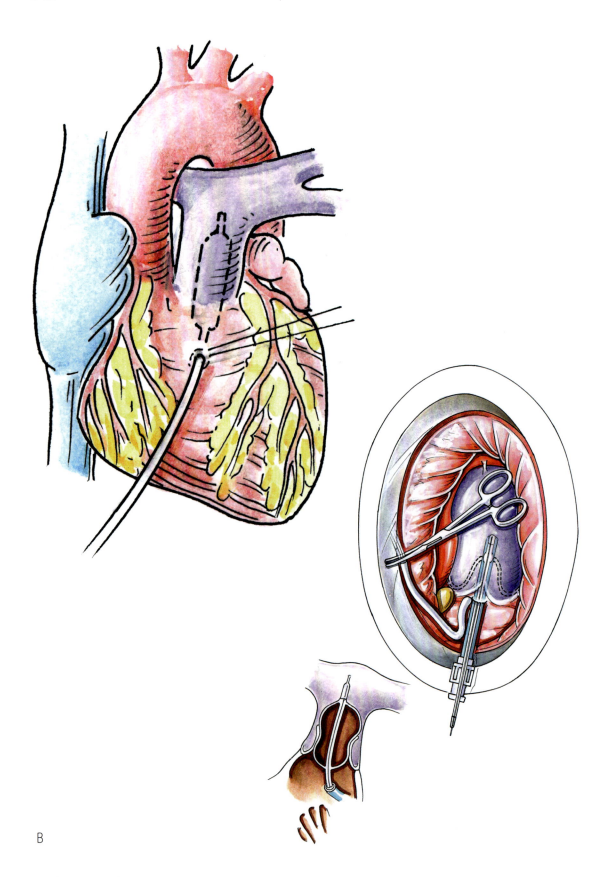

B

图 22-1 (续)

C. 扩张后再做跨瓣两侧压力测试, 压差小于 30mmHg 即表示扩张成功。

Figure 22-1 cont'd

C. After enlargement, a pressure test on both sides of the transvalvular valve is performed, and the pressure gradient less than 30mmHg indicates successful enlargement.

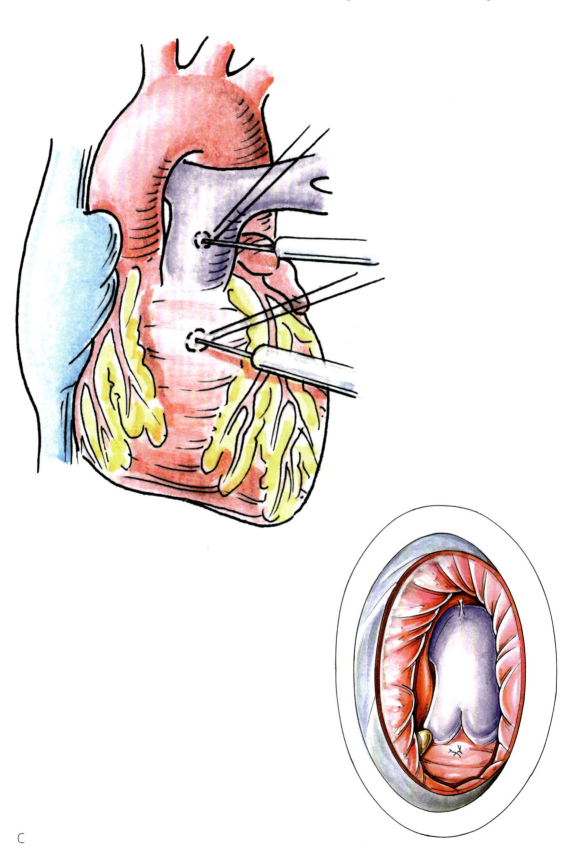

C

（2）非心肺转流术时直视下肺动脉瓣叶切开（图 22-2）

(2) Pulmonary valve leaflet is incised under direct view without cardiopulmonary bypass (Figure 22-2)

图 22-2　非心肺转流术时直视下肺动脉瓣叶切开

A. 正中胸骨切开，在上腔静脉和下腔静脉处分别置圈套控制带，在肺动脉瓣环上 1cm 处做两根牵引线。

Figure 22-2　Pulmonary valve leaflet is incised under direct view without cardiopulmonary bypass

A. Median sternotomy is performed with a loop control band respectively placed in the superior vena cava and inferior vena cava, and two traction wires are made 1 cm above the pulmonary annulus.

Continued

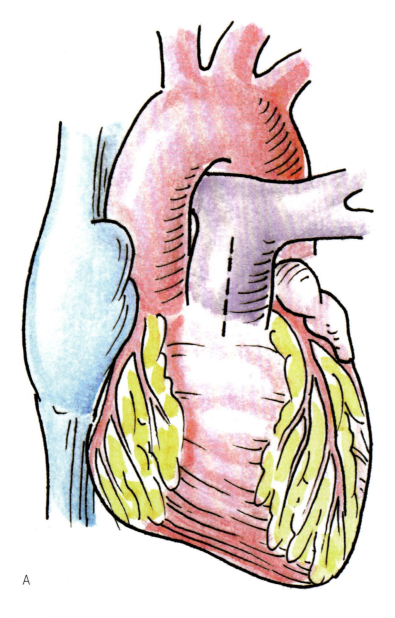

A

图 22-2（续）

B、C. 分别收紧上下腔静脉处的控制带，在肺动脉前壁做一纵行切口，暴露融合狭窄的肺动脉，做交界切开术。

Figure 22-2 cont'd

B, C. Tighten control bands placed in the superior vena cava and inferior vena cava respectively, make a longitudinal incision on the anterior wall of the pulmonary artery, expose the fused and stenotic pulmonary artery, and perform a commissurotomy.

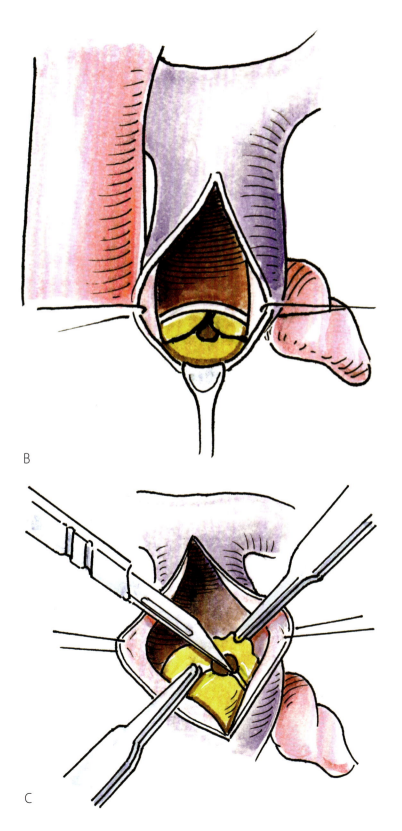

B

C

图 22-2（续）

D. 术毕将肺动脉壁牵引线拉起,用小的侧壁钳或心房钳将肺动脉切口钳夹。

Figure 22-2 cont'd

D. Pull up the guide wires from pulmonary artery wall after commissurotomy, clamp the pulmonary artery incision with a small anastomosis clamp or atrial clamp.

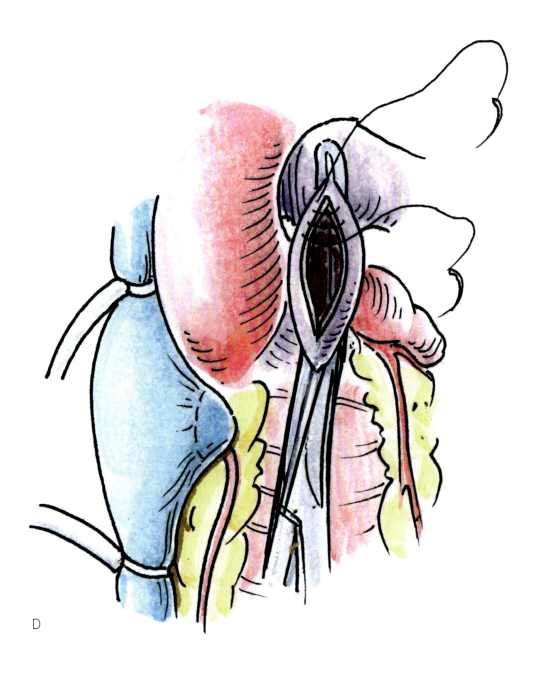

D

图 22-2（续）

E. 分别开放上下腔静脉处的控制带，6-0 Prolene 缝线连续缝合关闭肺动脉切口。

Figure 22-2 cont'd

E. The control bands placed in the superior vena cava and inferior vena cava are respectively released, and the pulmonary artery incision is closed with running sutures of 6-0 Prolene.

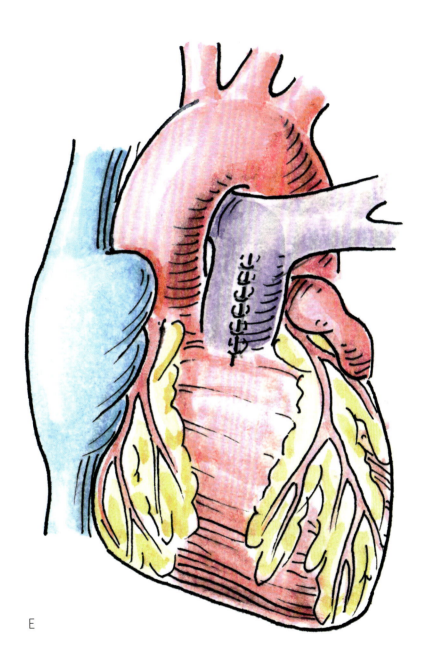

E

2. 婴儿和儿童肺动脉狭窄 这类患儿大多需要心肺转流术辅助下手术切开狭窄肺动脉瓣,有些新生儿危重患儿也可用此技术。

(1)心肺转流术直视下肺动脉瓣切开术(图 22-3)

2. Pulmonary stenosis in infants and children Infants and children with pulmonary stenosis require an incision in the stenotic pulmonary valve under cardiopulmonary bypass, and this technique may be used in some critically ill neonates.

(1) Pulmonary valvulotomy under direct vision with cardiopulmonary bypass (Figure 22-3)

图 22-3　心肺转流术直视下肺动脉瓣切开术

A. 主动脉、右心房插管行心肺转流术,可在常温不停搏情况下操作。

Figure 22-3　Pulmonary valvulotomy under direct vision with cardiopulmonary bypass

A. The aorta and right atrium are catheterized to establish cardiopulmonary bypass in the situation where the heart is beating at room temperature.

Continued

A

图 22-3（续）

B. 肺动脉瓣交界切开，方法同前。

Figure 22-3 cont'd

B. A pulmonary valvulotomy is performed following the aforementioned method.

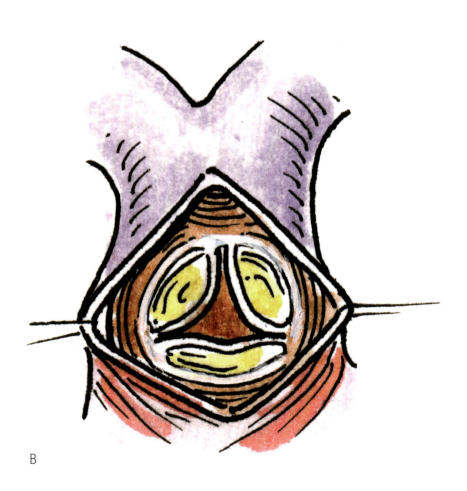

B

（2）合并肺动脉瓣环狭窄的手术方法：对单纯瓣膜狭窄切开加跨瓣环补片扩大的患者，无须心脏停搏（图 22-4）。

(2) Surgical procedures for pulmonary stenosis associated with ulmonary annular stenosis: For the patients with isolated valvular stenosis incision and enlargement of the trans-annular patch, there is no need to stop the heart beating (Figure 22-4).

图 22-4　**合并肺动脉瓣环狭窄的手术方法**

A. 行心肺转流术，将肺动脉瓣交界切开并切开瓣环向右心室延伸。

Figure 22-4　Surgical procedures for pulmonary stenosis associated with pulmonary annular stenosis

A. Establish cardiopulmonary bypass. The leaflet commissure is incised beginning at the pulmonary valve and extending to the right ventricle.

Continued

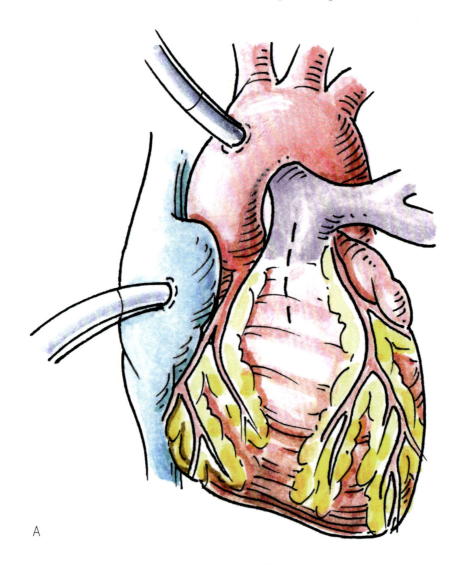

A

图 22-4（续）

B. 切断部分漏斗部肥厚性肌束，解除右心室流出道梗阻。

Figure 22-4 cont'd

B. Transect part of infundibular hypertrophic muscle bundle to relieve right ventricular outflow tract obstruction.

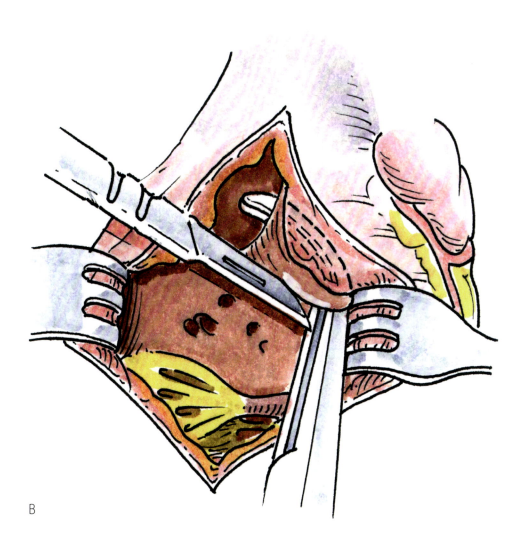

B

图 22-4（续）

Figure 22-4 cont'd

C. 用自身心包补片扩大肺动脉和右心
室流出道。

C. Enlarge pulmonary artery and right ventricular outflow
tract with an autologous pericardial patch.

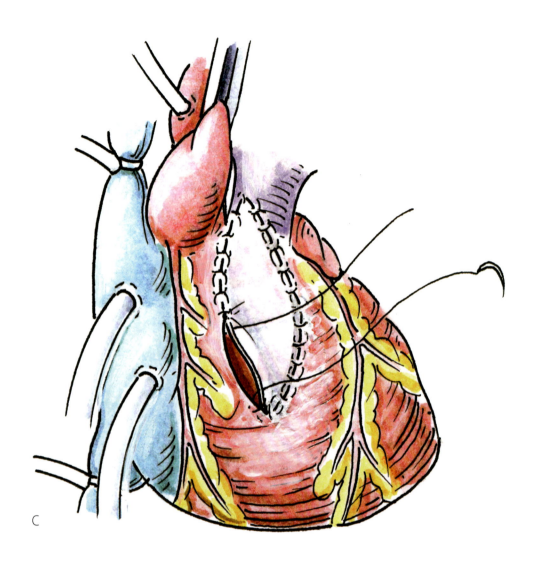

C

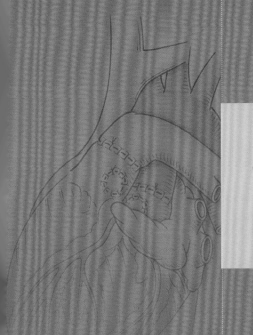

23　Pulmonary Atresia with Intact Ventricular Septum

一、解剖分型

肺动脉闭锁合并室间隔完整的患儿常伴有不同程度的右心室发育不全。三尖瓣直径（Z值）可反映右心室发育的状况。Z值为0表示三尖瓣直径的正常平均值，不同的三尖瓣Z值其治疗方法选择不同。所以术前对右心室的评估十分重要。

1. 轻度右心室发育不良 三尖瓣Z值为 -2~0。其治疗原则是建立右心室到肺动脉的连续性，达到右心室减压、肺血管床发育的目的。

2. 中度右心室发育不良 三尖瓣Z值为 -3~-2。这类患者将来有可能达到双心室矫治，取决于右心室的发育。其手术方法通常选择建立右心室到肺动脉的连续性加体肺分流术。

3. 重度右心室发育不良 三尖瓣Z值小于 -3。这类患者将来可能只能做单心室或一个半心室矫治。而且这组患者右心室依赖性冠状动脉循环的概率大大增加。早期多选择做 B-T 分流，以后视肺血管床发育情况选择做保留肺动脉前向

I. Anatomical Typing

Patients with pulmonary atresia with intact ventricular septum (PA-IVS) often have varying degrees of right ventricular dysplasia. A tricuspid valve's diameter (Z score) can reflect the growth of the right ventricle. Z score of zero represents the normal mean value of the diameter of the tricuspid valve, while different tricuspid valve Z scores indicate various treatment options. Therefore, preoperative assessment of the right ventricle is of significance.

1. Mild right ventricular dysplasia Tricuspid valve Z score ranges from –2 to 0. The therapeutic principle is to decompress the right ventricle and promote pulmonary vascular bed development by establishing right ventricle-pulmonary artery continuity.

2. Moderate right ventricular dysplasia Tricuspid valve Z score ranges from –3 to –2. These patients can potentially be treated by biventricular repair, and the probability of this outcome depends on the growth of the right ventricle. In addition to establishing right ventricle-pulmonary artery continuity, a systemic-pulmonary shunt is usually added in the repair.

3. Severe right ventricular dysplasia Tricuspid valve Z score <–3. Such patients may be treated by single ventricular or one and a half ventricle repair in the future. And they have an increasing risk of right ventricular-dependent coronary circulation. B-T shunts are usually performed for most patients in the early stage, and

血流的 Glenn 手术(一个半心室矫治)或选择做 Glenn 或 Fontan 手术(单心室矫治)。

4. 右心室依赖型冠状动脉循环 对这类患者不能做右心室减压手术。通常需做三期手术,初期做体肺分流手术,1 岁左右做双向 Glenn 手术,3 岁再做 Fontan 手术。

then, depending on the growth of the pulmonary vascular bed, the Glenn procedure with anterograde pulmonary blood flow (one and a half ventricle repair) can be applied. Glenn or Fontan procedures (single ventricle repair) is also an alternative.

4. Right ventricle-dependent coronary circulation (RVDCC) The patients with RVDCC cannot undergo right ventricular decompression. They usually undergo three-stage operations: systemic-pulmonary shunt in the early stage, bidirectional Glenn procedure generally around the age of one, and Fontan procedure at the age of three years old.

二、手术方法

II. Surgical Methods

1. 肺动脉瓣切开疏通术(图 23-1)

1. Pulmonary valvotomy (Figure 23-1)

图 23-1　肺动脉瓣切开术

A. 胸骨正中切口,切开心包悬吊固定,该手术可在非心肺转流术时直视下操作。

Figure 23-1　Pulmonary valvotomy

A. A median sternotomy is performed and the pericardium is opened and suspended. The procedure can be performed under direct vision without cardiopulmonary bypass.

Continued

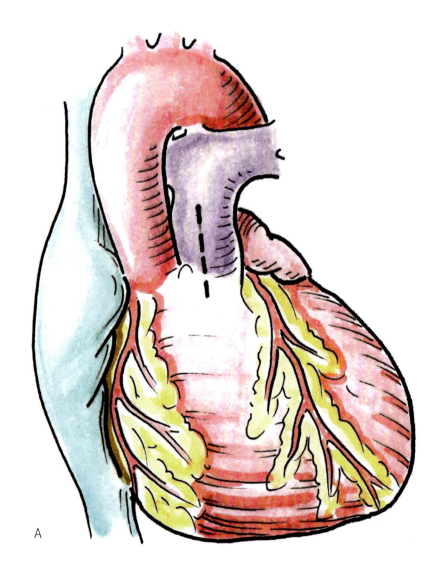

A

图 23-1（续）

B. 分离主肺动脉和动脉导管，在肺动脉分叉处将远端肺动脉夹闭，保留动脉导管至肺的血流，6-0 Prolene 缝线两根做悬吊牵引，纵行切开主肺动脉暴露膜状闭锁的肺动脉瓣。

Figure 23-1 cont'd

B. Dissociate the main pulmonary artery and ductus arteriosus. The distal pulmonary artery is clamped to the pulmonary artery bifurcation to maintain blood flow from the ductus arteriosus to the lung. Two 6-0 Prolene sutures are used for suspension and traction, and the main pulmonary artery is longitudinally incised to expose the membranous atresia of the pulmonary valve.

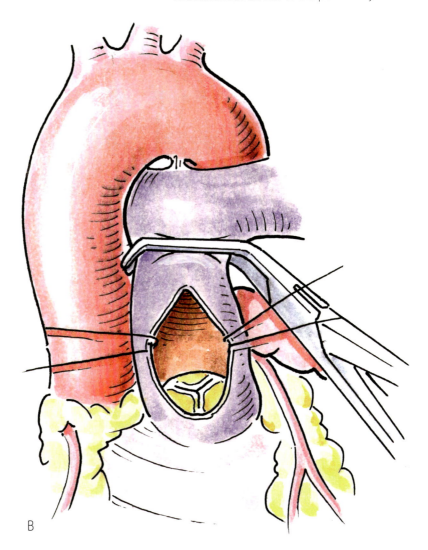

B

图 23-1（续）

C. 用尖头刀片戳开瓣膜并小心切开，也可用血管钳对瓣环进行扩张。

Figure 23-1 cont'd

C. The valve is penetrated with a sharp-pointed blade and carefully further opened, and the valve annulus can also be dilated with a vessel clamp.

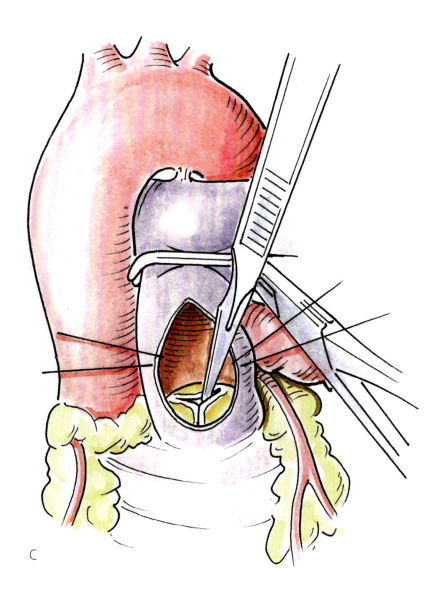

C

图 23-1（续）

Figure 23-1 cont'd

D. 用侧壁钳控制住肺动脉切口，去除远端肺动脉阻断钳，缝合肺动脉前壁切口。

D. An anastomosis clamp is applied to control the pulmonary artery incision, the distal pulmonary artery blocking clamp is released, and then the incision in the anterior wall of the pulmonary artery is closed.

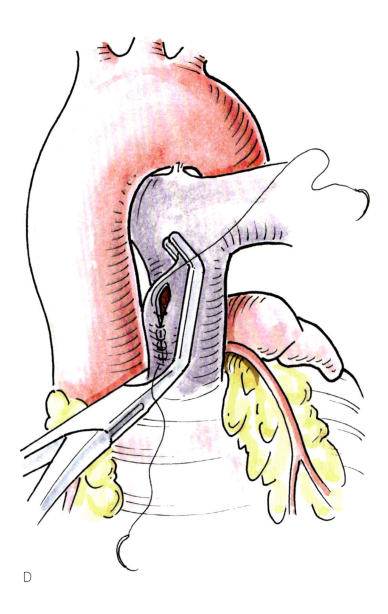

D

2. 右心室流出道跨瓣补片扩大术　可有两种方法。一种是非心肺转流术时做补片扩大术，另一种方法是常规行心肺转流术（图23-2）。

2. Transannular patch enlargement of right ventricular outflow tract　This condition is usually treated by two kinds of approaches. One is the technique of patch enlargement without cardiopulmonary bypass. Another approach is routinely under cardiopulmonary bypass (Figure 23-2).

图 23-2　**右心室流出道跨瓣补片扩大术**

A. 非心肺转流术时，先用心包补片扩大主肺动脉和右心室流出道。

Figure 23-2　Transannular patch enlargement of right ventricular outflow tract

A. The main pulmonary artery and the right ventricular outflow tract are augmented with pericardial patches without cardiopulmonary bypass.

Continued

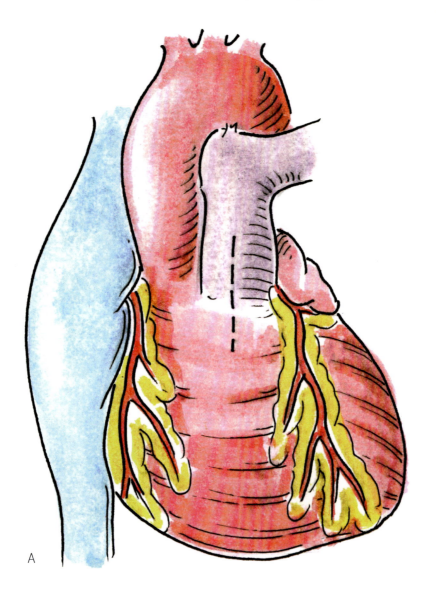

A

图 23-2（续）

Figure 23-2 cont'd

B. 在主肺动脉上阻断钳，用刀片将肺动脉瓣环和部分右心室流出道肌肉切开。

B. Block the main pulmonary artery with coarctation forceps and cut the pulmonary annulus and partial right ventricular outflow tract muscles open with a blade.

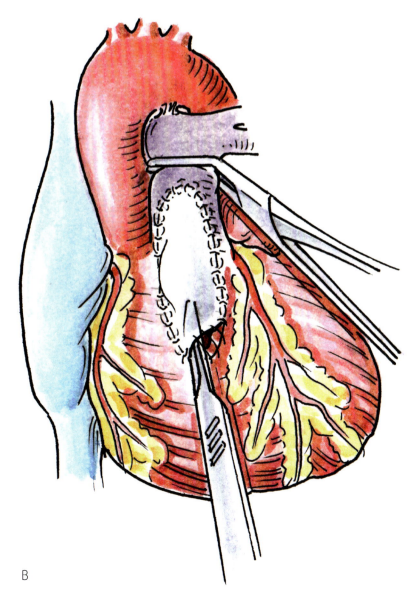

B

图 23-2（续）

Figure 23-2 cont'd

C. 最后将缝线收紧打结。

C. The suture is tightened to tie the knot.

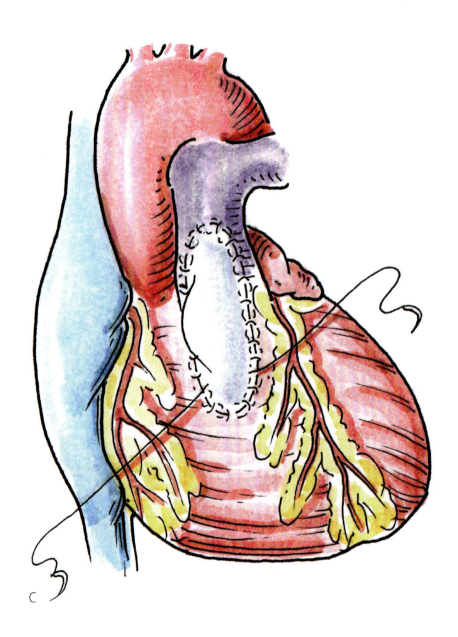

图 23-2（续）

Figure 23-2 cont'd

D. 另一种方法是常规行心肺转流术,若房间隔缺损够大,只需做单根右心房插管,圈套并控制动脉导管,也可采用阻断钳夹主肺动脉远端。

D. Another approach is routinely under cardiopulmonary bypass, and if the atrial defect is large enough, only a single right atrial intubation is needed. The ductus arteriosus is constricted, or the distal main pulmonary artery is blocked by coarctation forceps.

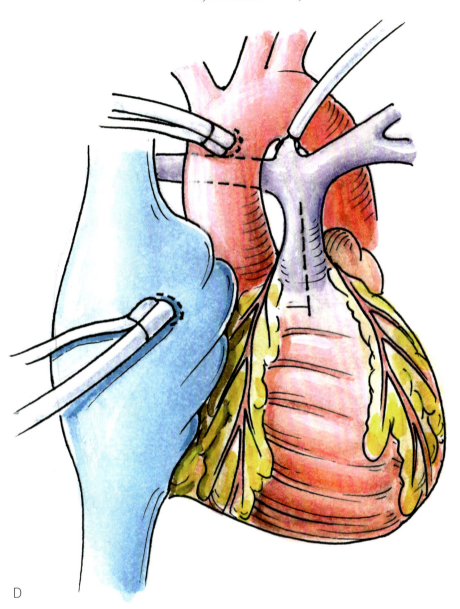

D

图 23-2（续）

Figure 23-2 cont'd

E. 纵行切开肺动脉，切开闭锁的肺动脉瓣，跨过瓣环向近心端延长，切口不宜太长，新生儿能置入 7~8mm 直径探条即可。

E. A longitudinal incision is performed in the pulmonary artery. The atretic pulmonary valve is incised and the incision is extended to the proximal part across the valve annulus. Care must be taken not to make a too long incision: an opening is enough for the neonate if a Hegar dilator of 7-8mm (diameter) can be placed through it.

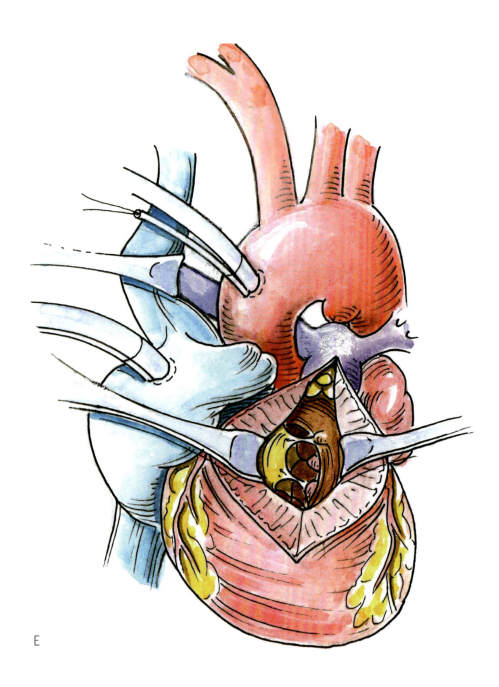

E

图 23-2（续）

F. 取戊二醛固定后的自身心包做跨瓣环补片扩大肺动脉及右心室流出道,若右室腔发育较小,必须再做 B-T 分流。

Figure 23-2 cont'd

F. A glutaraldehyde-fixed autologous pericardium is cut into the transannular patch to enlarge the pulmonary artery and right ventricular outflow tract. In the case of a small right ventricle, the B-T shunt must be performed.

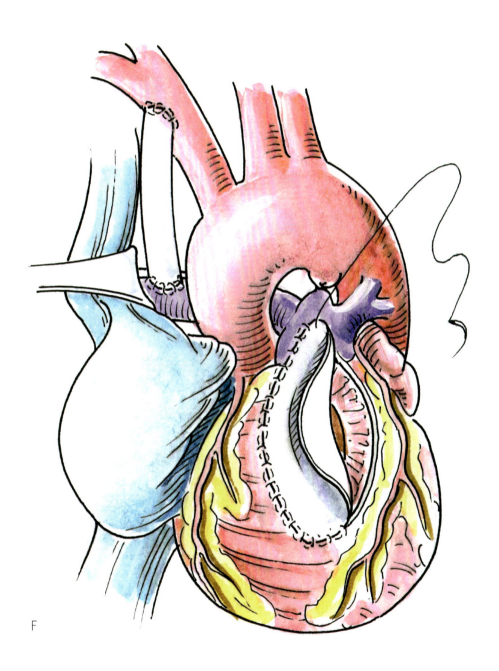

F

3. B-T 分流　对肺动脉发育很差或疑有右心室依赖型冠状动脉循环,则需选择分期手术。第一期做B-T分流术(前面姑息性手术方法一章已有详细描述)。

4. 一个半心室矫治手术　对右心室发育不良,Ⅰ期已做B-T分流加右心室流出道疏通术的患儿,6个月以后若右心室和肺动脉发育好,可考虑做一个半心室矫治手术(图23-3)。

3. B-T shunt　Staged procedures are indicated for patients with poorly developed pulmonary arteries or suspected RVDCC. B-T shunt is performed in the first stage (as described in detail in the chapter of *Palliative Surgery*).

4. One-and-a-half ventricular repair　For the children with right ventricular dysplasia who have undergone B-T shunt and right ventricular outflow tract dredging in the first stage, a one-and-a-half ventricular repair is considered if their right ventricles and pulmonary arteries are well developed after six months (Figure 23-3).

图 23-3 一个半心室矫治手术

A. 原正中胸骨切开进胸,主动脉、右心房插管行心肺转流术。

Figure 23-3 One-and-a-half ventricular repair

A. The chest is accessed through original median sternotomy, aortic and right atrial cannulae are conducted to establish cardiopulmonary bypass.

Continued

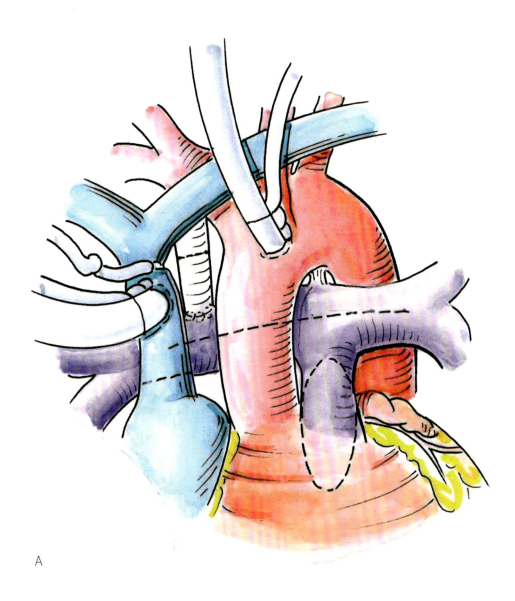

A

图 23-3（续）

Figure 23-3 cont'd

B. 将原 B-T 分流管钳闭切断，缝合关闭靠动脉侧管道，将肺动脉侧人工血管剪除，若有肺动脉狭窄，可用心包补片扩大。

B. The original B-T shunt should be blocked and severed, the conduit adjacent to the artery should be closed, and the artificial blood conduit around the pulmonary artery should be cut off. If there is pulmonary artery stenosis, the pulmonary artery can be enlarged by a pericardial patch.

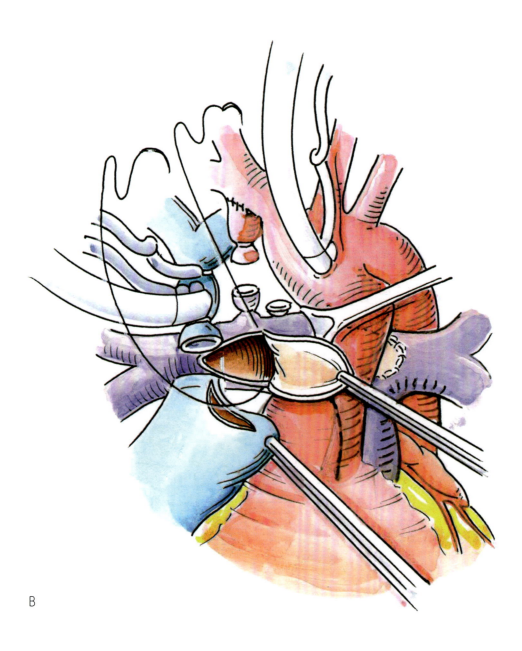

B

图 23-3（续）

C. 上腔静脉入右心房口处 5mm 横断，近端 6-0 Prolene 缝线连续缝合关闭，上腔静脉远端插入引流管作为上腔静脉回流。

Figure 23-3 cont'd

C. Make a transection on SVC 5mm to the entrance of the right atrium. The proximal end of SVC is closed by running sutures with a 6-0 Prolene suture. A drainage tube is inserted into the distal end of the SVC for blood retrograding into the SVC.

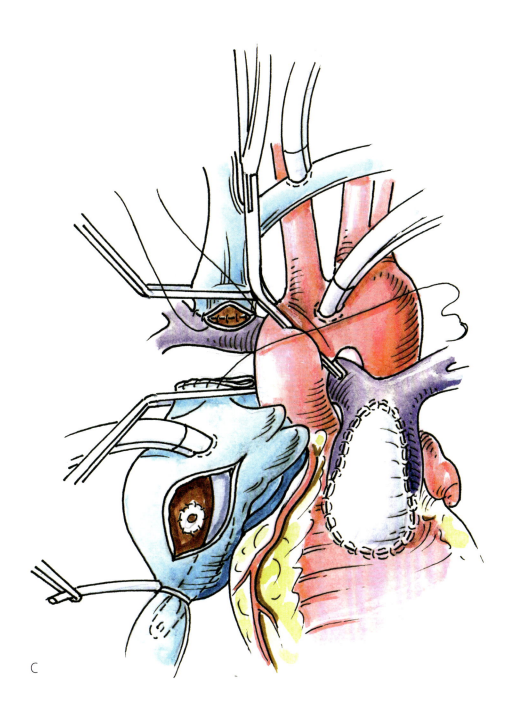

C

图 23-3（续）

D. 用 6-0 Prolene 缝线做上腔静脉 - 右肺动脉端侧吻合。

Figure 23-3 cont'd

D. SVC is end-to-side anastomosed to the right pulmonary artery with a 6-0 Prolene suture.

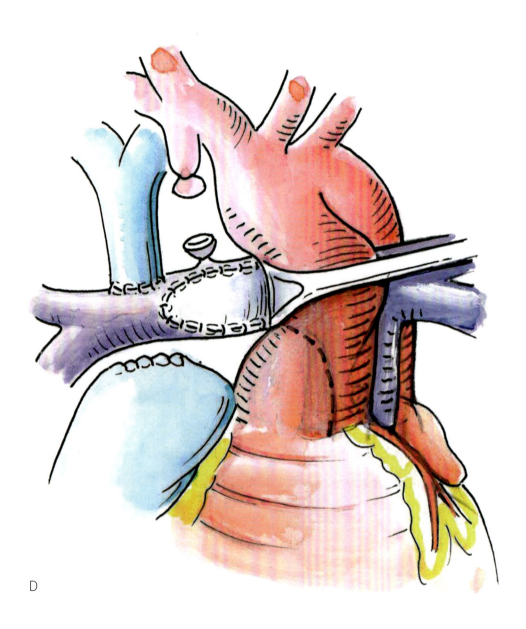

D

图 23-3（续）

E. 术毕肺动脉压力偏高（>20mmHg）或食管超声提示 Glenn 吻合口有逆向血流，可在主肺动脉或右肺动脉 Glenn 吻合口近端做肺动脉环束术。环束标准依据远端肺动脉压力、吻合口血流方向和动脉血氧饱和度三者之间的平衡。

Figure 23-3 cont'd

E. Patients are considered to undergo pulmonary artery banding at the proximal end of the main pulmonary artery or right pulmonary artery Glenn anastomosis, if they have an elevated high pulmonary artery pressure (>20mmHg) after surgery or retrograde blood flow as implicated in an esophageal ultrasound. The degree of banding is determined based on the balance among distal pulmonary artery pressure, anastomotic flow direction, and arterial oxygen saturation.

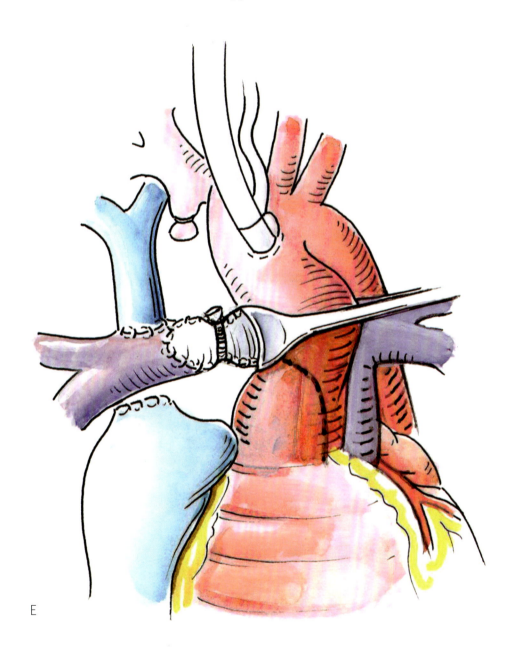

E

5. Fontan 手术　对重度右心室发育不良的患儿,最终仅能选择做单心室矫治(手术方法详见Fontan 手术图解,《功能性单心室与左心发育不全综合征手术图谱》,乔彬、刘中民、翁渝国主编,人民卫生出版社,2015)。

5. Fontan procedure　For children with severe right ventricular dysplasia, single ventricle repair is the only option.(See the diagram of Fontan procedure for the details of the surgical method, *Surgical Atlas of Functional Single Ventricle and Hypoplastic Left Heart Syndrome*. Edited by Qiao Bin, Liu Zhongmin, Weng Yuguo. People's Medical Publishing House, 2015.)

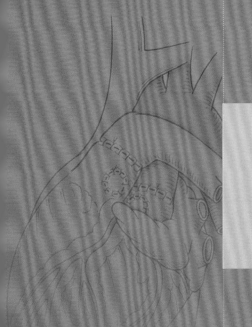

24 肺动脉闭锁合并室间隔缺损

24 Pulmonary Atresia with Ventricular Septal Defect

一、解剖分型

通常根据肺动脉的发育程度和体循环侧支血管的分布分成四大类型(图 24-1)。

Ⅰ型：主肺动脉存在,单纯的肺动脉瓣和漏斗部闭锁。动脉导管开通,提供肺循环血流。

Ⅱ型：主肺动脉缺如,左肺动脉和右肺动脉存在,肺循环仍为动脉导管依赖性。

Ⅲ型：肺动脉严重发育不良,并存在多发性主动脉肺动脉侧支血管。

Ⅳ型：原生肺动脉缺如,肺循环的血流来自主动脉肺动脉侧支血管。

I. Anatomical Typing

Pulmonary atresia with ventricular septal defect (PA/VSD) is usually divided into four types according to the degree of development of the pulmonary arteries and the distribution of collateral vessels in the systemic circulation (Figure 24-1) .

Type Ⅰ: The main pulmonary artery is present, but the pulmonary valve and infundibulum are atresia. The blood is supplied to pulmonary circulation through the ductus arteriosus.

Type Ⅱ: The main pulmonary artery is absent, the left and right pulmonary arteries are present, and the pulmonary circulation remains duct-dependent.

Type Ⅲ: There is a severe dysplasia of the pulmonary artery complicated with multiple aortopulmonary collateral arteries.

Type Ⅳ: Native pulmonary arteries are absent, and pulmonary blood comes from major aortopulmonary collateral arteries.

图 24-1　肺动脉闭锁合并室间隔
　　　　缺损解剖分型

A. Ⅰ型；B. Ⅱ型；C. Ⅲ型；D. Ⅳ型。

Figure 24-1　Anatomical typing of pulmonary atresia
　　　　　　　with ventricular septal defect

A. Type Ⅰ. B. Type Ⅱ. C. Type Ⅲ. D. Type Ⅳ .

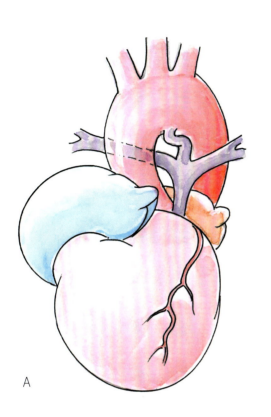

A

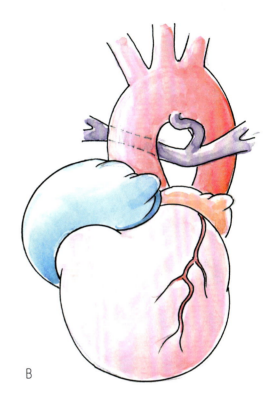

B

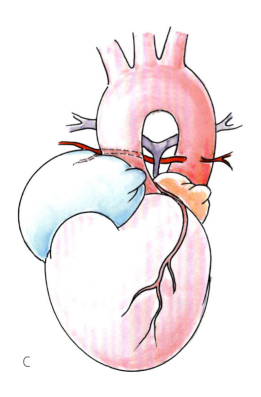

C

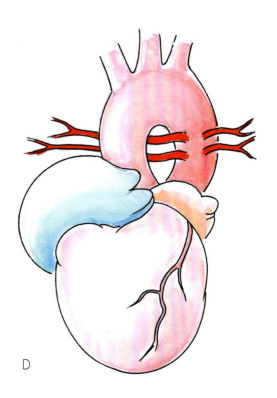

D

二、手术方法

II. Surgical Methods

手术治疗原则是根据原生肺动脉发育状况和侧支血管分布情况来考虑手术方法。

The principle of surgical treatment is to consider the surgical approaches based on the development of the native pulmonary arteries and the distribution of collateral arteries.

1. PA/VSD 合并动脉导管依赖性肺血流（图 24-2）

1. PA/VSD with duct-dependent pulmonary blood flow (Figure 24-2)

图 24-2　PA/VSD 合并动脉导管依赖性肺血流

Figure 24-2　PA/VSD with duct-dependent pulmonary blood flow

A. 常规正中胸骨切口行心肺转流术，转流前圈套动脉导管，并结扎切断，主动脉侧还需加强缝合。

A. Routine median sternotomy is performed to establish cardiopulmonary bypass. After the institution of bypass, the ductus arteriosus is constricted, ligated and cut off. Reinforced sutures are also required on the aortic side.

Continued

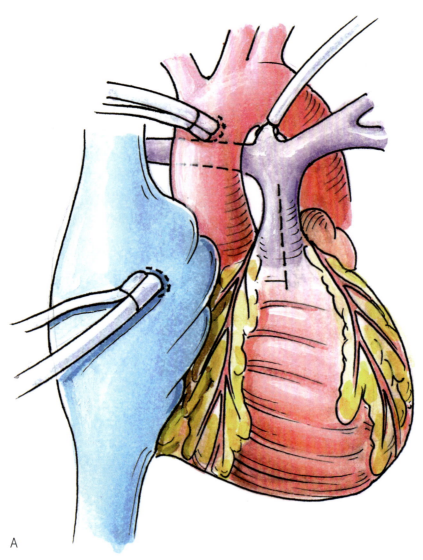

A

图 24-2（续）

Figure 24-2 cont'd

B. 切开右心室流出道,将膜性闭锁肺动脉瓣切开,若肺动脉瓣环小,则切开瓣环向上延伸至主肺动脉。

B. Open the right ventricular outflow tract and cut the pulmonary valve with membranous atresia, and if the pulmonary annulus is small, open the annulus and extend upward to the common pulmonary artery.

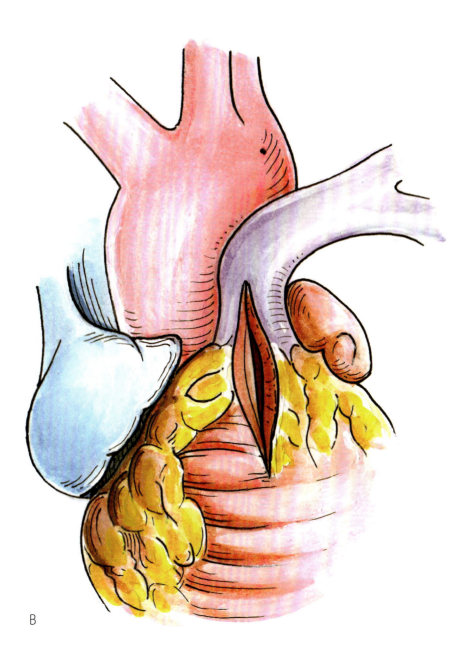

B

图 24-2（续）

Figure 24-2 cont'd

C. 暴露 VSD，大多为双动脉下，取心包或 ePTFE 补片连续缝合修补。

C. Exposed VSD is mostly subarterial and is to be closed with a pericardial or ePTFE patch using continuous sutures.

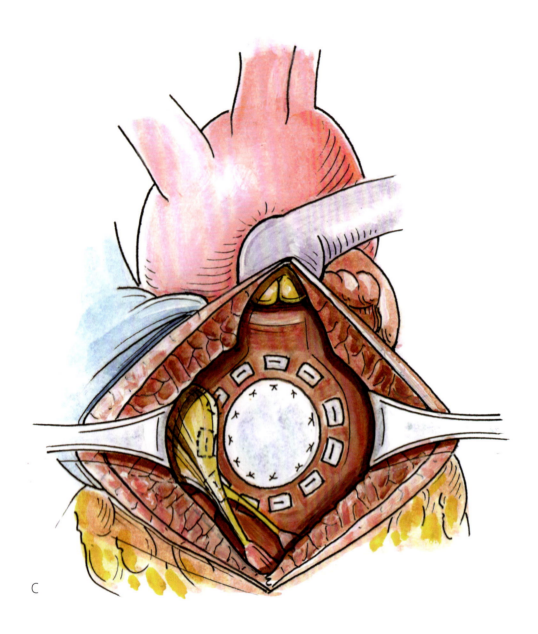

C

图 24-2（续）

Figure 24-2 cont'd

D. 取心包补片做右心室流出道跨瓣环补片扩大缝合。

D. Take a pericardial patch as a transannular patch for extended sutures of the right ventricular outflow tract.

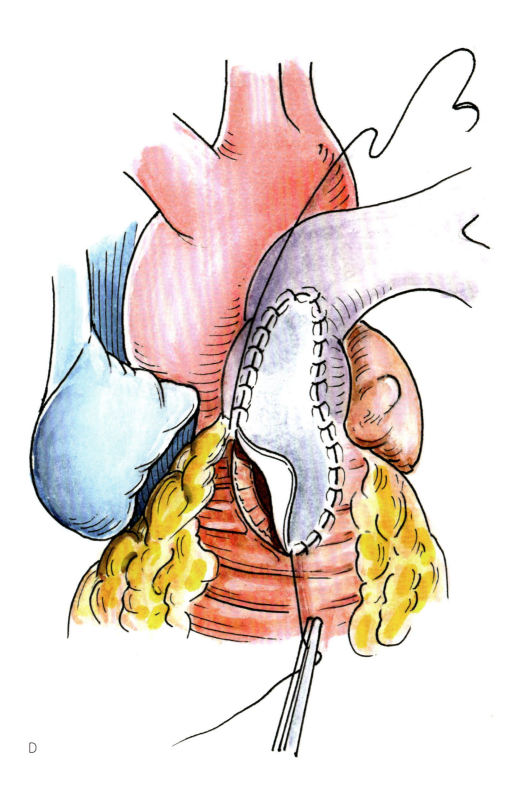

D

2. PA/VSD 合并肺血管发育不良（第一期手术）（图 24-3）

2. PA/VSD with hypoplastic pulmonary arteries (first stage surgery)(Figure 24-3)

图 24-3　PA/VSD 合并肺血管发育不良的第一期手术

A. 常规行心肺转流术后，仔细分离发育不全的主肺动脉和分支。

Figure 24-3　First stage surgery of PA/VSD with hypoplastic pulmonary arteries

A. After routine cardiopulmonary bypass is instituted, care should be taken to dissect hypoplastic common pulmonary arteries and branches.

Continued

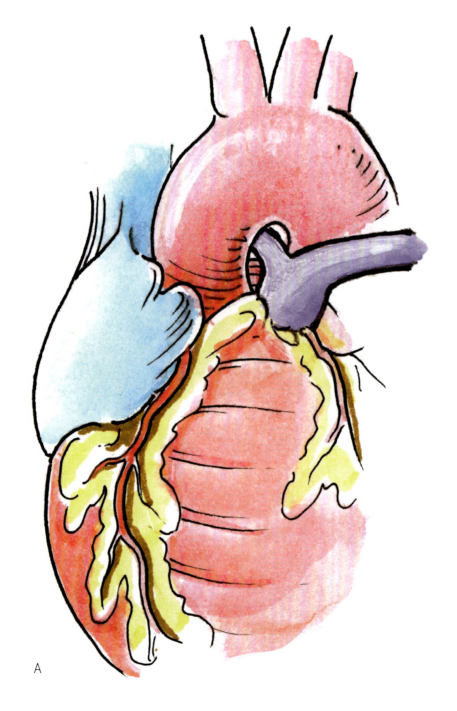

A

图 24-3（续）

Figure 24-3 cont'd

B. 取相应尺寸的外管道（可以使用同种异体带瓣管道、牛颈静脉管道或是ePTFE管道）。将管道远端与发育不全的主肺动脉用 6-0 Prolene 缝线做端端吻合。

B. Select the conduit of appropriate size (which can be valved homograft conduit, bovine jugular vein conduit, or ePTFE conduit). The distal end of the duct is end-to-end anastomosed to the dysplastic main pulmonary artery with 6-0 Prolene sutures.

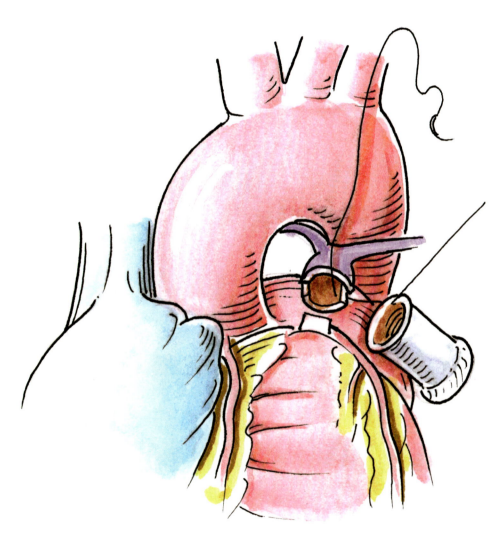

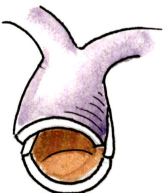

B

图 24-3(续)

C. 右心室漏斗部做一纵行切口,将管道的近端修剪成斜形,与右心室切口做连续缝合。

Figure 24-3 cont'd

C. A longitudinal incision is made in the infundibulum of the right ventricle. The proximal end of the duct is trimmed to an oblique fashion and sutured continuously with the right ventricular incision.

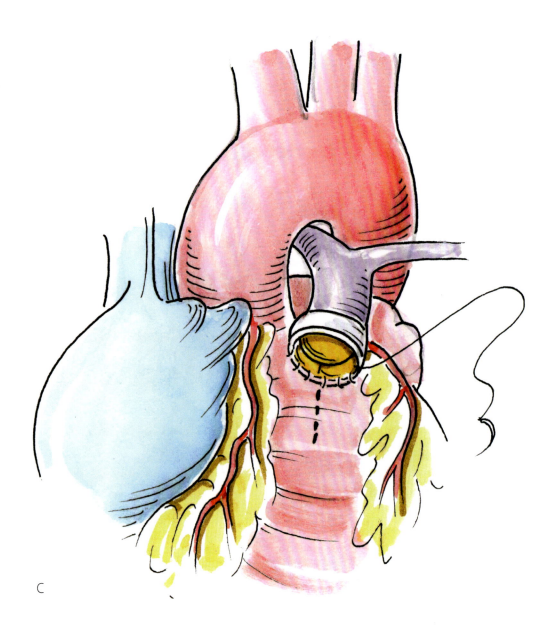

C

图 24-3（续）

Figure 24-3 cont'd

D. 也可在管道近端与右心室上缘做连续缝合。

D. Running sutures can also be made between the proximal end of the duct and the upper edge of the right ventricle.

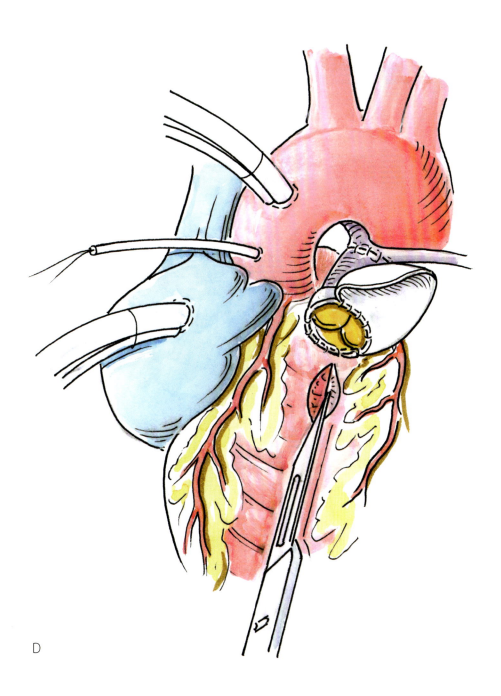

D

图 24-3（续）

Figure 24-3 cont'd

E. 取一块心包补片修剪成三角状覆盖在管道和右心室切口，形成一个"风帽状"补片，这样有助于瓣膜关闭。

E. Then a pericardial patch is trimmed into a triangle to cover the conduit and the right ventricular incision and form a cap-shaped patch. All of the above will facilitate valve closure.

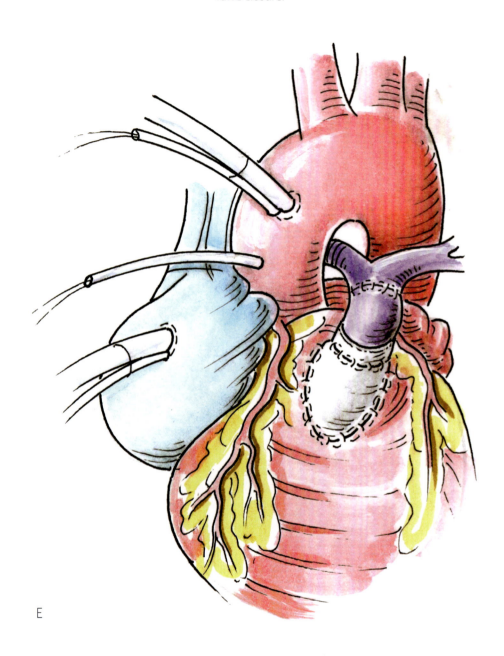

E

3. PA/VSD 肺血管发育不良（第二期手术） 第二期手术前通常要做心导管造影检查，判断患儿肺血管发育是否达到根治手术的标准或者首次手术放置的管道是否已经狭窄梗阻需要更换或扩大（图24-4）。

3. PA/VSD with hypoplastic pulmonary arteries (second stage surgery) Cineangiography with cardiac catheterization is usually performed before the second stage of surgery to determine whether the patient's pulmonary arteries have developed enough to the standard of radical surgery or whether the conduit placed in the one-stage surgery has stenosis and obstruction and needs to be replaced or expanded (Figure 24-4).

图 24-4　PA/VSD 合并肺血管发育不良的第二期手术

A. 正中胸骨锯开，原切口进胸。这种患者右心室及第一次连接的管道紧贴胸骨下缘，进胸分离需特别注意。术前胸片提示管道与胸骨下缘完全粘连，可采用股动脉转流技术，再做胸骨锯开分离，这样更安全。

Figure 24-4　Second stage surgery of PA/VSD with hypoplastic pulmonary arteries

A. The chest is accessed through the original incision with median sternotomy. The patient's right ventricle and the conduit connected in the first stage surgery are close to the lower edge of the sternum, so special attention should be paid when thoracotomy and separation are performed. If the preoperative chest radiographs suggest complete adhesion of the conduit to the lower edge of the sternum, the femoral artery bypass technique can be used, followed by sternotomy and separation. This way is much safer.

Continued

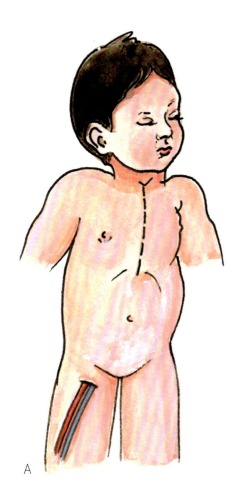

A

图 24-4（续）

B. CPB 后分离肺动脉至左右肺动脉分叉，将原钙化或狭窄的管道去除。通过原右心室切口暴露 VSD。

Figure 24-4 cont'd

B. Separate the pulmonary artery to the bifurcation of the left and right pulmonary artery after CPB and remove the primary calcified or stenotic conduit. The VSD is exposed through the original right ventricular incision.

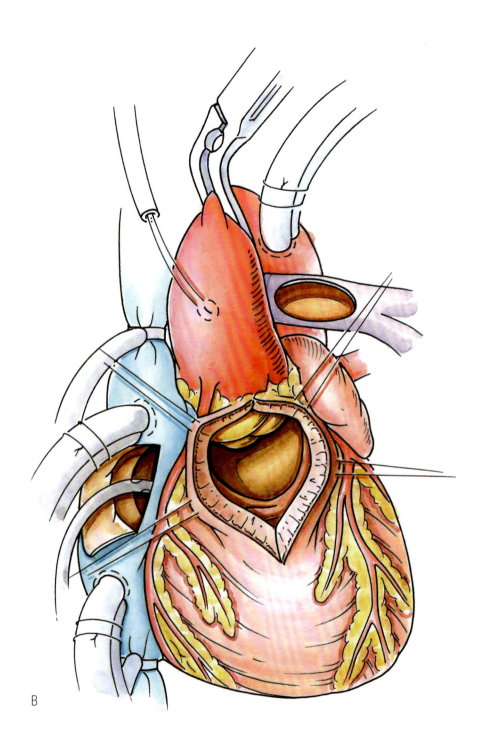

B

图 24-4（续）

C. 取牛心包或 ePTFE 补片修补 VSD。通常用 5-0 Prolene 缝线做连续缝合。

Figure 24-4 cont'd

C. Repair the VSD with a bovine pericardial or ePTFE patch. Running sutures are usually performed with a 5-0 Prolene suture.

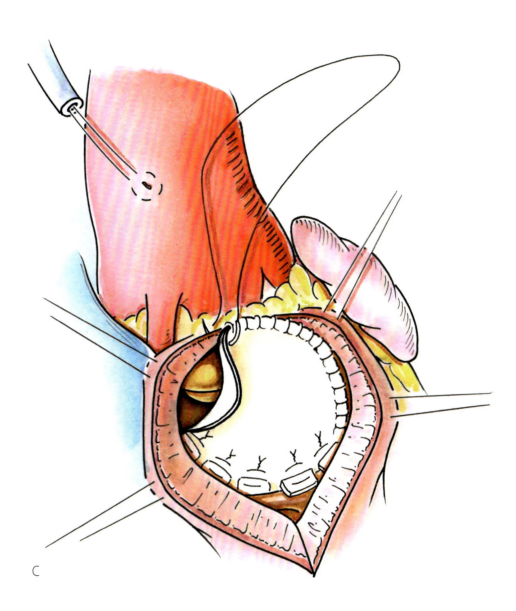

C

图 24-4（续）

Figure 24-4 cont'd

D. 如左、右肺动脉有狭窄,取心包补片扩大。

D. If there is stenosis in the left and right pulmonary arteries, a pericardial patch can be used to enlarge it.

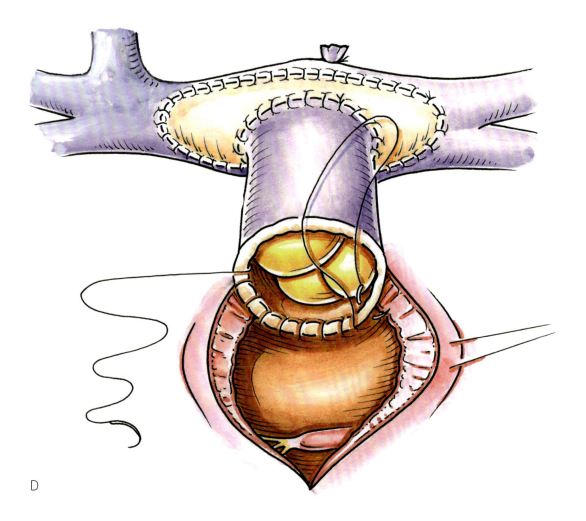

D

图 24-4(续)

E. 取合适大小的 ePTFE 管道(可自行缝制的三叶瓣)重建右心室流出道与肺动脉的连接,也可再取一块三角形补片扩大右心室与流出道。

Figure 24-4 cont'd

E. An appropriately sized ePTFE conduit (or a self-sewn trileaflet conduit) is used to reconstruct the connection between the right ventricular outflow tract and pulmonary artery, and another triangular patch can be used to expand the right ventricle and outflow tract.

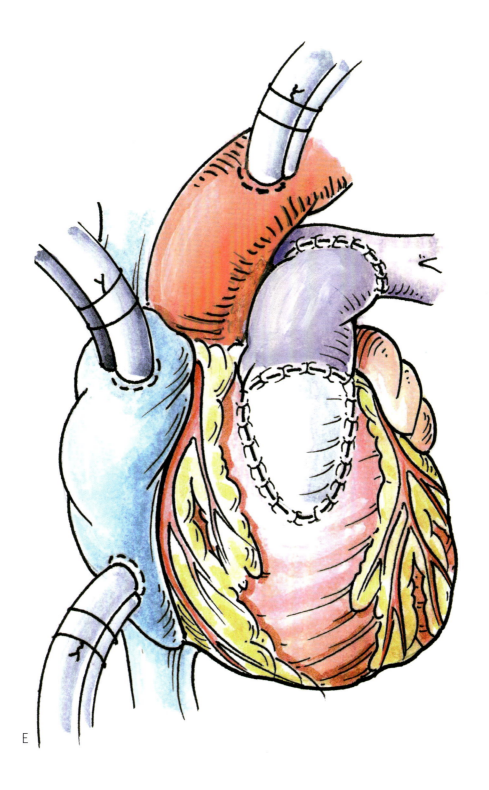

E

4. PA/VSD 合并粗大侧支行单元化手术技术 根据自然肺动脉的发育和侧支血管的大小分布选择不同的手术方法。尽可能用自身血管组织之间吻合来实现单元化目的（图 24-5）。

4. Unifocalization surgical techniques for PA/VSD with main aortopulmonary collateral arteries (MAPCAs) Select different surgical methods according to the development of natural pulmonary arteries and the size distribution of collateral vessels. Whenever possible, the purpose of unifocalization is achieved by anastomosis between self-vascular tissues (Figure 24-5).

图 24-5 **PA/VSD 合并粗大侧支行单元化手术技术**

A、B. 自然肺动脉发育好。侧支血管靠近肺动脉，可经胸骨正中切口分离侧支血管，离断并与自然肺动脉做端侧或侧侧吻合。

Figure 24-5 Unifocalization surgical techniques for PA/VSD with thick large collaterals

A, B. Natural pulmonary arteries develop well. The collateral vessels are close to the pulmonary artery and can be dissected through a median sternotomy to divide the collateral vessels and make end-to-side or side-to-side anastomoses with the natural pulmonary arteries.

Continued

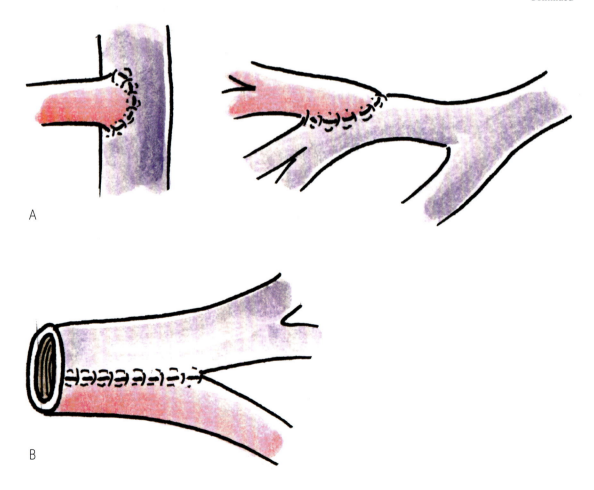

图 24-5（续）

C. 若肺动脉局部有狭窄，可取心包补片将其扩大。

D. 也可将侧支血管取下后，与自身的肺动脉做端端或端侧吻合。

Figure 24-5 cont'd

C. If there is local stenosis in the pulmonary artery, the pericardial patch can be used to enlarge it.

D. In addition, the collateral vessels can also be removed and anastomosed end-to-end or end-to-side with their own pulmonary artery.

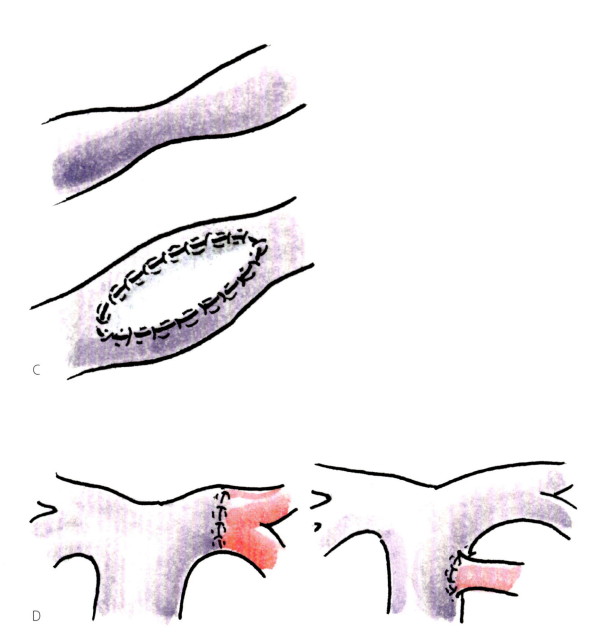

图 24-5（续）

E. 降主动脉发出无梗阻侧支,可以将其与部分降主动脉组织一起取下(带纽扣状),并直接与自身肺动脉做端侧吻合。

F. 若有需要可将上述几种方法联合使用,并可用自身心包组织扩大肺动脉以增加吻合口直径。

Figure 24-5 cont'd

E. Unobstructed collateral vessels arising from the descending aorta may be removed together with a portion of the descending aorta tissue (button-like) and anastomosed directly to their own pulmonary arteries.

F. If necessary, the above methods can be used in combination, and the pulmonary artery can be enlarged with autologous pericardium tissue to increase the anastomotic diameter.

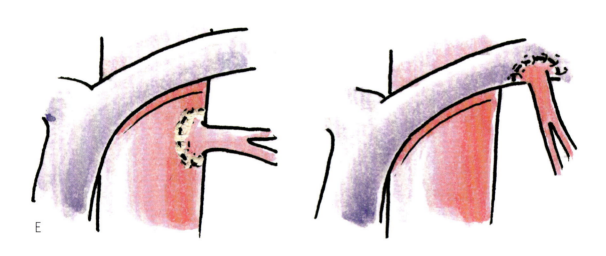

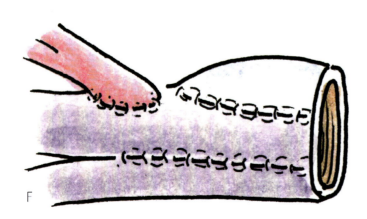

5. PA/VSD 合并肺动脉发育细小行中央分流术（图 24-6）

5. PA/VSD with small pulmonary artery development for central shunt (Figure 24-6)

图 24-6　PA/VSD 合并肺动脉发育细小行中央分流术

A. 肺动脉有汇合，但发育很差。对这类患者可选择做中央分流手术。正中胸骨切口径路分离肺动脉。在主肺动脉近端与右心室流出道闭锁处切断缝合，将主肺动脉近端与升主动脉侧壁或主动脉弓下部做端侧吻合。

Figure 24-6　PA/VSD with small pulmonary artery development for central shunt

A. Pulmonary arteries are confluent but poorly developed. Central shunt surgery is an option for such patients. A median sternotomy approach is performed to separate the pulmonary arteries. The proximal end of the pulmonary artery and the atresia right ventricular outflow tract are cut and sutured. An end-to-side anastomosis is performed between the proximal main pulmonary artery and the lateral wall of the ascending aorta or the lower part of the aortic arch.

Continued

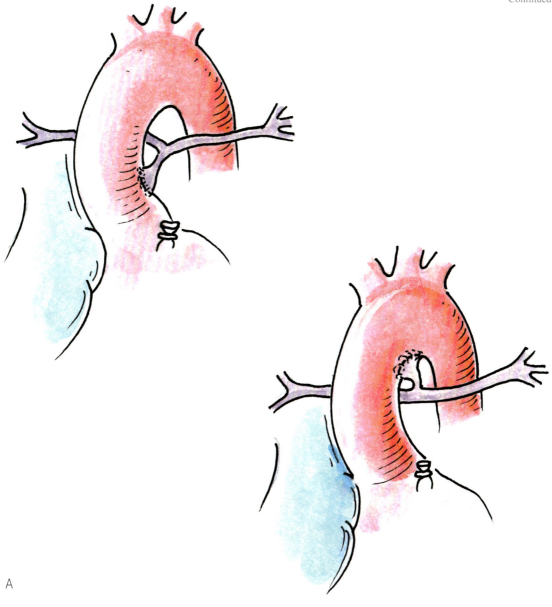

A

图 24-6（续）

B. 对肺动脉很短的患者，也可采用一根直径 3.5mm 或 4.0mm ePTFE 管道连接肺动脉和升主动脉，构建一个主 - 肺动脉窗。

Figure 24-6 cont'd

B. For patients with very short pulmonary arteries, an ePTFE conduit with a diameter of 3.5mm or 4.0mm may also be used to connect the pulmonary artery with the ascending aorta to construct an aorto-pulmonary window.

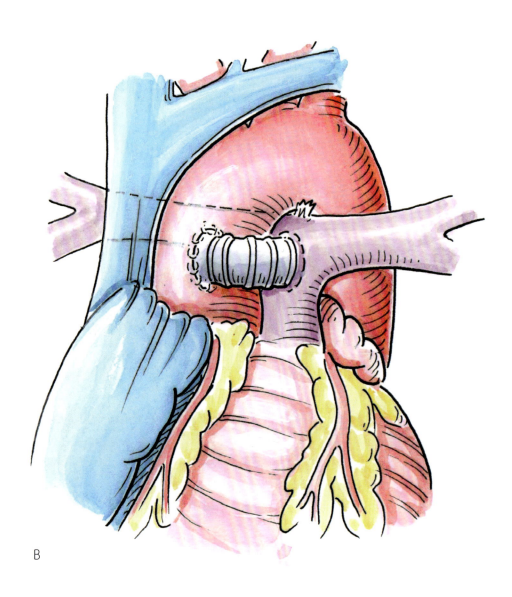

B

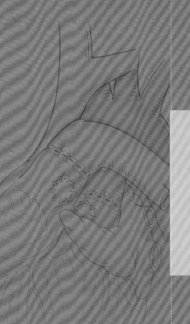

25　法洛四联症

25　Tetralogy of Fallot

一、解剖分型

法洛四联症包括肺动脉狭窄、室间隔缺损、主动脉骑跨和右心室肥大。法洛四联症的肺动脉狭窄，包括漏斗部狭窄、流出道狭窄，或同时合并肺动脉瓣狭窄，也可能合并主肺动脉或分支的狭窄。肺动脉瓣狭窄可能由于二瓣化或者三个交界相互融合而狭窄。

法洛四联症右心室漏斗部狭窄一般可以分为三型（图 25-1）。

1. 漏斗部近端狭窄较局限，有较大的第三心室，肺动脉瓣和瓣环发育良好。单纯切除肥厚的室上嵴往往可以达到疏通流出道。

2. 漏斗部弥漫性狭窄，漏斗部长管状狭窄，第三心室不明显，肺动脉瓣环也发育不全。修补时需要跨瓣补片，或带瓣管道扩大。

3. 漏斗部发育不全、短小，肺动脉瓣狭小甚至闭锁，肺动脉瓣可闭锁形成假性共同动脉干。主肺动脉及分支狭小，肺血靠动脉导管或主动脉侧支供应，外科矫治要用到

I. Anatomical Typing

Tetralogy of Fallot (TOF) consists of pulmonary artery stenosis, ventricular septal defect (VSD), overriding aorta, and right ventricular hypertrophy. Pulmonary stenosis in tetralogy of Fallot includes infundibulum stenosis, outflow tract stenosis, or may be associated with stenosis of pulmonary valvular or stenosis of main pulmonary artery or branches. Pulmonary stenosis may occur as a result of bileaflet or fusion of the three junctions.

Right ventricular infundibular stenosis in tetralogy of Fallot is generally classified into three types (Figure 25-1).

1. The stenosis of the proximal infundibulum is limited, and there is a large third ventricle with a well-developed pulmonary valve and annulus. Simply removing the hypertrophic supraventricular crest can often clear the outflow tract.

2. If there is diffuse stenosis of the infundibulum, long tubular stenosis of the infundibulum, unremarkable third ventricle, and dysplasia of the pulmonary annulus, a transvalvular patch, or enlargement of the valved conduit is required during the repair.

3. The infundibulum is hypoplastic and short, the pulmonary valve is stenotic or even atretic, and the pulmonary valve can be atretic and form a pseudo truncus arteriosus. The main pulmonary artery and its branches are

带瓣管道连接右心室及肺动脉。

stenotic, and pulmonary blood flow is dependent on ductus arteriosus or aortic collaterals. Under such circumstances, a valved external conduit is required to connect the right ventricle and pulmonary artery during the surgical repair.

图 25-1　**法洛四联症解剖分型**
A. 法洛四联症。

Figure 25-1　Anatomical typing of tetralogy of Fallot
A. Tetralogy of Fallot.

Continued

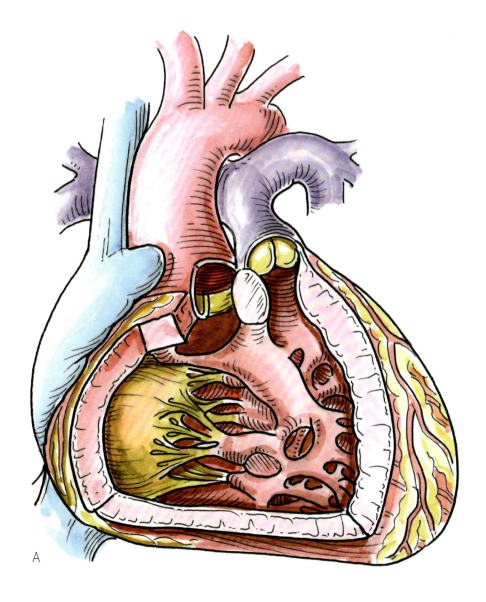

A

图 25-1（续）

Figure 25-1 cont'd

B. 漏斗部近端局限狭窄。

B. Limited stenosis of the proximal infundibulum.

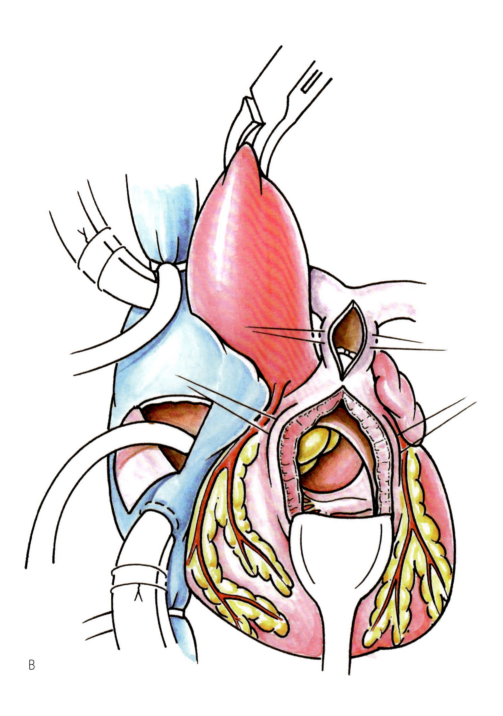

B

图 25-1（续）

Figure 25-1 cont'd

C. 漏斗部弥漫性狭窄。

C. Diffuse stenosis of the infundibulum.

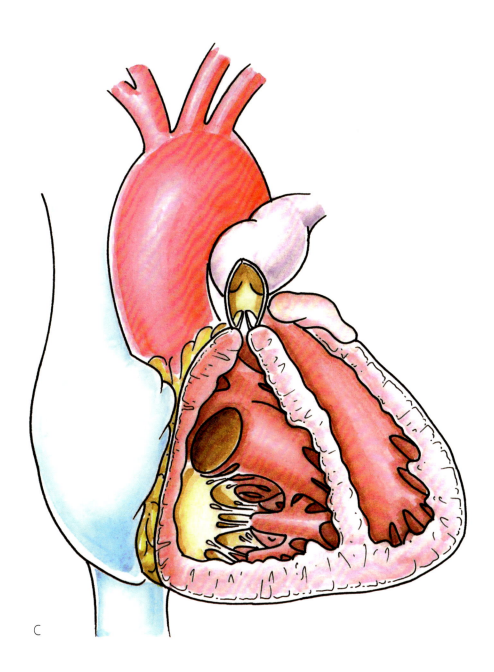

C

图 25-1（续）

Figure 25-1 cont'd

D. 漏斗部发育不全。

D. Hypoplastic infundibulum.

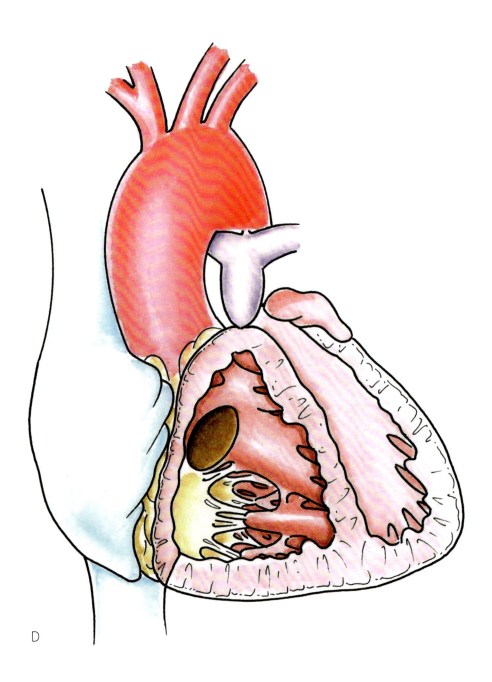

D

二、手术方法

II. Surgical Methods

1. 经心房修补 经右心房途径矫治法洛四联症适用于肺动脉发育良好,瓣环没有明显狭窄,肺动脉瓣二叶或者三叶,瓣叶发育基本正常,仅有交界融合。漏斗部足够大(图 25-2)。

1. Transatrial repair Treatment of tetralogy of Fallot via the right atrial approach is suitable for the following conditions: The pulmonary artery is well developed, the annulus is not significantly stenotic, the pulmonary valve is either bicuspid or tricuspid, and the development of the valve leaflets is basically normal, with only junctional fusion. The infundibulum is large enough (Figure 25-2).

图 25-2　**经心房修补室间隔缺损**

A. 行心肺转流术,主动脉和上下腔静脉插管,常温或中低温(32℃),阻断升主动脉,常规使用心肌保护液。弧线形切开右心房,通过未闭卵圆孔或房间隔切开放置左心房引流管。经三尖瓣暴露右心室流出道及室间隔缺损,注意探查室间隔缺损前缘及主动脉瓣位置,探查室间隔缺损与三尖瓣之间的右心室流出道是否存在粗大的肌束。

Figure 25-2　Transatrial repair of VSD

A. Cardiopulmonary bypass is established, and cannulation of the aorta, superior and inferior vena cava is performed under normothermic or moderate hypothermia (32℃). The ascending aorta is blocked, and a cardioplegic solution is routinely used. The right atriotomy is made in a curved line, and the left atrium drainage tube is placed through the patent foramen ovale or atrial septal incision. Expose the right ventricular outflow tract and VSD through the tricuspid valve. Explore the front edge of the VSD and the position of the aortic valve, and identify whether there is a thick muscle bundle in the right ventricular outflow tract between the VSD and the tricuspid valve.

Continued

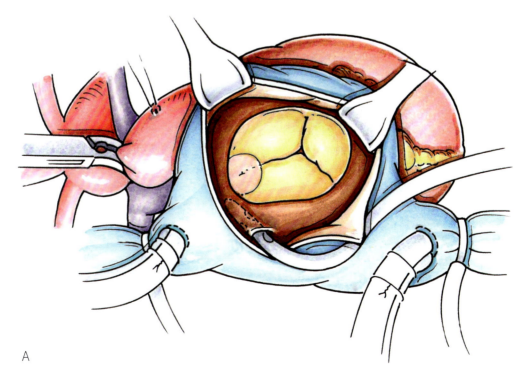

A

图 25-2（续）

B. 沿隔束前支切除右心室流出道肥厚肌束,疏通右心室流出道。有时隔束还有分支也可以一并切断或者切除。法洛四联症的室间隔缺损都在主动脉瓣下,三尖瓣后面。牵开三尖瓣叶,避免损伤三尖瓣叶和瓣下结构。尽可能清晰地显露室间隔缺损和主动脉瓣膜。

Figure 25-2 cont'd

B. Excise the hypertrophic muscle bundles in the right ventricular outflow tract along the anterior branch of the septal band and relieve obstruction in the right ventricular outflow tract. The septal band may have branches, which may also be severed or excised. The ventricular defect of tetralogy are all under the aortic valve and behind the tricuspid valve. Retract the tricuspid valve leaflets to avoid damaging the tricuspid valve leaflets and subvalvular structures. Expose the VSD and aortic valve as clearly as possible.

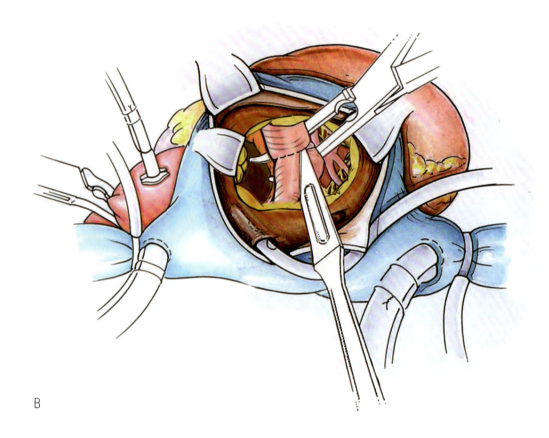

B

图 25-2（续）

C. 切除流出道肥厚肌束后，可用经戊二醛处理后的自身心包或牛心包补片修补室间隔缺损。法洛四联症的室间隔缺损都在主动脉瓣下，一般分为嵴下型和嵴内型。如果嵴下型的室间隔缺损，房室传导束走行于膜部间隔的左侧缘上。在补片修补时，下缘缝线缝在室间隔缺损右侧缘上，通常 5-0 Prolene 带垫片连续缝合。

Figure 25-2 cont'd

C. After excision of the hypertrophic muscle bundles in the outflow tract, the VSD may be repaired with a glutaraldehyde-treated autologous pericardial or bovine pericardial patch. The VSD in the tetralogy of Fallot are all under the aortic valve, and they are generally divided into infracristal type and intracristal type. If the ventricular defect is infracristal, the atrioventricular conduction bundles run on the left edge of the membranous septum. In the patch repair, the lower edge sutures are stitched on the right edge of the ventricular defect, usually with pledget-supported running sutures of 5-0 Prolene.

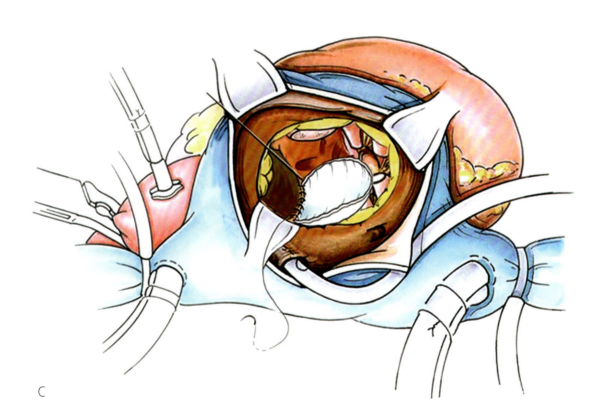

C

图 25-2 (续)

D. 经肺动脉瓣置入探条,如果肺动脉瓣有狭窄,瓣环大小正常,可以经肺动脉切口进行交界切开,必要时主肺动脉补片扩大。

Figure 25-2 cont'd

D. Insert the Hegar dilator through the pulmonary valve. If the pulmonary valve has stenosis and the valve annulus is of normal size, a junctional incision is made through a pulmonary artery incision. If necessary, enlarge the patch of the main pulmonary artery trunk.

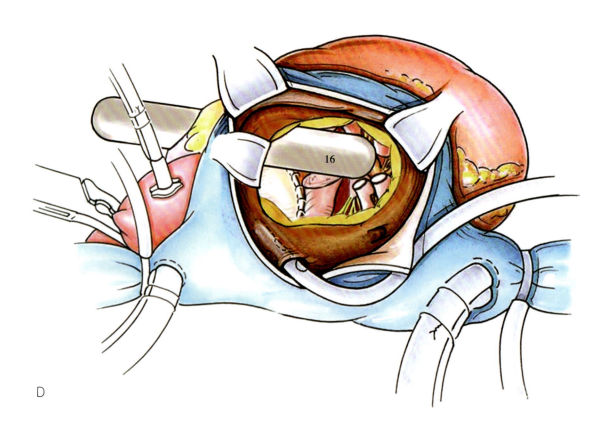

D

2. 经心室修补（图 25-3）

2. Transventricular repair (Figure 25-3)

图 25-3　经心室修补室间隔缺损

A. 在右心室流出道做纵行切口，注意避开冠状动脉分支，切口不宜过长，以免影响右心室收缩功能。

Figure 25-3　Transventricular repair of VSD

A. Make a longitudinal incision in the right ventricular outflow tract, avoiding coronary artery branches, and the incision should not be too long so as not to affect the systolic function of the right ventricle.

Continued

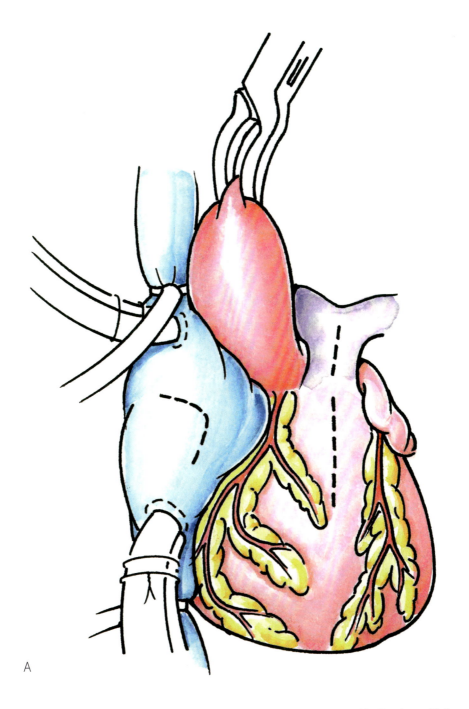

A

图 25-3（续）

Figure 25-3 cont'd

B. 根据狭窄情况离断隔、壁束，注意避免损伤主动脉瓣。

B. Dissect the septal band and the parietal band based on varying degrees of stenosis, taking care not to damage the aortic valve.

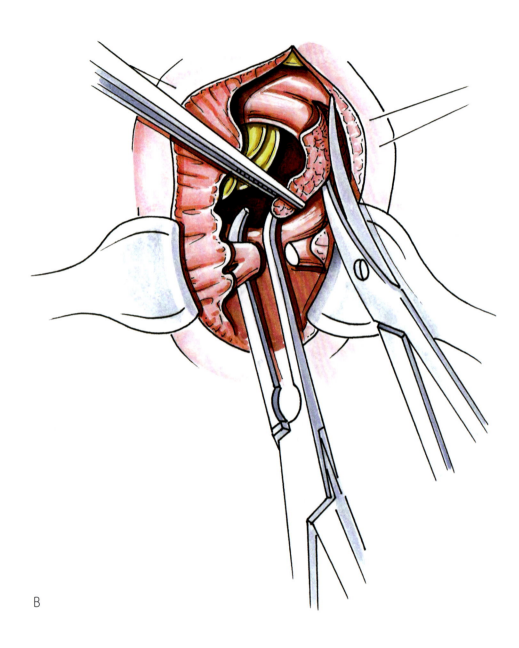

B

图 25-3（续）

C. 虚线显示的是室间隔缺损边缘，包括肺动脉瓣下切除的残留圆锥体。补片盖过主动脉瓣，缝合在右心室的内膜。若主动脉瓣骑跨严重，为避免左心室流出道狭窄，补片应稍大，略呈穹状。经右心室切口修补室间隔缺损，室间隔缺损暴露清楚，一般可以连续缝合。

Figure 25-3 cont'd

C. The dotted liney indicates the edge of the ventricular defect, including the residual cone resected under the pulmonary valve. The patch covers the aortic valve and is sutured to the inner membrane of the right ventricle. If the aortic valve severely overrides, to avoid stenosis of the left ventricular outflow tract, the patch should be slightly larger and dome-shaped. When the ventricular defect is repaired through a right ventricular incision, the ventricular defect is clearly exposed and may usually be sutured continuously.

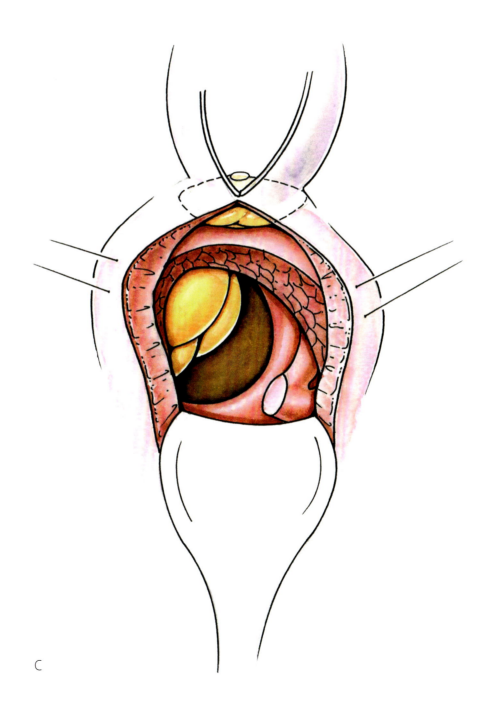

C

图 25-3（续）

D. 补片在右心室流出道肺动脉瓣下圆锥体打结。由于圆锥体部分已经被切除或者切开，为防止圆锥体部分撕裂，缝线脱落。建议在此加几针间断缝线，加固补片。

Figure 25-3 cont'd

D. The patch is knotted at the arterial cone under the pulmonary valve of the right ventricular outflow tract. Since the arterial cone portion has been excised or incised, in order to prevent the arterial cone from partial tearing and the suture from falling off, it is recommended that several interrupted stitches be added here to reinforce the patch.

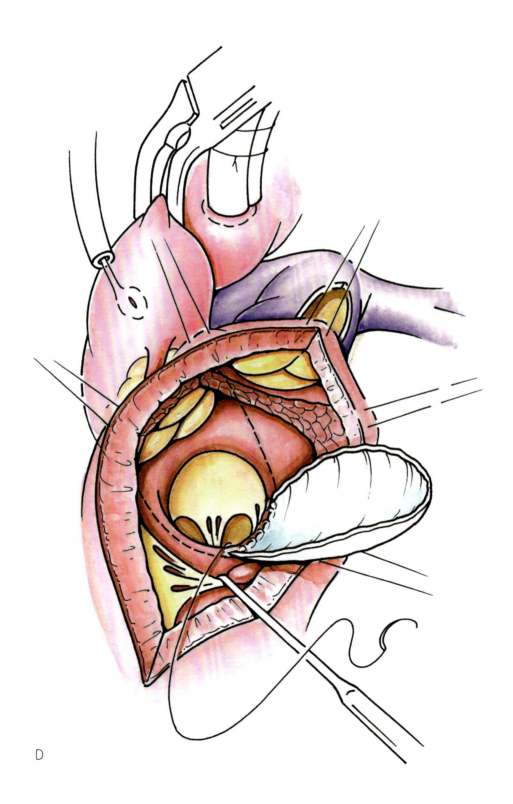

D

图 25-3 (续)

E. 肺动脉和瓣环基本正常大小,可以经肺动脉切口进行处理。①做肺动脉纵行切口,避免切断肺动脉瓣环。肺动脉瓣无论是二叶还是三叶,交界多有和肺动脉壁粘连。②在交界切开前,先沿交界处锐性从肺动脉壁分开。③再切开交界。

Figure 25-3 cont'd

E. If the pulmonary artery and valve annulus are generally of normal size, pulmonary stenosis may be managed through a pulmonary artery incision. ① The pulmonary artery is longitudinally incised to avoid severing the pulmonary annulus. Whether the pulmonary valve is either bicuspid or tricuspid, the commissure often adheres to the pulmonary artery wall. ② Prior to the incision into the commissure, the pulmonary valve is separated from the pulmonary artery wall along the commissure sharpness. ③ The commissure is then cut.

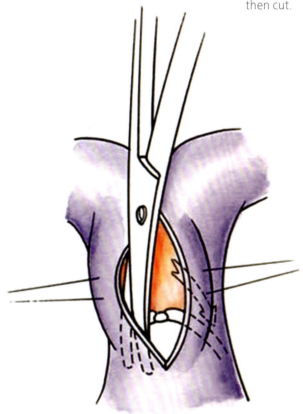

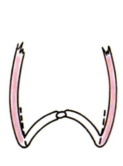

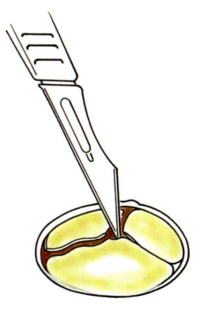

E

图 25-3（续）

Figure 25-3 cont'd

F. 再测量右心室流出道，肺动脉瓣环和肺动脉，确定没有狭窄，可以直接缝合右心室切口和肺动脉，反之则需补片扩大。

F. After the measurement, if the right ventricular outflow tract, the pulmonary annulus, and the pulmonary artery are not stenotic, the right ventricular incision and the pulmonary artery may be sutured directly. Otherwise, the right ventricular outflow tract, the pulmonary annulus, and the pulmonary artery need to be enlarged by patch.

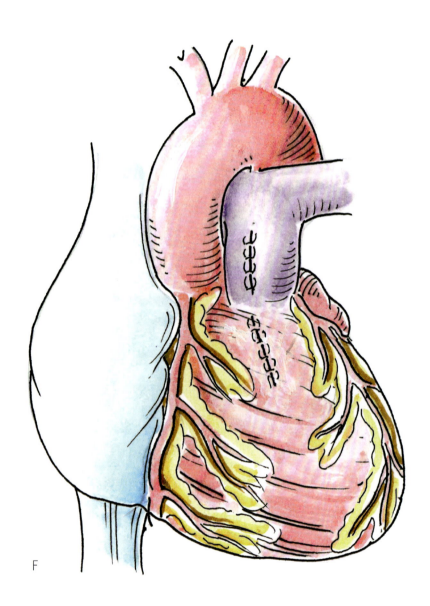

F

3. 右心室流出道和肺动脉扩大术（不跨瓣补片扩大） 法洛四联症选择经主肺动脉纵行切口和经右心室修补的病例，如果肺动脉环直径正常，肺动脉和右心室流出道可以用适当大小补片闭合切口（图 25-4）。

3. Enlargement of right ventricular outflow tract and pulmonary artery (non-transvalvular patch enlargement) For patients with tetralogy of Fallot who have undergone the longitudinal incision through the main pulmonary arter and the repair through the right ventricle, if the diameter of the pulmonary artery annulus is normal, the pulmonary artery and right ventricular outflow tract may be closed with a patch of appropriate size (Figure 25-4).

图 25-4 **右心室流出道和肺动脉扩大术（不跨瓣补片扩大）**
A. 肺动脉和右心室纵行切口。

Figure 25-4 Enlargement of right ventricular outflow tract and pulmonary artery (non-transvalvular patch enlargement)

A. A longitudinal incision of the pulmonary artery and right ventricle.

Continued

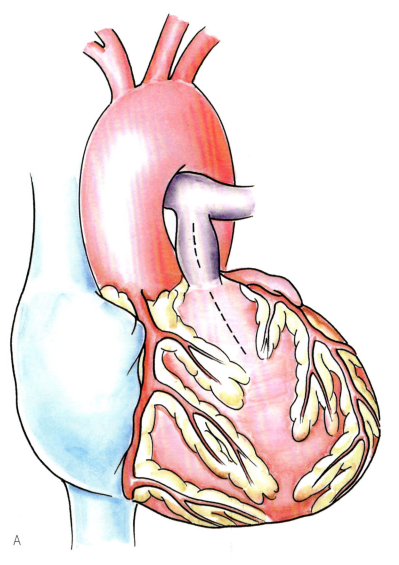

A

图 25-4（续）

Figure 25-4 cont'd

B. 右心室流出道有众多冠状动脉分支，为避免损伤冠状动脉采用了横切口。

B. A transverse incision is made to avoid damage to the coronary arteries due to so many coronary artery branches in the right ventricular outflow tract.

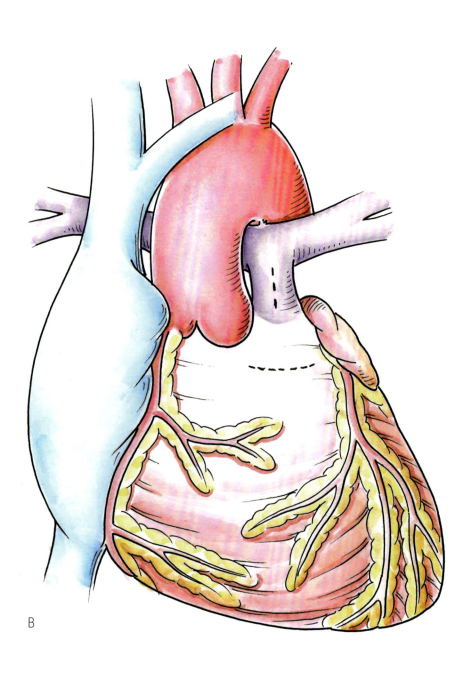

B

图 25-4（续）

C. 图中所示为修补前肺动脉和瓣膜,瓣环和右心室流出道。按前述方法分别切断异常肌束,松解右心室流出道。

Figure 25-4 cont'd

C. Pulmonary artery, valve, annulus, and right ventricular outflow tract before repairing shown in the figure. The abnormal muscle bundles are severed, and the right ventricular outflow tract is released, as previously described.

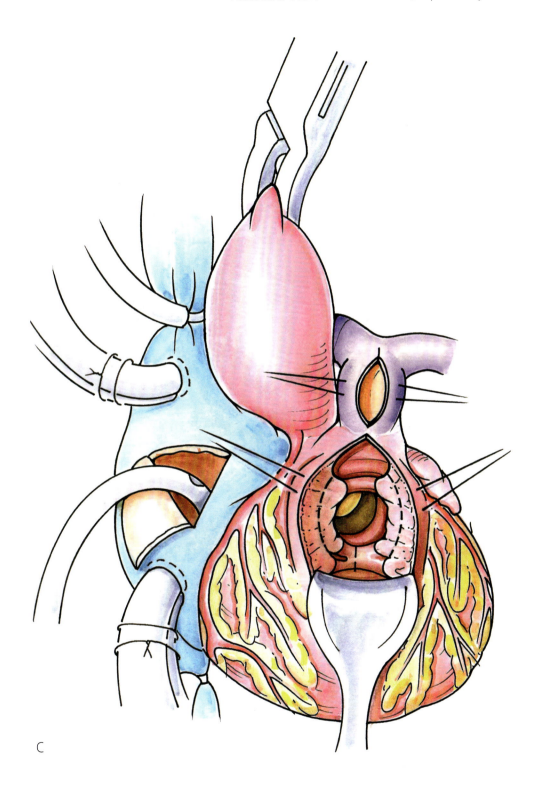

C

图 25-4（续）

Figure 25-4 cont'd

D. 先行室间隔缺损修补, 再用补片闭合右心室流出道和主肺动脉。由于右心室压力不大, 补片材料可采用自身心包或牛心包, 也可用 ePTFE。使用 Prolene 缝线连续缝合。

D. The ventricular defect is repaired first, and then the right ventricular outflow tract and main pulmonary artery are closed with a patch. Since the right ventricular pressure is not high, the patch material may be the patient's own pericardium, bovine pericardium, or ePTFE. A running suture of Prolene is made.

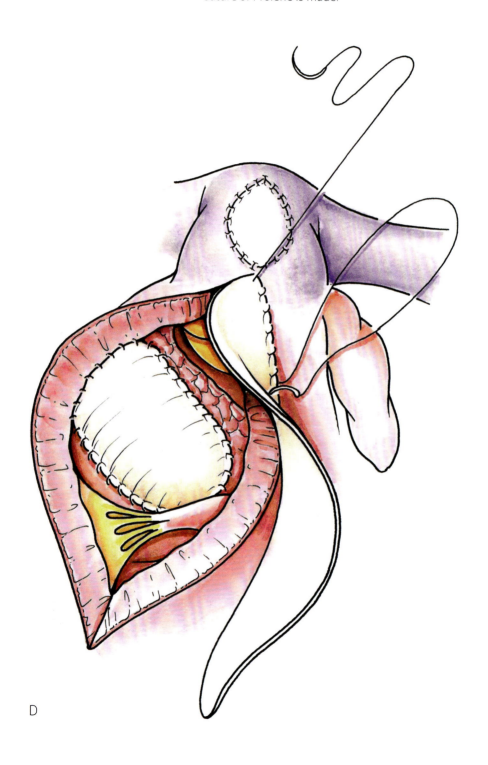

D

图 25-4(续)

Figure 25-4 cont'd

E. 完成法洛四联症的"双片法"不跨瓣补片扩大术。

E. The two-patch method of non-transvalvular patch enlargement for tetralogy of Fallot is accomplished.

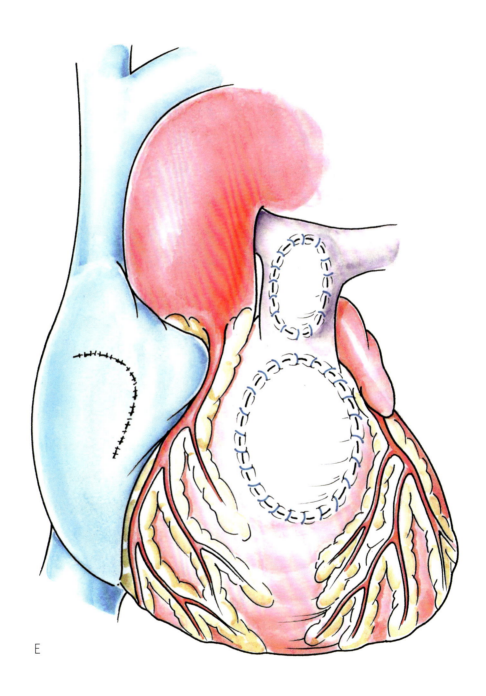

E

4. 右心室流出道和肺动脉扩大术（跨瓣补片扩大）（图 25-5）

4. Right ventricular outflow tract and pulmonary artery enlargement (transvalvular patch enlargement)(Figure 25-5)

图 25-5　右心室流出道和肺动脉扩大术（跨瓣补片扩大）

A. 如果肺动脉瓣环直径不够大，造成右心室流出道狭窄严重，则可进行跨环修补，以确保彻底解除梗阻。切开肺动脉瓣环，不管是二叶的肺动脉瓣，还是切开瓣环后的一叶瓣膜，可以把部分残留的瓣叶切除。使用自体心包或者异种心包片扩大右心室和肺动脉切口，甚至可扩大至左肺动脉开口处。

Figure 25-5　Right ventricular outflow tract and pulmonary artery enlargement (transvalvular patch enlargement)

A. In the case of severe stenosis of the right ventricular outflow tract due to the small diameter of the pulmonary annulus, a transannular repair may be performed to ensure complete resolution of the obstruction. A pulmonary annulus valvulotomy is made. Whether it is a bicuspid pulmonary valve or a one-leaf valve after annulus valvulotomy, some residual leaflets may be excised. The right ventricular and pulmonary artery incisions are enlarged with autologous or heterologous pericardial patches, even extended to the left pulmonary artery ostium.

Continued

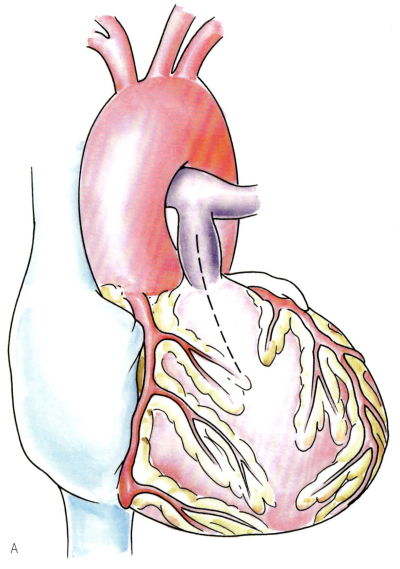

A

图 25-5（续）
B. 跨瓣补片可选用自身心包或牛心包材料补修右心室流出道、肺动脉瓣环和肺动脉。

Figure 25-5 cont'd
B. The autologous pericardium or bovine pericardium material may be used as a transvalvular patch to repair the right ventricular outflow tract, pulmonary annulus, and pulmonary artery.

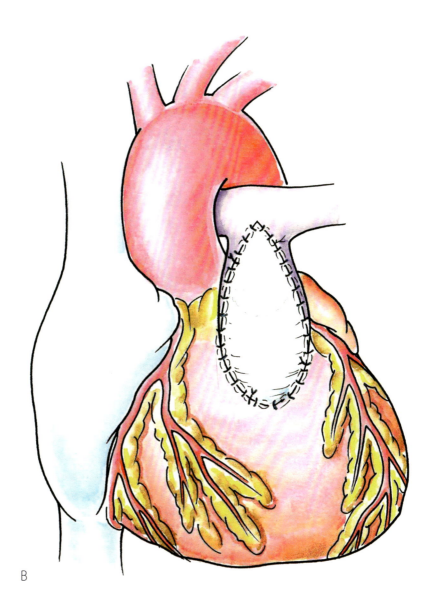

B

图 25-5（续）

C. 使用不带瓣叶的跨环补片后，常会导致肺动脉瓣反流，不管肺动脉瓣反流轻重，久而久之会加重右心室负担，导致右心衰竭，影响患者术后的远期生活质量。使用带单瓣的生物材料，或在补片材料上缝合一个单瓣以减轻肺动脉瓣反流，可保护右心功能。

Figure 25-5 cont'd

C. The use of transannular patch without a leaflet often results in incomplete closure of the pulmonary valve regurgitation. Regardless of the severity of pulmonary regurgitation, it will increase the burden on the right ventricle over time, leading to right heart failure. The patient's long-term quality of life after surgery is adversely affected. The use of biomaterials with a single valve, or the use of patch sutured with a single valve may reduce pulmonary regurgitation and protect the normal function of the right heart.

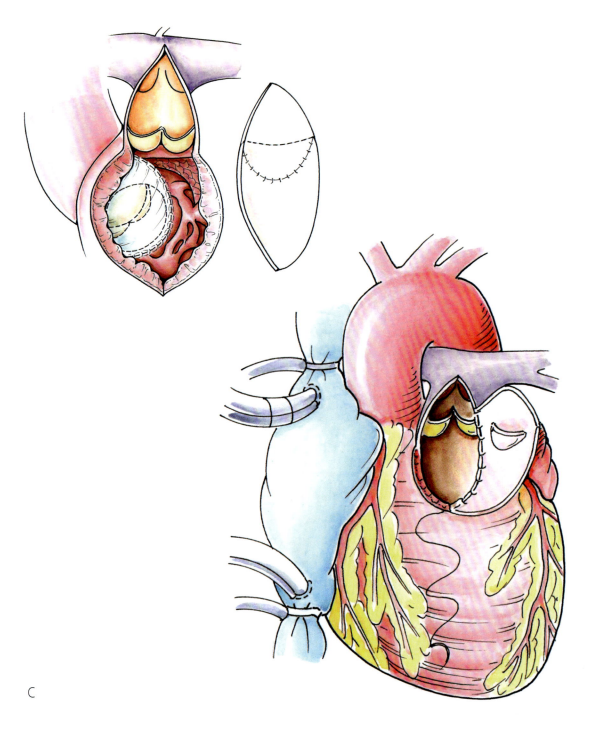

C

图 25-5（续）

Figure 25-5 cont'd

D. 把带瓣的补片连续缝合在右心室流出道、瓣环和肺动脉。通过缝合的补片扩大了狭窄的流出道、肺动脉瓣环，同时保证了肺动脉瓣的完整性。

D. Running suture the valved patch to the right ventricular outflow tract, annulus and pulmonary artery. The sutured patch enlarges the stenotic outflow tract, the pulmonary annulus, and at the same time ensures the integrity of the pulmonary valve.

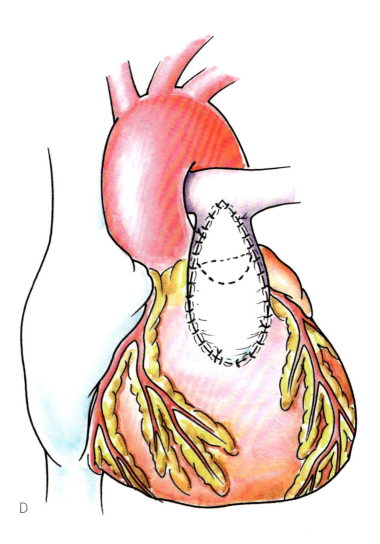

D

图 25-5（续）

E. 自制带瓣补片植入后保证了流出道
通畅。

Figure 25-5 cont'd

E. After the self-made valved patch is implanted, the outflow tract is unobstructed.

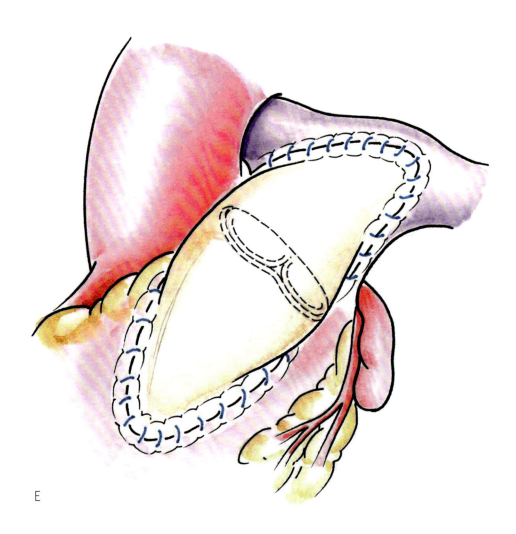

E

图 25-5（续）

F. 自制的单瓣随时间推移会发生纤维化或钙化,导致瓣口梗阻或反流,目前可以通过介入治疗进行带肺动脉瓣膜支架植入,降低再手术的风险。

Figure 25-5 cont'd

F. Fibrosis or calcification of the self-made single valve occurs over time, leading to valve obstruction or regurgitation. At present, a stent with a pulmonary valve may be implanted through intervention, reducing the risk of reoperation.

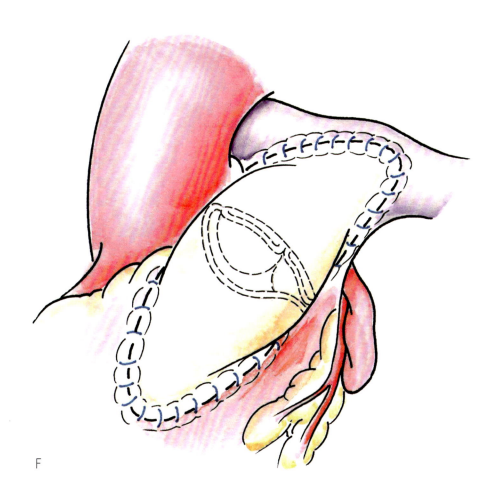

F

图 25-6 带瓣管道重建右心室流出道

A. 法洛四联症漏斗部、肺动脉发育不全或一侧肺动脉闭锁,漏斗部短小,肺动脉瓣口狭小甚至闭锁,形成假性共同动脉干。外科矫治要用到带瓣管道连接右心室及肺动脉。

Figure 25-6 Reconstruction of right ventricular outflow tract with valved conduit

A. TOF is usually associated with hypoplastic infundibulum, hypoplastic PA, or atretic PA on either side, and hence, the short infundibulum and stenotic or even atretic pulmonary valve form a pseudo truncus arteriosus. For surgical repair, a valved conduit is needed to connect the right ventricle and the pulmonary artery.

Continued

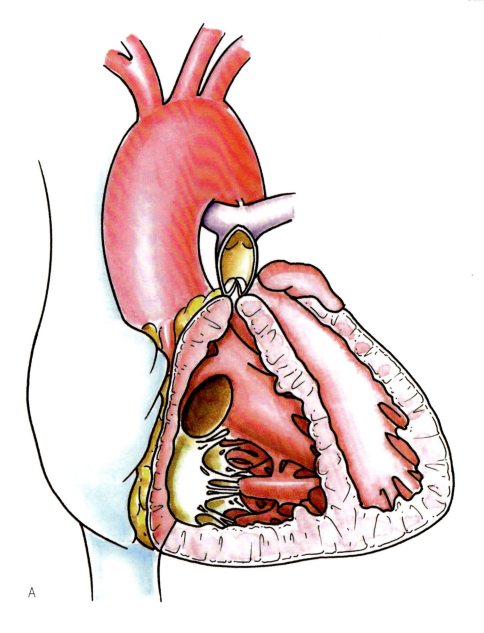

A

图 25-6（续）

B. 带瓣管道有以下三大种类：①同种异体带瓣管道，生物相容性好，使用寿命长，国外已商品化，国内来源有限，少有应用；②牛颈静脉管道，目前国内已有产品，可选用不同规格尺寸，其缺点是极易钙化，使用寿命较短；③ ePTFE 管道，应用 ePTFE 薄膜在管道内腔缝制三个瓣叶，开闭功能良好，但太小的管道不易缝制，并容易产生梗阻。

Figure 25-6 cont'd

B. Valved conduit may be divided into the following three categories. ① Homograft valved conduit. It has good biocompatibility and long service life. It has been commercialized abroad, but it has limited domestic sources and few applications. ② Bovine jugular vein conduit. At present, products with different specifications and sizes are available in China, but they are easy to calcify and have a short service life. ③ ePTFE conduit. Three leaflets are sutured inside the conduit with ePTFE membranes, which usually open and close well. However, a conduit that is too small is not easy to suture and is prone to obstruction.

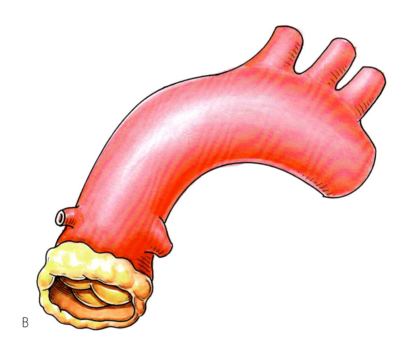

B

图 25-6（续）

C. 取适当尺寸管道,注意瓣口开放的方向。牛颈静脉管道通常产品上有绿线箭头,指示血流方向。使用 5-0 Prolene 线进行连续缝合。一般从远端肺动脉端开始缝合。

Figure 25-6 cont'd

C. Take the conduit of the appropriate size and pay attention to the direction of the valve. Usually, there is a green arrow on the product of the bovine jugular vein conduit, indicating the direction of blood flow. A running suture of 5-0 Prolene is made, usually starting from the distal end of the pulmonary artery.

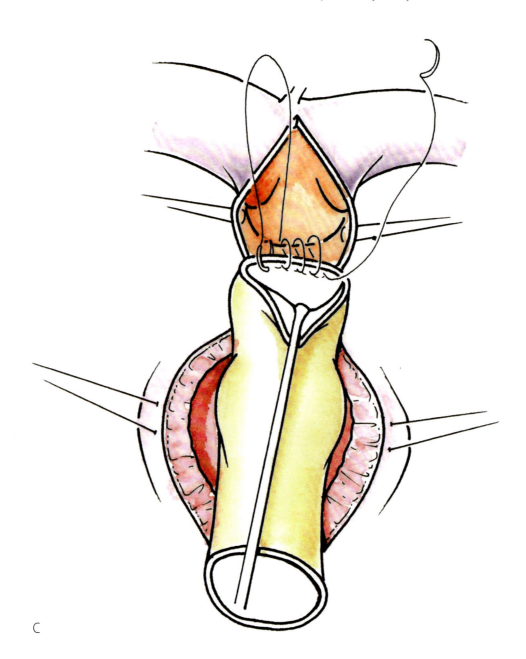

C

图 25-6（续）

D. 再完成近端吻合，进行流出道的吻合。

Figure 25-6 cont'd

D. Anastomosis in the proximal end of the pulmonary artery is then made to accomplish anastomosis of the outflow tract.

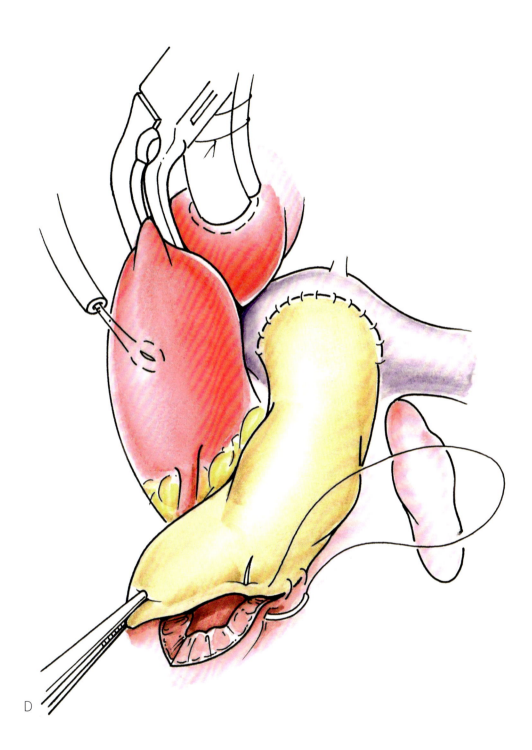

图 25-6（续）
E. 完成带瓣管道与右心室切口吻合。

Figure 25-6 cont'd
E. The anastomosis of the valved conduit and the right ventricular incision is accomplished.

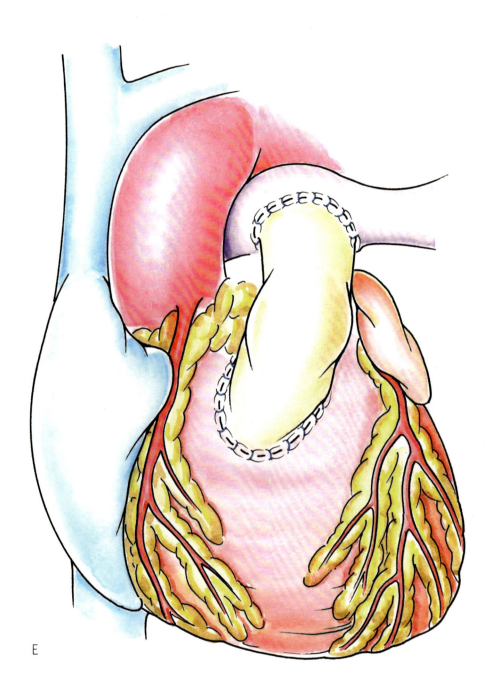

E

26 右心室双出口

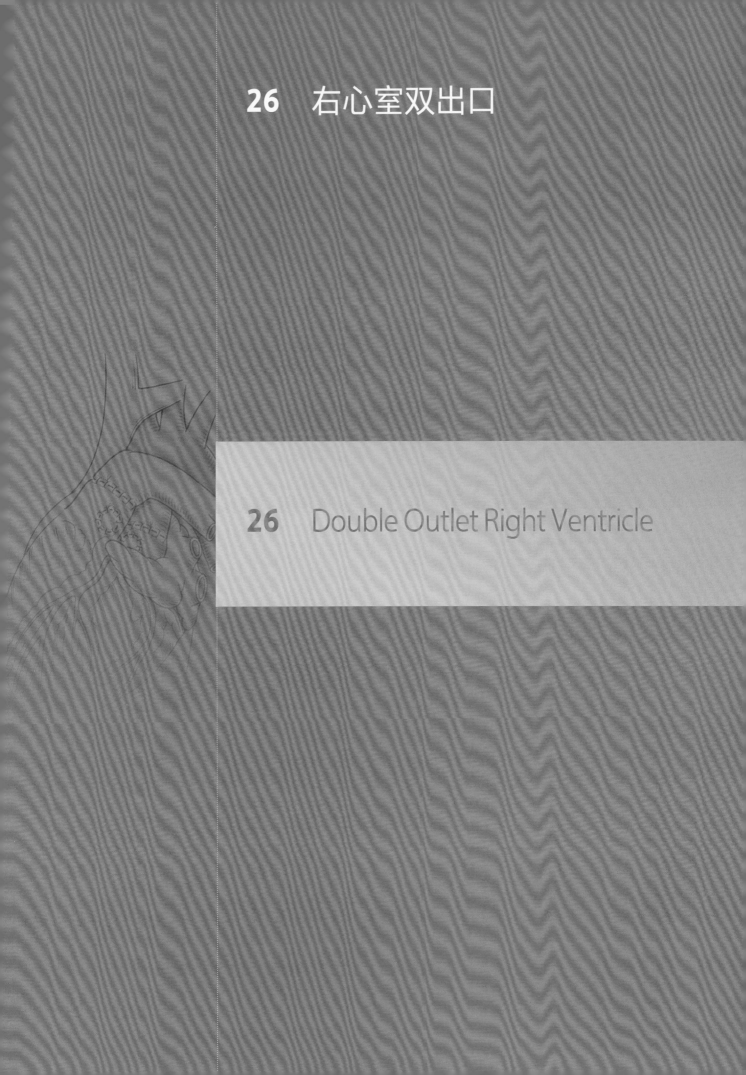

26 Double Outlet Right Ventricle

一、解剖分型

右心室双出口(double outlet right ventricle,DORV)属于圆锥动脉干发育畸形,由于大动脉瓣下的圆锥没有正常的吸收和旋转,主动脉瓣和肺动脉瓣都未能和左心室和二尖瓣完全连接,所以 DORV 的定义是:①主动脉和肺动脉都起源于右心室;②半月瓣和房室瓣被肌性圆锥结构分隔,无纤维联系;③室间隔缺损是左心室唯一的出口。

DORV 传统的分类由 Lev 医生于 1972 年提出,其分类的依据是室间隔缺损的位置和是否合并肺动脉狭窄(图 26-1):①室间隔缺损位于主动脉瓣下;②室间隔缺损位于肺动脉瓣下;③室间隔缺损位于双动脉瓣下;④室间隔缺损远离两大动脉。再根据是否合并肺动脉狭窄分成另外四型,故总共有八大类型。

2000 年美国胸外科医师协会(Society of Thoracic Surgeons,STS)和欧洲心胸外科协会(European Association for Cardio-thoracic Surgery,EACTS)数据库提出了一种新的分类方法:①室间隔缺损型,包括传统分型中主动脉瓣下和双动脉瓣下的室间隔缺损类型;②法洛四联症型,包括主动脉下和双动脉下室间隔缺损,合并有肺动脉狭窄;③大动脉错位型,传统分类的肺动

I. Anatomical Typing

Double outlet right ventricle (DORV) belongs to conotruncal anomalies in which aortic and pulmonary valves do not completely connect to the left ventricle and mitral valve because of abnormal absorption and rotation of arterial conus below the great artery valves. Therefore, DORV is defined as that: ① Both the aortic and pulmonary arteries originate from the right ventricle; ② The semilunar and atrioventricular valves are separated by a muscular conus structure and have no fibrous connections; ③ The ventricular septal defect is the only outlet of the left ventricle.

The traditional classification of DORV was proposed by Dr. Lev in 1972 based on the location of VSD and the presence of pulmonary artery stenosis (Figure 26-1): ① subaortic VSD; ② subpulmonary VSD; ③ doubly committed VSD; ④ remote (or noncommitted) VSD (distal to both great arteries). Based on the presence or absence of pulmonary artery stenosis, four subtypes are distinguished, so a total of eight types are classified.

In 2000, the STS database in the United States and the EACTS database in Europe proposed a new classification method. ① VSD type: the subaortic VSD and the doubly committed VSD in the conventional classification; ② Tetralogy of Fallot type: the subaortic VSD and doubly committed VSD, with pulmonary artery stenosis; ③ transposition of great arteries type: subpulmonary VSD in the classic classification; ④ Remote (or noncommitted) VSD type: uncommitted VSD with or without pulmonary artery stenosis; ⑤ Other

脉瓣下型室间隔缺损；④远离大动脉型，室间隔缺损位置远离两大动脉，合并有或无肺动脉狭窄；⑤其他亚型，右心室双出口合并单心室、心房异构、房室瓣畸形等。

subtypes: DORV combined with single ventricle, atrial isomerism, atrioventricular malformation, etc.

该分类的最大特点是解剖特征与临床手术风险密切相关，也有利于临床数据采集和分析。

The distinguishing feature of this anatomical classification lies in its close relation to the risks of the clinical procedure and its role in helping clinical data collection and analysis.

图 26-1　**右心室双出口解剖分型**
A. 室间隔缺损位于主动脉瓣下。

Figure 26-1　Anatomical typing of double outlet right ventricle
A. Subaortic VSD.

Continued

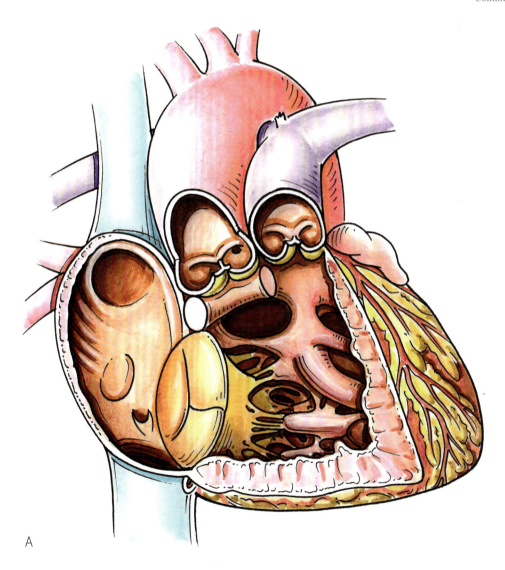

A

图 26-1（续）

Figure 26-1 cont'd

B. 室间隔缺损位于肺动脉瓣下。

B. Subpulmonary VSD.

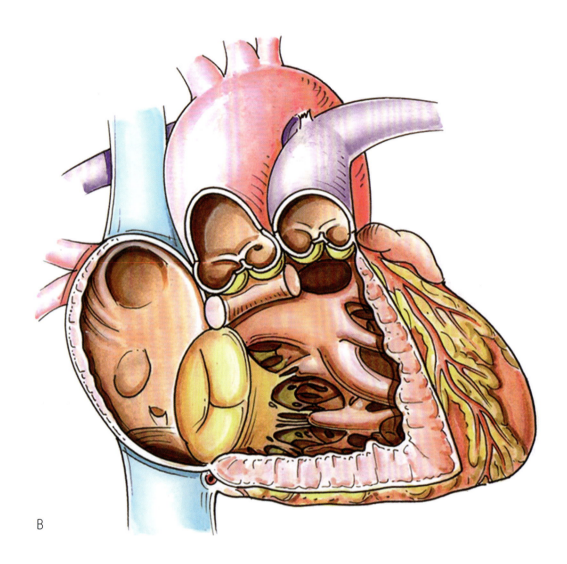

B

图 26-1（续）

Figure 26-1 cont'd

C. 室间隔缺损位于双动脉瓣下。

C. Doubly committed VSD.

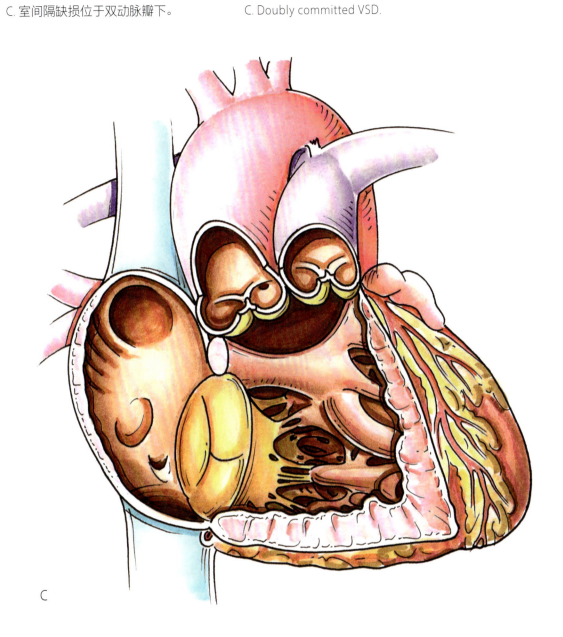

C

图 26-1（续）

Figure 26-1 cont'd

D. 室间隔缺损远离两大动脉。

D. Remote (or noncommitted) VSD (distal to both great arteries).

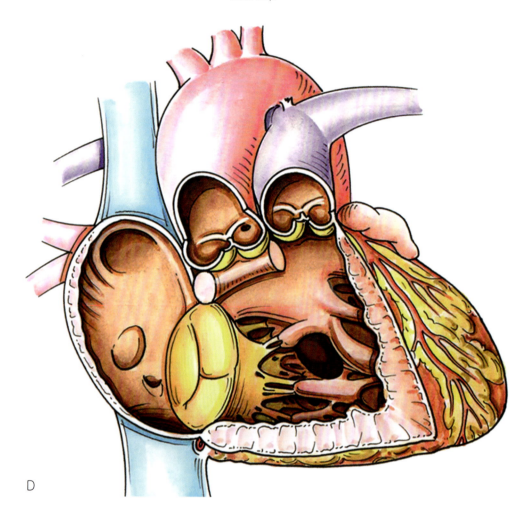

D

二、手术方法

II. Surgical Methods

本章手术方法主要介绍双心室矫治技术。对不适宜做双心室矫治的患者则需考虑做单心室手术矫治（Glenn 或 Fontan 类手术）。

The surgical method section of this chapter mainly introduces the biventricular repair technique. Univentricle repair (the Glenn procedure or the Fontan procedure) should be considered in patients who are not suitable for biventricular repair.

1. 主动脉瓣下室间隔缺损无肺动脉狭窄,补片修补(图 26-2)。

1. Subaortic VSD without pulmonary artery stenosis are closed with patches (Figure 26-2).

图 26-2　**主动脉瓣下室间隔缺损无肺动脉狭窄,补片修补**

A. 主动脉瓣下 VSD 不合并肺动脉狭窄的 DORV 心内隧道修复术:右心室切口,暴露并探查 VSD 与主动脉瓣的位置,VSD 的大小与主动脉瓣及三尖瓣相互位置关系。

Figure 26-2　Subaortic VSD without pulmonary artery stenosis are closed with patches

A. Baffle tunnel repair for DORV with subaortic VSD without pulmonary artery stenosis: A right ventricular incision is made to expose the position of VSD and the aortic valve, and then the VSD's size, as well as its position related to the aortic valve and the tricuspid valves are explored.

Continued

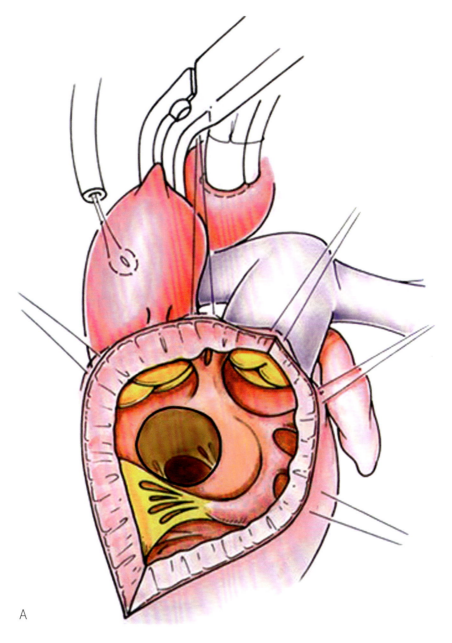

A

图 26-2（续）

B. 为保证左心室流出道通畅，依据 VSD 大小，VSD 与主动脉瓣位置关系，修补后是否影响右心室流出道等因素来决定补片大小。通常室间隔缺损离主动脉瓣近，室间隔缺损足够大，单纯用心包补片修补即可。如果三尖瓣到肺动脉瓣开口的距离大于主动脉瓣直径，流出道补片修补后，一般不会影响左心室流出道通畅。也可选用 ePTFE 管道剪成半隧道状补片修补，确保左心室流出道畅通。

Figure 26-2 cont'd

B. In order to ensure the patency of the left ventricular outflow tract, the size of the patch is determined according to the size of VSD, the relationship between VSD and the position of the aortic valve, and whether the repair affects the right ventricular outflow tract. Generally, the VSD is close to the aortic valve, and the ventricle is large enough, so a routine pericardial patch repair can be considered. If the distance from the tricuspid valve to the pulmonary valve exceeds the diameter of the aortic valve, the repair of the outflow tract with patches usually does not affect the patency of the left ventricular outflow tract. However, it is also feasible to use ePTFE conduit called a half-tunnel-shaped patch to maintain the patency of the left ventricular outflow tract.

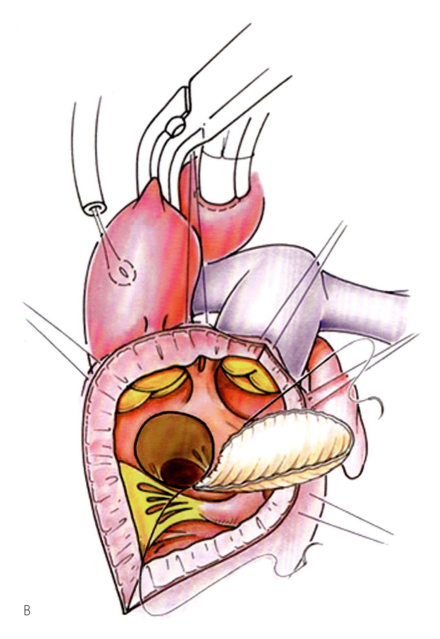

B

图 26-2（续）

C. 对于限制性 VSD，术中应予以 VSD
前上缘肌肉部分切除扩大后，再用相应
大小的探条测量合适再行补片修补。
室间隔缺损修补的补片要足够大，确保
左心室流出道通畅。

Figure 26-2 cont'd

C. For the restrictive VSD, the anterior superior muscle of
the VSD shall be partially excised and enlarged during
operation, and then the defect is closed with a patch after
measuring the length of the defect with a Hegar dilator. The
patch for closing the VSD shall be large enough to ensure
the patency of the left ventricular outflow tract.

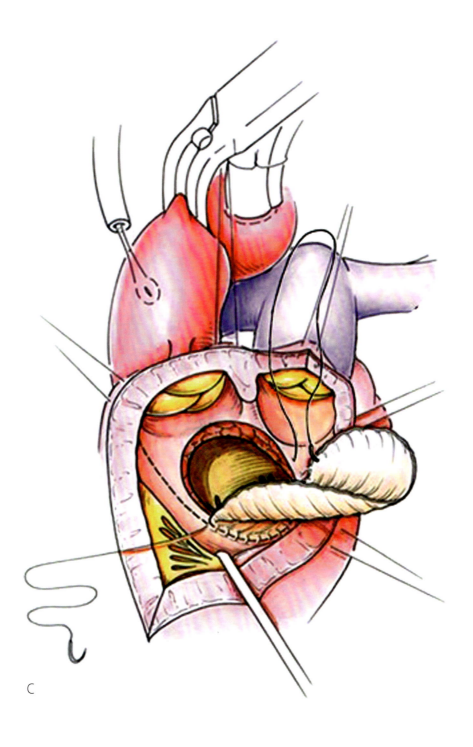

C

图 26-2（续）

Figure 26-2 cont'd

D. VSD 补片修补后左心室到主动脉的
连接形成心内隧道。

D. baffle tunnel from the left ventricle to the aorta is formed
after closure of the VSD with a patch.

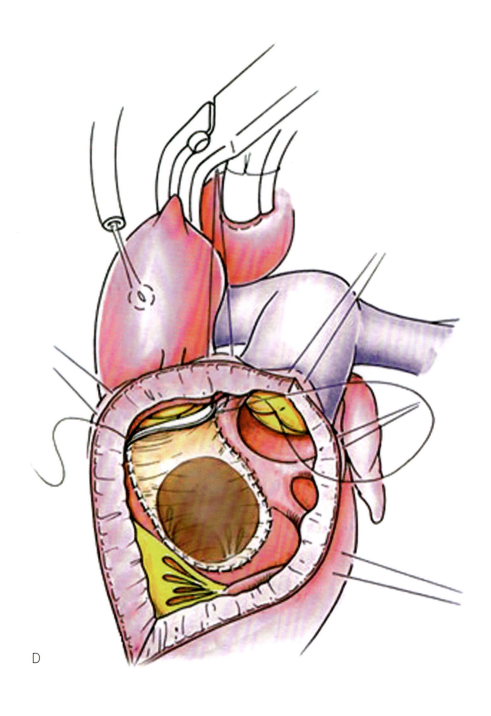

D

图 26-2（续）

Figure 26-2 cont'd

E. 右心室流出道切口一般采用补片予以加宽扩大修补。补片材料可采用心包补片或者 ePTFE 人工血管，也剪成穹形。保证右心室流出道畅通。

E. The right ventricular outflow tract incision is usually augmented and closed with a pericardial patch or an ePTFE graft, which can be cut into a dome shape. Ensure the right ventricular outflow tract is unobstructed.

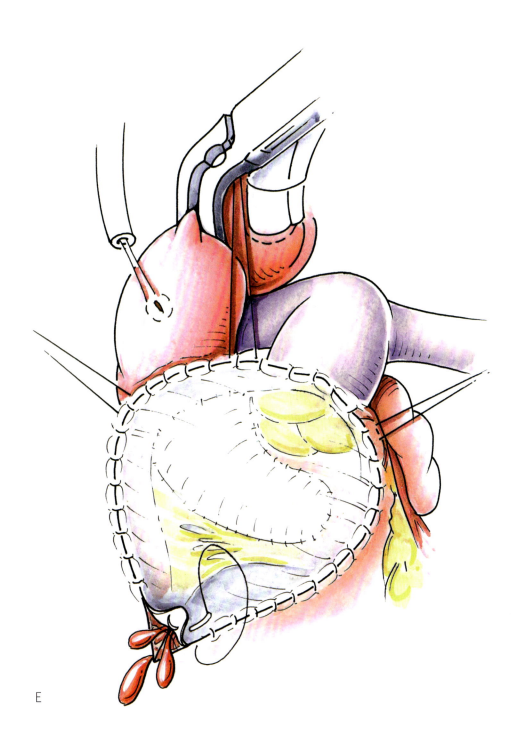

E

图 26-2（续）

F. 右心室双出口主动脉瓣下 VSD 的心内隧道的矫治。

Figure 26-2 cont'd

F. Repair of intracardiac baffles in the DORV with a subaortic VSD.

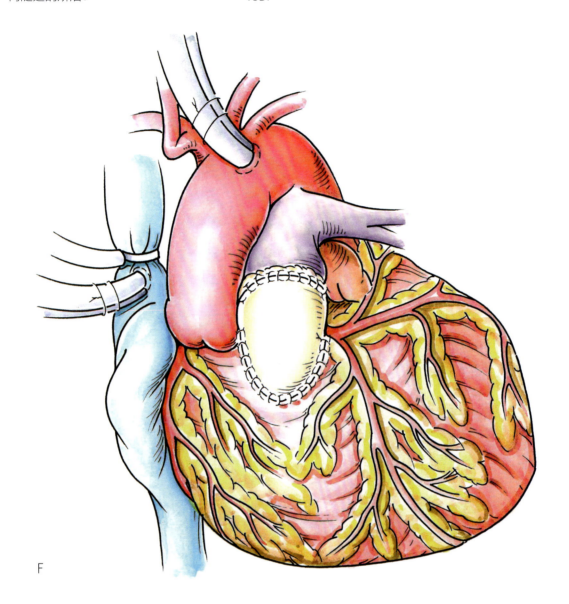

F

2. 肺动脉下室间隔缺损，无肺动脉狭窄：大动脉调转术（动脉转位术） 虽然外科治疗右心室双出口合并肺动脉下室间隔缺损有多种方法，但是大动脉调转术（或者 Lecompte 手术）同时修补室间隔缺损仍是常用的结构治疗。大动脉调转术和其他心内直视手术一样常规

2. Subpulmonary VSD without pulmonary artery stenosis: transposition of great arteries (Arterial Switch operation) Although there are many methods for surgical treatment of DORV with the subpulmonary VSD, transposition of great arteries (or the Lecompte maneuver) with the closure of the VSD is still commonly used structural therapy. As in other open-heart

采用心肺转流术、中低温。心肺转流和心脏停搏后首先修补室间隔缺损,视室间隔缺损大小和在肺动脉下的位置选用经不同途径的修补方法(图 26-3)。

surgeries, transposition of great arteries is also performed under routine cardiopulmonary bypass and moderate hypothermia. The VSD should be repaired at first after cardiopulmonary bypass and cardiac arrest, and based on the size of the VSD and its location under the pulmonary artery, the repair can be performed with different approaches (Figure 26-3).

图 26-3　**肺动脉下室间隔缺损,无肺动脉狭窄:大动脉调转术(动脉转位术)**

A. 右心室双出口合并肺动脉下室间隔缺损。

Figure 26-3　Subpulmonary VSD without pulmonary artery stenosis: transposition of great arteries (arterial switch operation)

A. DORV with the subpulmonary VSD.

Continued

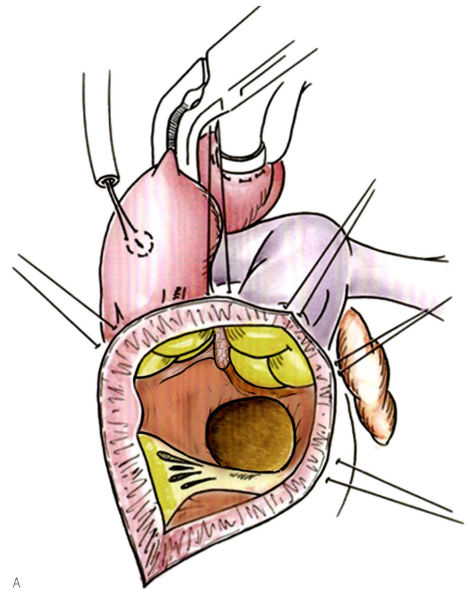

A

图 26-3（续）

Figure 26-3 cont'd

B. 经右心房修补室间隔缺损。

B. VSD repair via the right atrial approach.

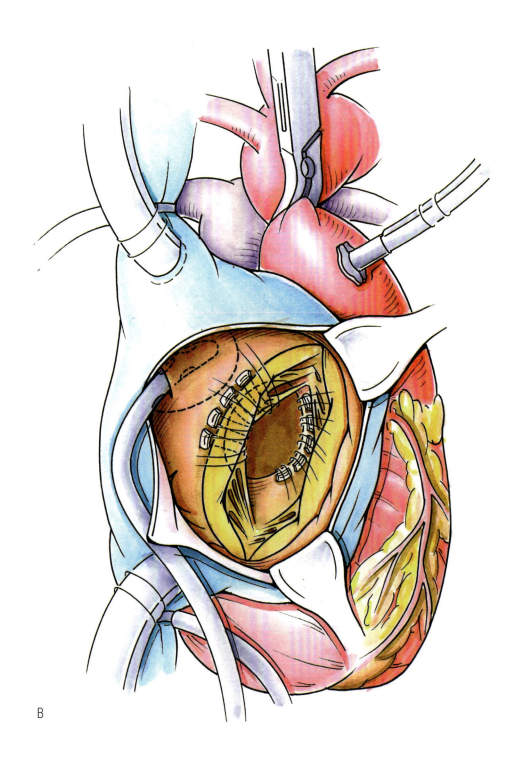

B

图 26-3（续）

Figure 26-3 cont'd

C. 经肺动脉修补室间隔缺损。

C. VSD repair via the transpulmonary arterial approach.

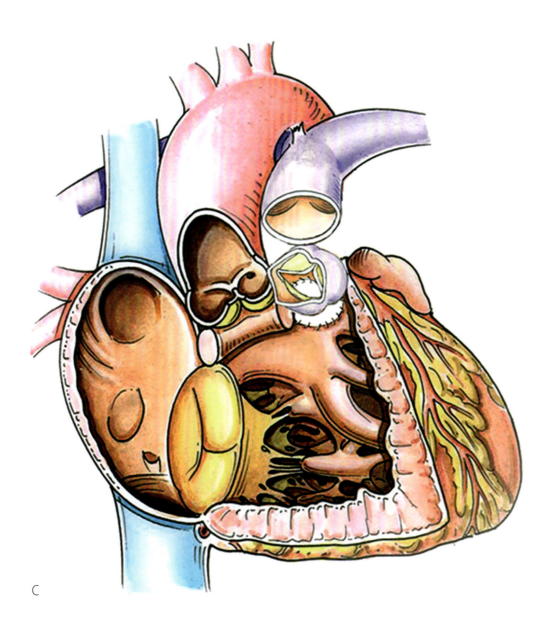

C

图 26-3（续）

D. 经右心室切口修补室间隔缺损。

Figure 26-3 cont'd

D. VSD repair via right ventricular incision.

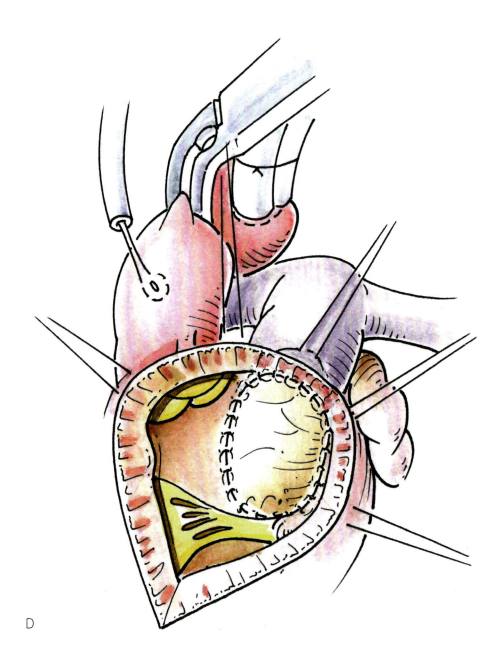

D

图 26-3（续）

E. 右心室双出口的大动脉位置都在右心室，而且多数并行排列，所以在大动脉调转时要考虑是否进行 Lecompte 换位。如果不做 Lecompte 换位，升主动脉横断的位置要高于肺动脉数毫米（虚线显示）。

Figure 26-3 cont'd

E. Since the great arteries of DORV are located at the right ventricle and most are in parallel, it is necessary to consider whether to perform the Lecompte maneuver for the transposition of great arteries. If the Lecompte transposition is not considered, the transverse incision in the ascending aorta should be made several millimeters above the pulmonary artery (the dotted line).

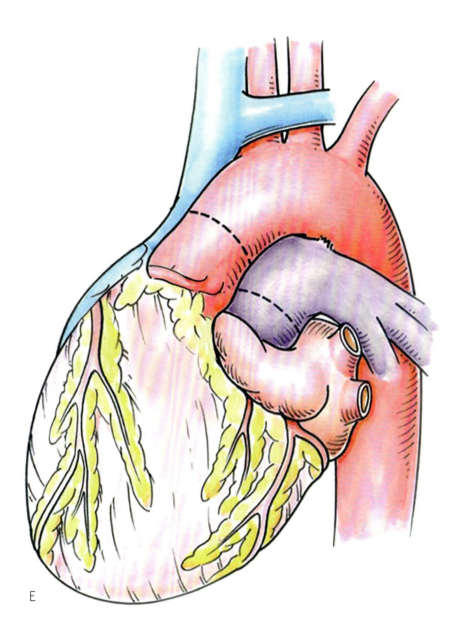

E

图 26-3（续）

F. 从主动脉根部纽扣状切下左右冠状动脉。由于升主动脉在肺动脉右侧，右冠状动脉移植到肺动脉需要一定的长度，因此右冠状动脉需要充分的游离段，避免冠状动脉移植后张力过大。相反，左冠状动脉从冠状动脉窦右侧移植到左侧，冠状动脉长度足够，吻合时要注意左冠状动脉在移植和充盈后不要因为过长而扭曲。主动脉被切下的左右冠状动脉窦口可用自身心包片或牛心包修补。

Figure 26-3 cont'd

F. Left and right coronary buttons are cut from the aortic root. Since the ascending aorta lies on the right side of the pulmonary artery, the right coronary artery grafting to the pulmonary artery requires a sufficient length, and the right coronary artery should be sufficiently freed to avoid excessive tension after grafting. In contrast, when the left coronary artery is grafted from the right side of the coronary sinus to the left side, the coronary artery shall be of sufficient length, and during anastomosis, attention should be paid to controlling the length of the left coronary artery to avoid distortion after implantation and inflation. The left and right coronary ostium from which the aorta is excised can be repaired with a pericardial patch or bovine pericardium.

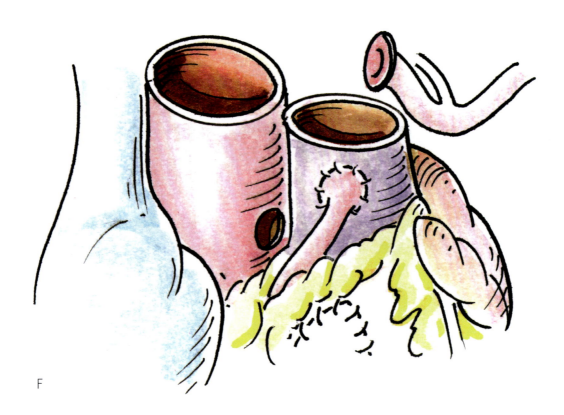

F

图 26-3（续）

G. 不做 Lecompte 换位的大动脉调转术可以直接把肺动脉远端切口和较长的升主动脉近端切口吻合。婴幼儿可以使用 6-0 的 Prolene 缝线，稍大的儿童可用 5-0 号缝线连续缝合。如果担心儿童成长后吻合口狭窄，吻合口的前 1/3 可采用间断吻合。

Figure 26-3 cont'd

G. In arterial switch operation without Lecompte operation, the incision in the distal pulmonary artery can be directly anastomosed to the incision in the proximal ascending aorta. The incision should be closed with 6-0 Prolene sutures in infants and young children, and closed by running sutures with 5-0 Prolene in slightly elder children. The first one-third of the anastomotic stoma can be closed with interrupted sutures if there is concern of anastomotic stenosis after children grow up.

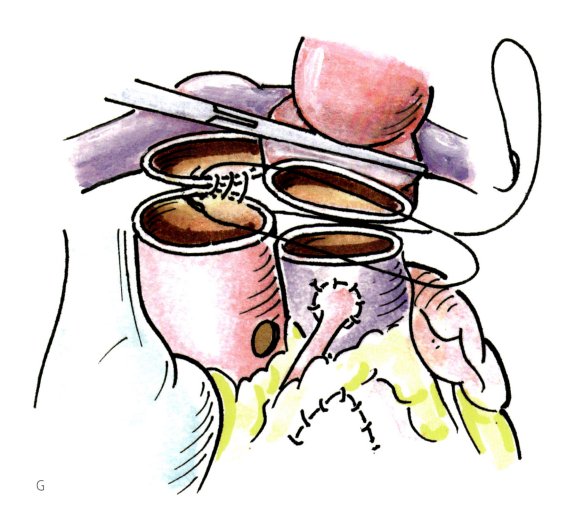

G

图 26-3（续）

H. 大动脉调转术后, 没有进行 Lecompte 操作, 升主动脉在肺动脉前侧。

Figure 26-3 cont'd

H. After arterial switch operation without Lecompte procedure, the ascending aorta lies anterior to the pulmonary artery.

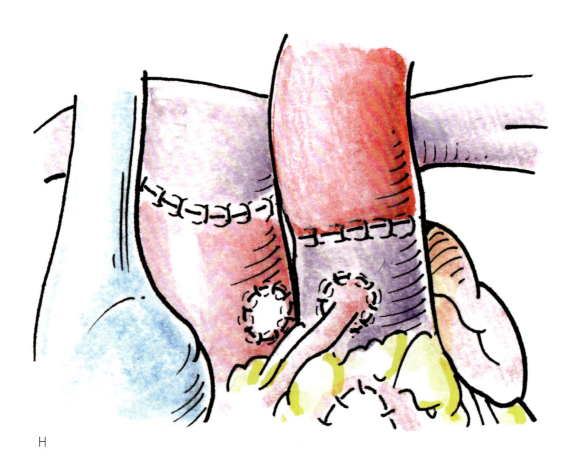

H

图 26-3（续）

Figure 26-3 cont'd

I. 大动脉调转和 Lecompte 换位手术后，肺动脉骑跨在升主动脉前。

I. After the arterial switch operation and Lecompte procedure, the pulmonary artery overrides the ascending aorta.

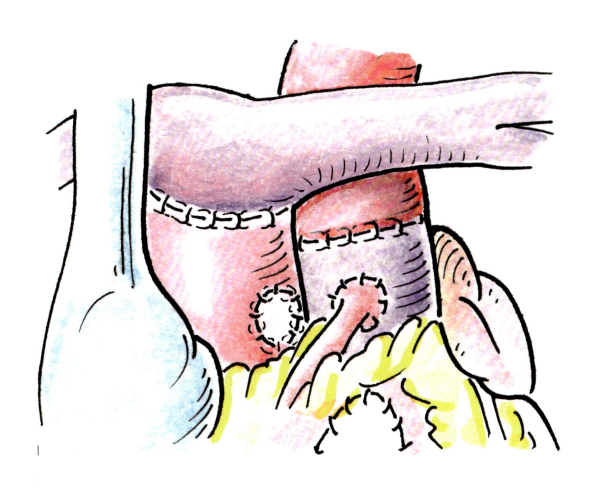

3. 肺动脉瓣下室间隔缺损，无肺动脉狭窄：室间隔缺损补片 - 左心室流出道重建（Kawashima 手术）

对于右心室双出口两大动脉侧侧位合并肺动脉下室间隔缺损的病例可以采用 Kawashima 手术。Kawashima 手术原则上切除漏斗部圆锥隔，扩大流出道，所以室间隔缺损必须扩大。由于隧道位于三尖瓣和肺动脉瓣之间，此两者间必须有足够的距离。如果三尖瓣腱索异常附着漏斗隔，则不能进行此手术。

3. Subpulmonary VSD without pulmonary artery stenosis: VSD patch-left ventricular outflow tract reconstruction (the Kawashima procedure)

A Kawashima procedure is appropriate for cases in which the side-by-side great arteries of DORV are associated with subpulmonary VSD. The Kawashima procedure, in principle, is to remove the infundibular septum and widen the outflow tract, so the VSD must be augmented. Since the tunnel is located between the tricuspid valve and the pulmonary valve, there must be a sufficient distance between both valves. If the tricuspid

右心室双出口两大动脉前后位合并肺动脉下室间隔缺损的病例也可以采用 Patrick-McGoon 手术治疗。即使用一个裤衩形复杂的心室内补片重建左心室流出道（图 26-4）。

chordae tendineae are abnormally attached to the infundibular septum, this procedure cannot be performed. Patrick-McGoon operation is applicable to the cases of DORV with antero-posterior relation of the great arteries complicated with subpulmonary VSD. Reconstruct the left ventricular outflow tract using a trouser-shaped complex intraventricular patch (Figure 26-4).

图 26-4　肺动脉瓣下室间隔缺损，无肺动脉狭窄：室间隔缺损补片 - 左心室流出道重建（Kawashima 手术）

A. 对于右心室双出口两大动脉侧侧位合并肺动脉下室间隔缺损的病例可以采用 Kawashima 手术，心内穹形补片重建左心室流出道。

Figure 26-4　Subpulmonary VSD without pulmonary artery stenosis: VSD patch-left ventricular outflow tract reconstruction (the Kawashima procedure)

A. Kawashima procedure is appropriate for cases in which the side-by-side great arteries of DORV are associated with subpulmonary VSD. The left ventricular outflow tract is to be reconstructed with an intracardiac dome-shaped patch.

Continued

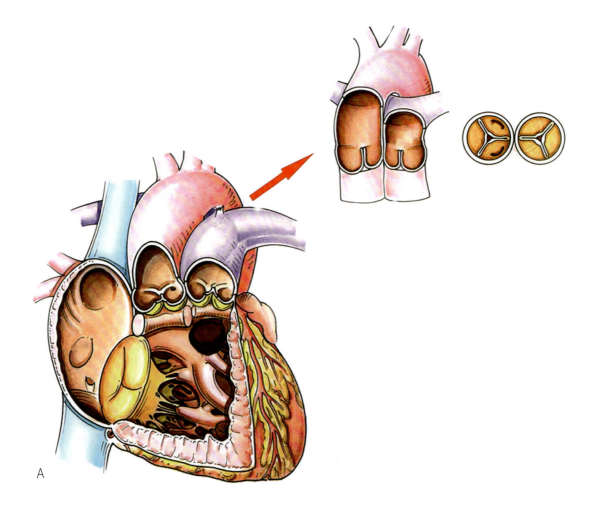

A

图 26-4（续）

Figure 26-4 cont'd

B. 右心室双出口两大动脉前后位合并肺动脉下室间隔缺损的病例可以采用Patrick-McGoon 手术治疗。补片隧道沿肺动脉瓣左前方走行，直接将室间隔缺损和主动脉连接起来。而静脉血流直接由三尖瓣进入肺动脉，不必考虑三尖瓣和肺动脉瓣之间的距离。如果室间隔缺损太小，需要扩大。

B. Patrick-McGoon operation is applicable to the cases of DORV with antero-posterior relation of the great arteries complicated with subpulmonary VSD. Intraventricular baffle which extends to the left anterior aspect of the pulmonary valve directly connects the VSD to the aorta. The venous blood flows directly from the tricuspid valve into the pulmonary artery, regardless of the distance between the tricuspid valve and the pulmonary valve. The VSD needs to be enlarged if it is too small.

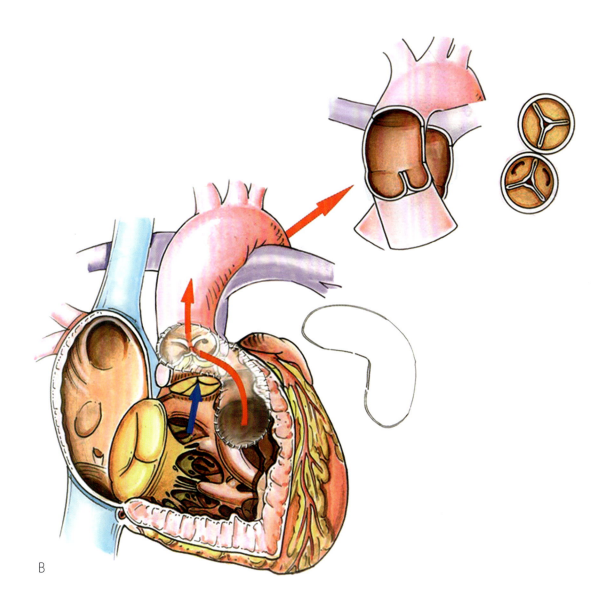

B

图 26-4（续）

Figure 26-4 cont'd

C. Kawashima 手术要切除两大动脉下的漏斗隔圆锥体，使内隧道补片无梗阻，虚线显示的是要切除的漏斗隔圆锥体和扩大室间隔缺损。

C. The Kawashima procedure is to remove the infundibular septum below two large arteries, which leaves the inner tunnel patch unobstructed. The dotted line indicates the infundibular septum to be removed and the enlarged VSD.

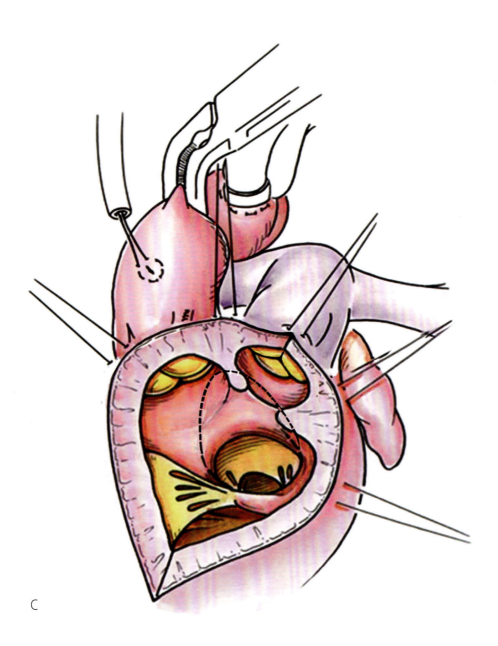

C

图 26-4（续）

Figure 26-4 cont'd

D. 两大动脉下漏斗隔圆锥体切除后，使用穹形补片连接室间隔缺损和升主动脉。

D. After the resection of the infundibular septum under the two great arteries, a dome-shaped patch is used to connect the VSD and the ascending aorta.

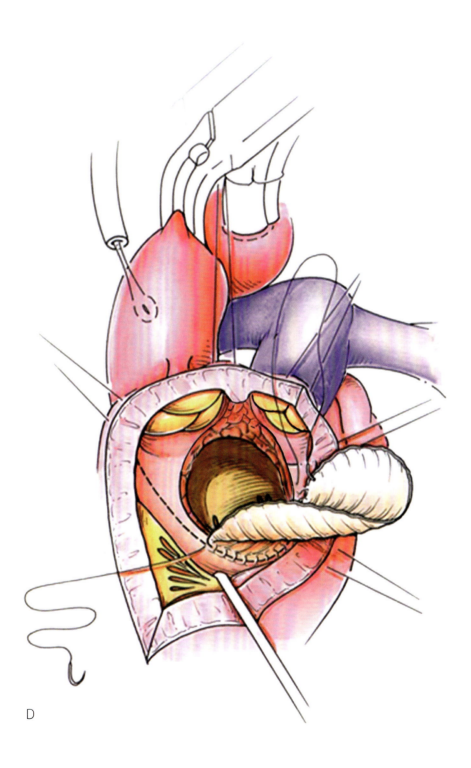

D

图 26-4（续）

Figure 26-4 cont'd

E. 动脉血从室间隔缺损经隧道进入主动脉。

E. Arterial blood enters the aorta from the VSD through the intraventricular tunnels.

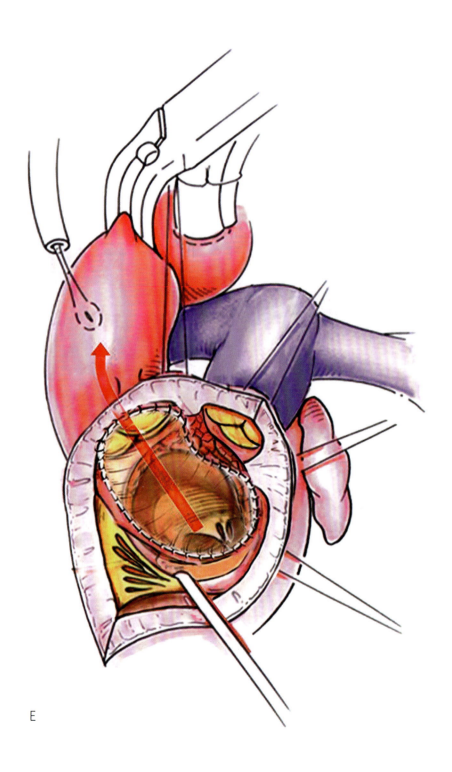

E

图 26-4（续）

Figure 26-4 cont'd

F. 右心室切口需要用补片扩大，必要时主肺动脉也可用补片扩大，避免流出道狭窄。

F. Right ventricular incision is to be widened with patches. If necessary, the main pulmonary artery can also be expanded with patches to avoid stenosis of the outflow tract.

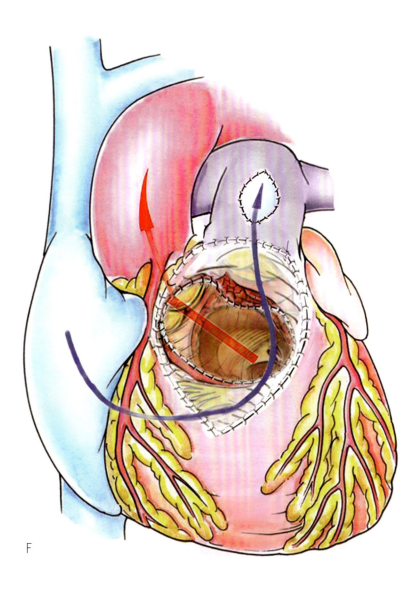

F

4. 肺动脉下室间隔缺损，合并肺动脉狭窄：Rastelli 手术（图 26-5）

4. Subpulmonary VSD complicated with pulmonary artery stenosis: the Rastelli procedure (Figure 26-5)

图 26-5　肺动脉下室间隔缺损，合并肺动脉狭窄：Rastelli 手术

A. 右心室双出口肺动脉瓣下室间隔缺损伴肺动脉狭窄：VSD 的上缘邻近肺动脉瓣，与主动脉瓣较远。如果室间隔缺损较小，虚线显示切除室间隔缺损上缘肌肉，扩大室间隔缺损，连接室间隔缺损和主动脉开口。

Figure 26-5　Subpulmonary VSD complicated with pulmonary artery stenosis: the Rastelli procedure

A. DORV with subpulmonary VSD and pulmonary stenosis: the upper edge of the VSD is adjacent to the pulmonary valve and distal to the aortic valve. If the VSD is small, the muscles attached on the superior border of the VSD are to be resected (as the dotted line shows), and the VSD should be enlarged to get close to the aortic opening.

Continued

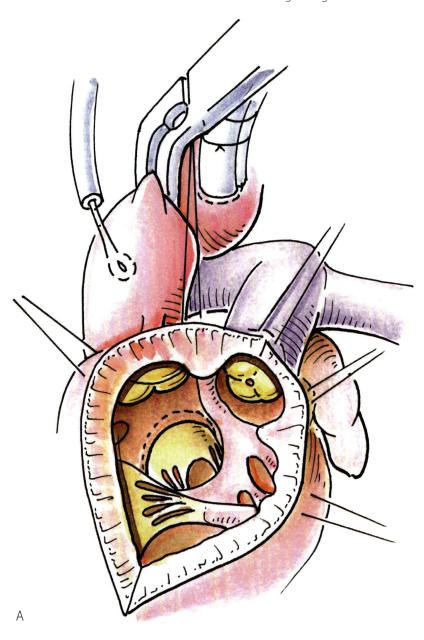

A

图 26-5（续）

Figure 26-5 cont'd

B. 剪去狭小的室间隔缺损上缘，下缘常有三尖瓣腱索，避免切断。扩大室间隔缺损成为左心室—主动脉的流出道。

B. Cut off the small upper edge of VSD and avoid cutting the tricuspid valve chordae which often appears on the lower edge. The VSD is to be enlarged into the outflow tract of the left ventricular.

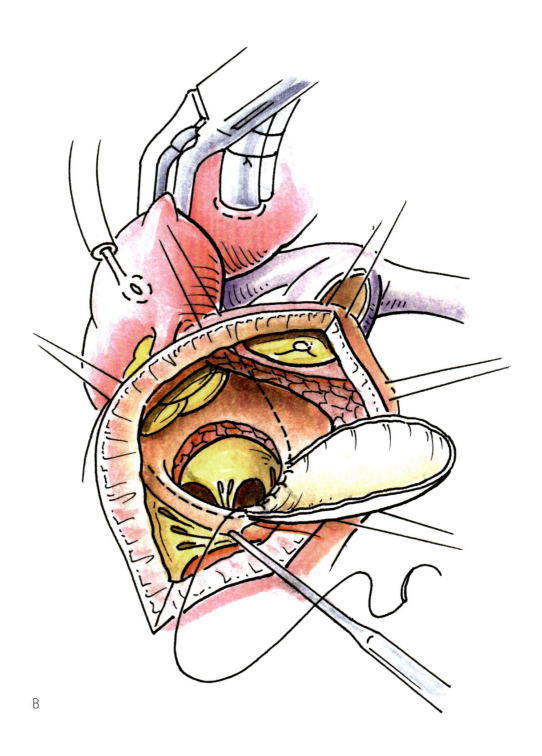

B

图 26-5（续）

C. 测量室间隔缺损的最下缘到升主动脉的距离和需要补片的穹形宽度，按测量的大小把人工血管剪成穹状补片，将补片沿虚线连续缝合在室间隔缺损边缘覆盖到主动脉口。选用 5-0 Prolene 缝线连续缝合。缝合一般从室间隔缺损的下缘开始，边缝边调整补片的位置和大小。

Figure 26-5 cont'd

C. Measure the distance from the lowest edge of the ventricular defect to the ascending aorta and the width of the dome-shaped patch required. The artificial vessel is cut into dome-shaped patches of sufficient size, and the patches are sutured continuously with 5-0 Prolene sutures along the dotted liney to cover the edge of the VSD to the aortic opening. The stitching generally starts from the lower edge of the VSD, and the position and size of the patch are adjusted when suturing.

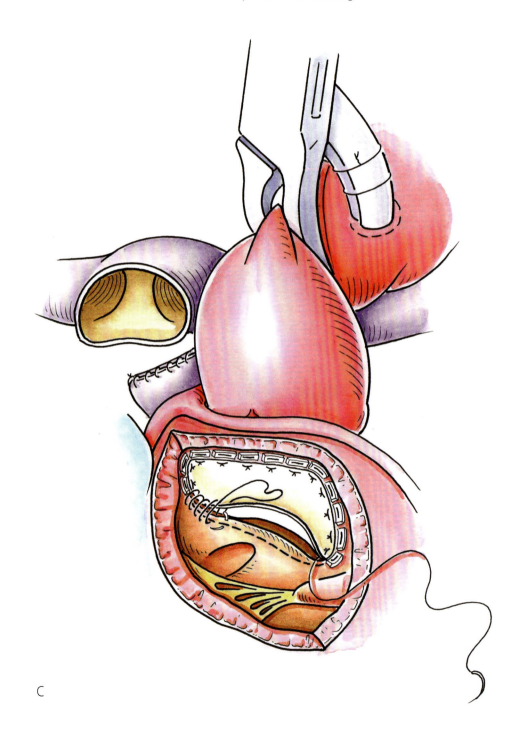

C

图 26-5（续）

D. 将狭窄的肺动脉近端横断，连续缝合关闭。使用同种或者异种肺动脉带瓣管道连接右心室流出道和肺动脉远端。

Figure 26-5 cont'd

D. Transversely incise the stenotic pulmonary artery and close the proximal end by running suture. The right ventricular outflow tract and the distal pulmonary artery are connected with the valved homograft or heterologous conduits.

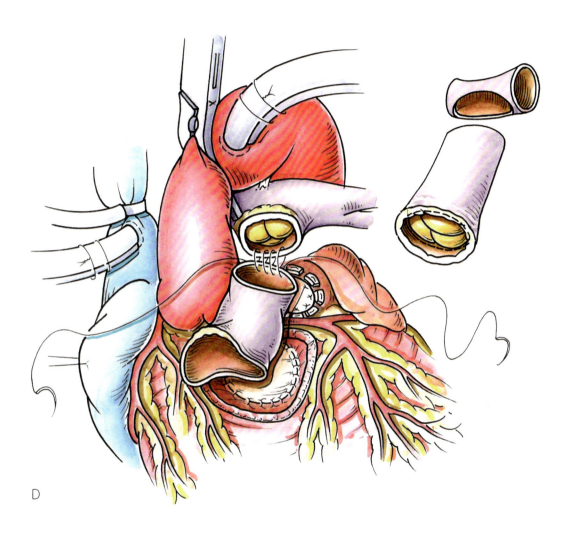

D

图 26-5（续）

Figure 26-5 cont'd

E. Rastelli 手术后,肺动脉带瓣移植物连接右心室。右心室流出道可再用补片加宽,保证左右心室流出道都畅通。

E. After the Rastelli procedure, the valved pulmonary artery graft is attached to the right ventricle. The right ventricular outflow tract can be widened with a patch again to ensure the patency of both ventricular outflow tracts.

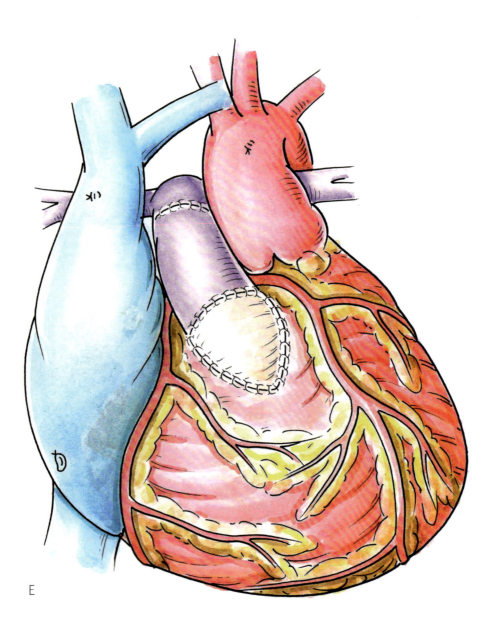

E

5. 肺动脉下室间隔缺损合并主动脉狭窄（Damus-Kaye-Stansel手术） 右心室双出口肺动脉下室间隔缺损合并主动脉狭窄，结构矫正手术的方法是左右流出道重建术，又称 Damus-Kaye-Stansel 手术。手术的原理是通过隧道样补片修补肺动脉下室间隔缺损并连接到肺动脉瓣。主肺动脉横断后和升主动脉连接成为左心室的新建流出道。右心室流出道将用带瓣移植物（多为同种或者异种管道）和肺动脉连接。手术的条件是室间隔缺损足够大，小的室间隔缺损要扩大，穹形补片的宽度相当于肺动脉瓣直径的 2/3。如果肺动脉瓣下圆锥影响新建流出道的通畅，必须切除（图 26-6）。

5. Subpulmonary VSD with aortic stenosis (the Damus-Kaye-Stansel procedure) Left and right ventricular outflow tract reconstruction, also known as Damus-Kaye-Stansel procedure, is the structural surgery for DORV with subpulmonary VSD and aortic stenosis. The principle of the procedure is to repair the subpulmonary VSD through a tunnel-like patch and connect it to the pulmonary valve. The main pulmonary artery is transversed and joined to the ascending aorta to create a new outflow tract in the left ventricle. The right ventricular outflow tract is to be connected to the pulmonary artery with a valved graft (mostly homograft or heterologous conduits). The operation conditions are that the VSD is large and it is to be widened if not large enough, and the width of the dome-shaped patches should be equal to 2/3 of the pulmonary valve diameter. If the subpulmonary conus affects the patency of the new outflow tract, it must be excised (Figure 26-6).

A. 右心室双出口肺动脉下室间隔缺损合并主动脉狭窄。

A. DORV with subpulmonary VSD with aortic stenosis.

Continued

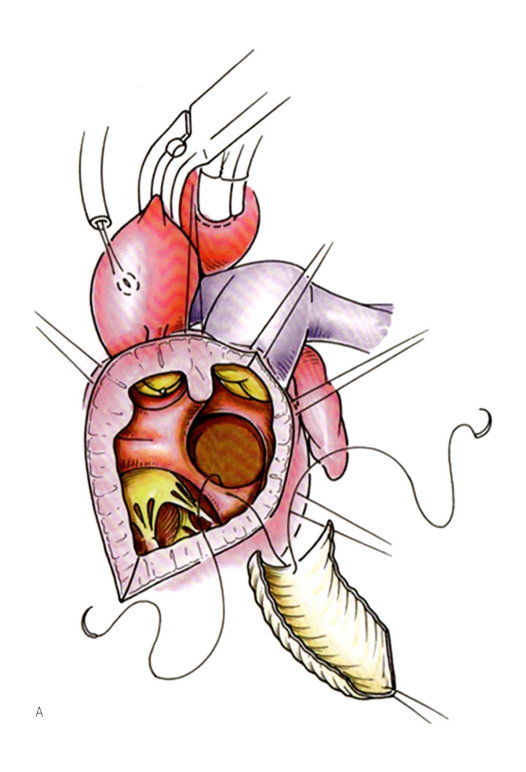

A

图 26-6（续）

B. 经右心室流出道切口用穹形补片覆盖室间隔缺损和肺动脉瓣。补片用 Prolene 线连续缝合。

Figure 26-6 cont'd

B. A dome-shaped patch is used to cover the VSD and the pulmonary valve through an incision in the right ventricular outflow. The patch is sutured continuously with Prolene suture.

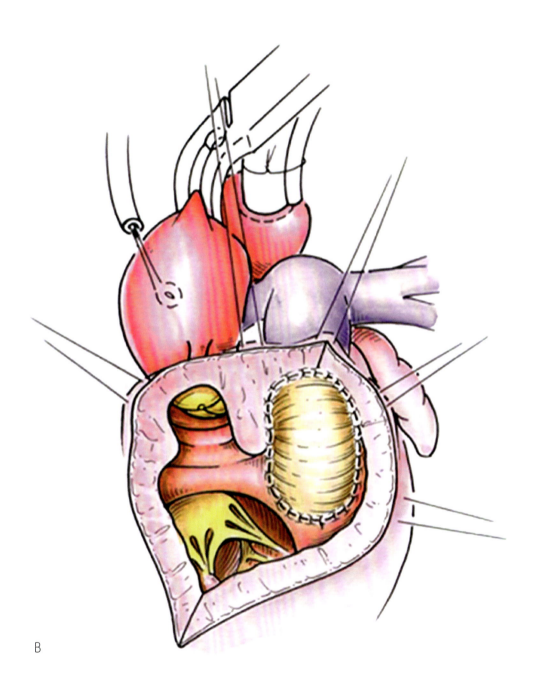

B

图 26-6（续）

C. 同样经右心室切口，若有主动脉瓣反流可利用补片缝闭主动脉瓣开口。主动脉瓣下的圆锥因为不影响新建流出道，可以和补片一起缝上。升主动脉和肺动脉分叉处虚线位置将成为主肺动脉和升主动脉的吻合口。

Figure 26-6 cont'd

C. If aortic regurgitation is present, the aortic valve can be closed with a patch also through the right ventricular incision, and the conus under the aortic valve can be sutured together as it does not interfere with the new outflow tract. The dotted line at the bifurcation of the ascending aorta and the pulmonary artery will serve as an anastomotic stoma between the main pulmonary artery and the ascending aorta.

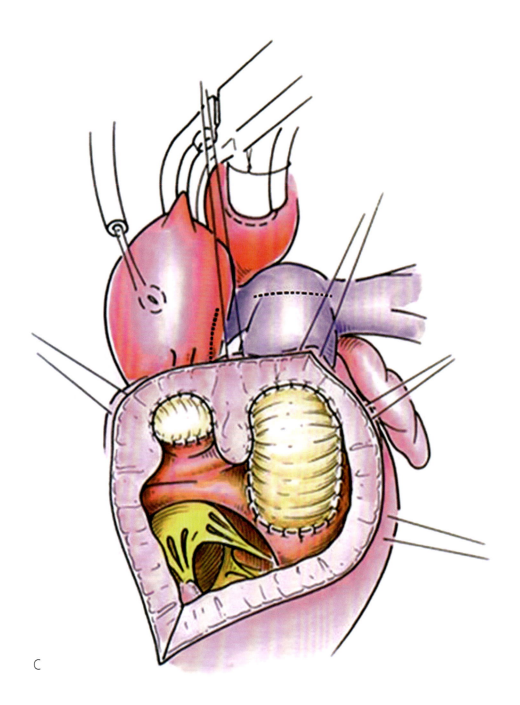

C

图 26-6（续）

D. 在肺动脉分叉处横断肺动脉，延长靠近主动脉侧的肺动脉切口。在升主动脉靠近肺动脉侧纵行切开升主动脉。

Figure 26-6 cont'd

D. The pulmonary artery is transversed at the pulmonary artery bifurcation, and the pulmonary artery incision close to the aortic side is extended. Dissect longitudinally the ascending aorta proximal to the anterior aspect of the pulmonary artery.

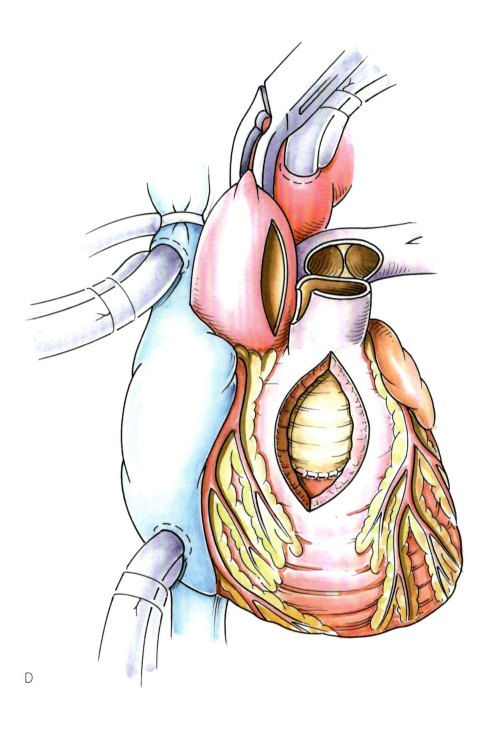

D

图 26-6（续）

E. 将主肺动脉近端切口修整与主动脉
侧壁切口行端侧吻合。

Figure 26-6 cont'd

E. Trim the proximal incision of the main pulmonary artery and connect it to the aortic sidewall with end-to-side anastomosis.

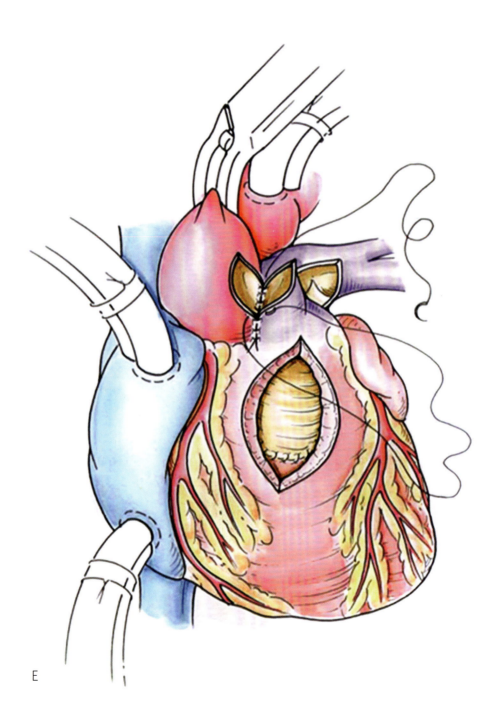

E

图 26-6（续）

Figure 26-6 cont'd

F. 在主肺动脉和升主动脉吻合时由于主肺动脉的长度不合适，或者过度扭曲使得新建的左心室流出道不通畅，可选取适当大小的心包补片或人工血管补片，剪成楔形与升主动脉侧切口、主肺动脉近端切口进一步吻合，形成左心室通过室间隔缺损、主肺动脉近端、升主动脉通道的"顶棚"吻合，形成新建左心室流出道。

F. In the anastomosis of the main pulmonary artery and the ascending aorta, a pericardial patch or artificial vascular patch of appropriate size can be selected in the presence of inappropriate length of the main pulmonary artery or the newly established left ventricular outflow tract obstruction caused by excessive distortion. The patch is cut into wedges and sewn to lateral incision of the ascending aorta and proximal end of the main pulmonary artery to form left ventricle-VSD-proximal end of the aorta-the ascending aorta channel, forming a new left ventricular outflow tract.

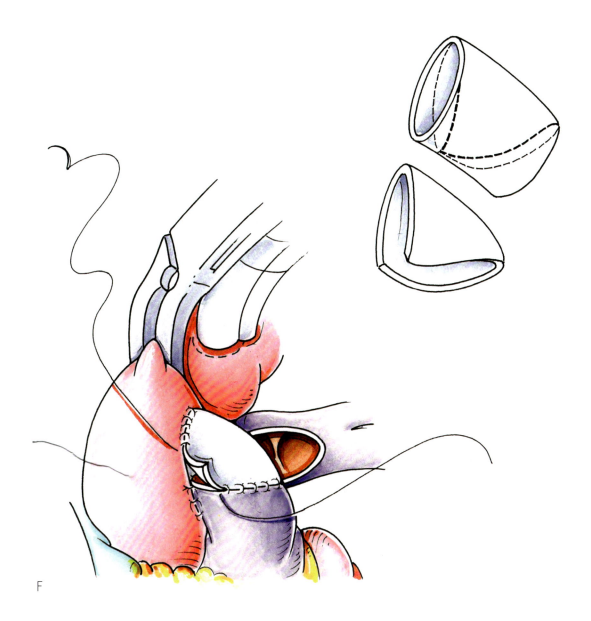

F

图 26-6（续）

G. 选择长度合适的带瓣同种或异种管道与肺动脉远端切口（左右肺动脉起始部）吻合。吻合从后缘开始，使用 Prolene 缝线，连续缝合。

Figure 26-6 cont'd

G. Select valved homograft or heterologous conduit of sufficient length to anastomose to the distal end of the pulmonary artery (left and right pulmonary artery origin) with running Prolene sutures, from the posterior margin.

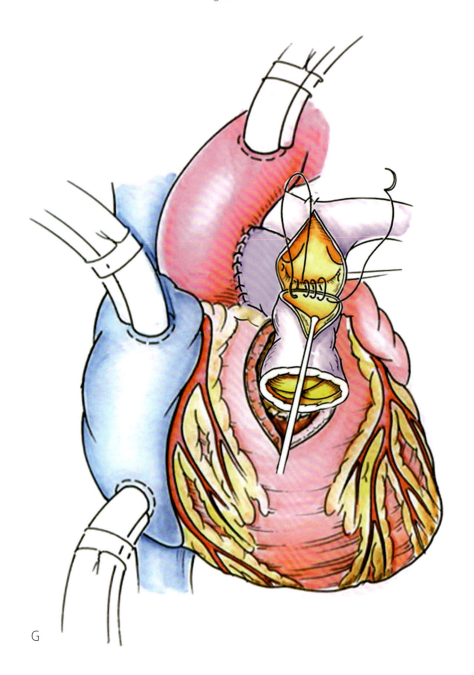

G

图 26-6（续）

H. 右心室切口上缘与带瓣管道近端下缘吻合，形成右心室流出道后壁。

Figure 26-6 cont'd

H. The upper edge of the right ventricular incision is anastomosed to the proximal lower edge of the valved conduit to form the posterior wall of the right ventricular outflow tract.

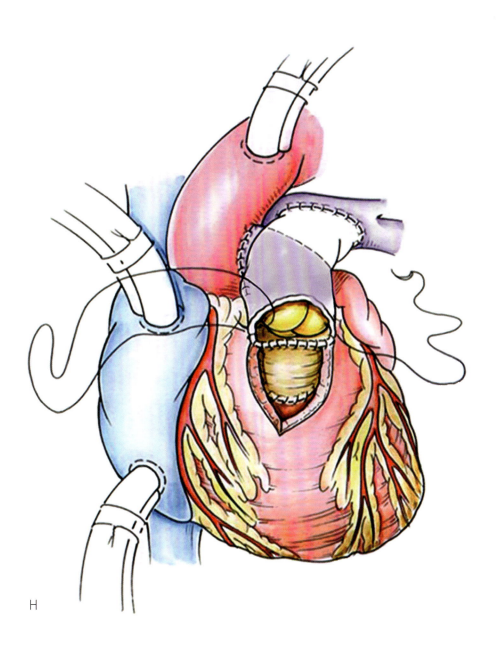

H

图 26-6(续)

I. 再将合适大小补片覆盖在带瓣肺动脉和右心室流出道,完成右心室流出道的重建。

Figure 26-6 cont'd

I. A patch of sufficient size is to cover the valved pulmonary artery and the right ventricular outflow tract to reconstruct the right ventricular outflow tract.

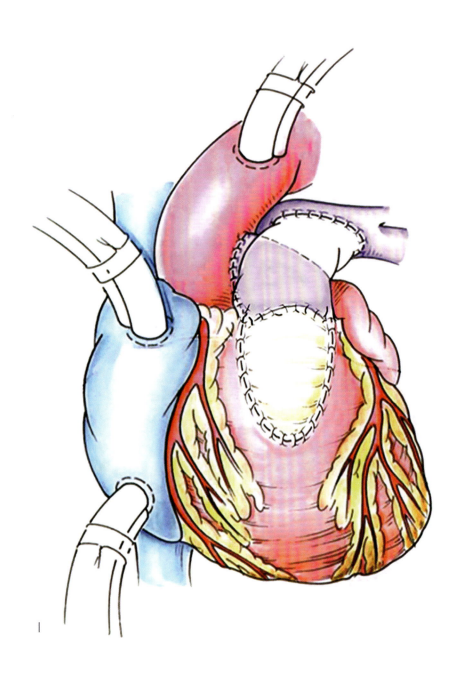

6. 肺动脉下室间隔缺损，三尖瓣腱索异常附着在漏斗圆锥隔（REV Lecompte 手术） 右心室双出口合并肺动脉下室间隔缺损、三尖瓣腱索异常附着在漏斗圆锥隔，无法直接采用心内隧道修补时，可以采用 REV Leompte 手术，该方法也适用肺动脉狭窄（左心室流出道）。切开右心室流出道前壁，暴露室间隔缺损位置（图 26-7）。

6. Subpulmonary VSD with abnormally attached tricuspid chordae tendineae on the infundibular septum (the REV Lecompte procedure) In cases of DORV with subpulmonary VSD and abnormally attached tricuspid chordae tendineae, the REV Lecompte procedure can be performed when the defect cannot be repaired directly by baffle tunnel or pulmonary artery stenosis is present (left ventricular outflow tract). Dissect the anterior wall of the right ventricular outflow tract to expose the location of the VSD (Figure 26-7).

图 26-7 　肺动脉下室间隔缺损，三尖瓣腱索异常附着在漏斗圆锥隔（REV Lecompte 手术）

A. 升主动脉远端插管，行心肺转流术。心脏停搏后，左心室引流管置入左心房，心肺转流术结束后关闭房间隔缺损。右心室下部行垂直右心室切口，三尖瓣腱索乳头肌在室间隔缺损上方附着于漏斗圆锥隔。分别在主动脉和肺动脉瓣上 5mm~1cm 处横断。REV Lecompte 手术类似大动脉调转术，把肺动脉换位至升主动脉前，因此要充分游离主动脉和肺动脉。肺动脉分离到左右肺动脉分叉处。

Figure 26-7 　Subpulmonary VSD with abnormally attached tricuspid chordae tendineae on the infundibular septum (the REV Lecompte procedure)

A. The distal end ascending aorta is cannulated to establish cardiopulmonary bypass. After the heart stops beating, the left heart drainage tube is placed into the left atrium, and the atrium is closed after the termination of the cardiopulmonary bypass. A vertical incision is made in the lower right ventricle, and the tricuspid chordae tendineae papillary muscle is attached to the infundibular septum above the ventricular defect. Transverse incisions are performed 5mm-1cm above the aortic and pulmonary valves, respectively. The REV Lecompte procedure resembles the transposition of great arteries. The pulmonary artery is translocated anterior to the ascending aorta, so the pulmonary artery is to be sufficiently freed from the aorta. The pulmonary artery is separated to the left and right pulmonary artery bifurcation.

Continued

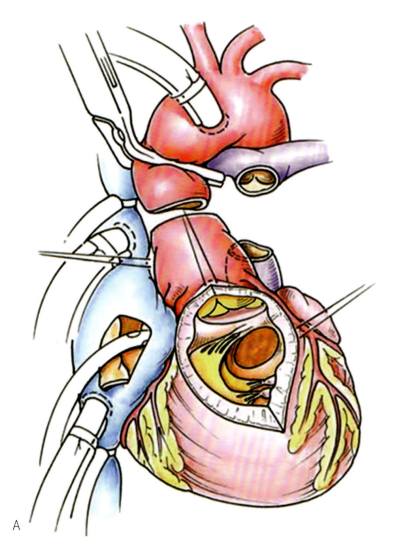

A

图 26-7（续）

B. 如果位于两个半月瓣之间的漏斗圆锥部妨碍室间隔缺损和主动脉之间建立隧道，可以将漏斗隔切断。通常主动脉位于肺动脉右后方时，漏斗隔并不妨碍建立内隧道，并可以形成其前壁。当大动脉处于前后位关系时，圆锥漏斗隔常位于室间隔缺损和主动脉之间。要切除漏斗隔，先做 2 个平行于主动脉轴的切口。在紧靠主动脉瓣下方做第 3 个切口，与前面 2 个切口会合。要非常注意避免损伤主动脉瓣。如果有三尖瓣腱索异常附着漏斗部，切断其漏斗隔附着处的乳头肌和腱索，但要保持附着部位完整，而不能切除，缝闭肺动脉近端。

Figure 26-7 cont'd

B. The infundibular septum can be cut off if the infundibulum between the two semilunar valves prevents the construction of a tunnel connecting VSD to the aorta. Generally, when the aorta is located at the right rear of the pulmonary artery, the infundibular septum does not preclude the construction of an internal tunnel but forms its anterior wall. With the anterior-to-posterior relation of the great arteries, the infundibular septum is often located between the VSD and the aorta. In order to resect the septum, two incisions are made parallel to the aortic axis and the third incision is performed just below the aortic valve, converging the first two incisions. Great care should be taken to avoid damaging the aortic valve. If the chordae tendineae are abnormally attached to the infundibula, cut off the papillary muscles and chordae tendineae at the attachment of the infundibula, but remain the attachment site instead of resection and close the proximal end of the pulmonary artery.

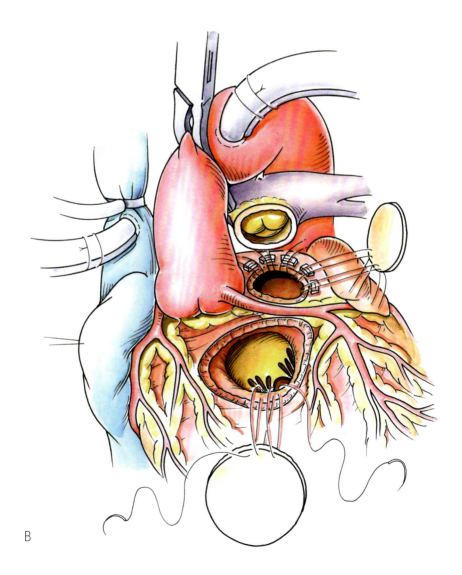

B

图 26-7（续）

C. 穹形补片修补室间隔缺损。补片闭合室间隔缺损后将包含有三尖瓣腱索附着处的漏斗隔缝合到内隧道补片的右心室面上。测试三尖瓣功能，Lecompte 换位把离断并充分游离的肺动脉向前提到主动脉前面。在肺动脉后连续缝合升主动脉。

Figure 26-7 cont'd

C. Close VSD with dome-shaped patches. When closing VSD with patches, the infundibular septum to which the tricuspid chordae tendineae attach should be sutured to the right ventricle. The tricuspid valve's function is tested, and the Lecompte maneuver is performed to advance the transected and fully dissected pulmonary artery to the anterior aspect of the aorta. The ascending aorta is sutured continuously behind the pulmonary artery.

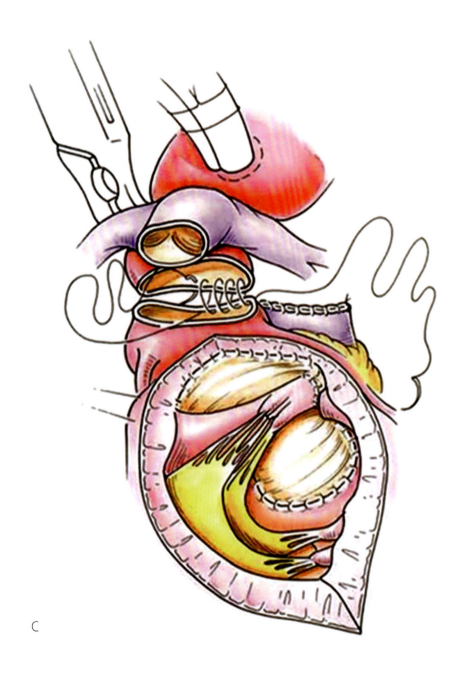

C

图 26-7 (续)
D. 用自制单瓣叶的补片连续缝合关闭右心室切口。

Figure 26-7 cont'd
D. Close the right ventricular incision using continuous suture with patches with a self-made single leaflet.

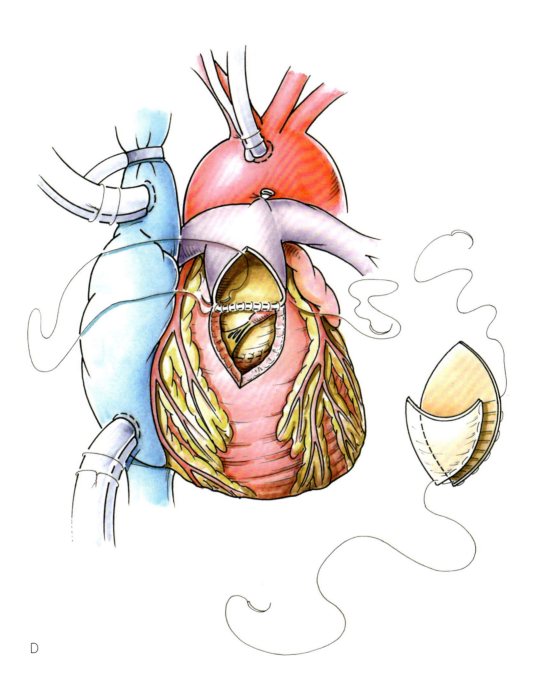

D

图 26-7（续）

Figure 26-7 cont'd

E. 也可使用同种异体带瓣管道关闭右心室流出道。

E. The right ventricular outflow tract can also be closed with the valved homograft conduit.

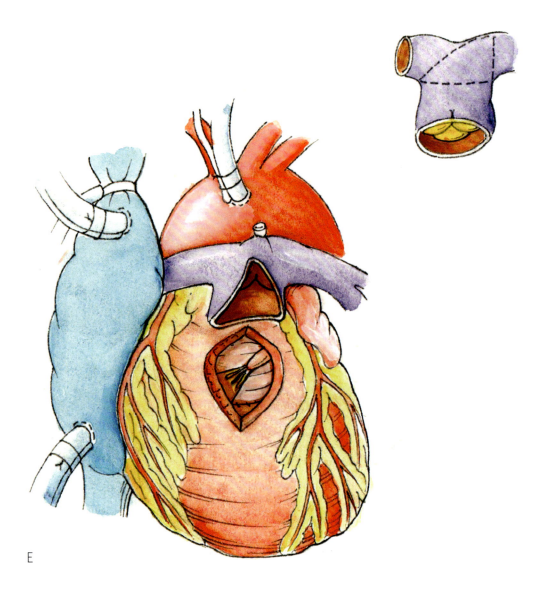

E

图 26-7（续）

Figure 26-7 cont'd

F. 必要时近端可加用心包补片扩大右心室流出道。

F. The pericardial patch can be placed on the proximal end to widen the right ventricular outflow tract if necessary.

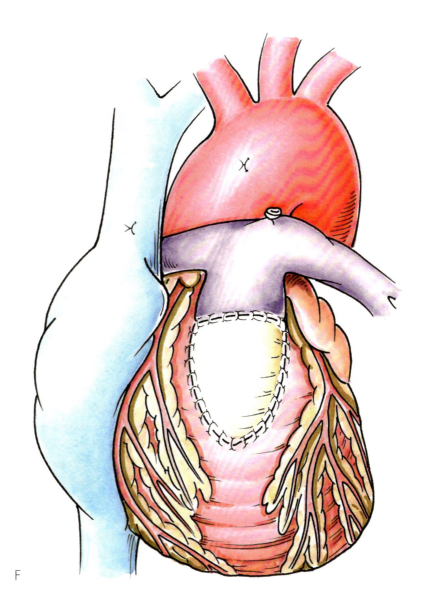

F

7. 双动脉下室间隔缺损 补片修补室间隔缺损,补片扩大右心室流出道或者 Rastelli 手术(图 26-8)。

7. Doubly committed VSD Patch repair for VSD, patch enlargement of right ventricular outflow tract, or the Rastelli procedure (Figure 26-8).

图 26-8 双动脉下室间隔缺损
A. 双动脉下室间隔缺损一般缺损较大,离双动脉开口不远。

Figure 26-8 Doubly committed VSD
A. Doubly committed VSD is often large, not far from the opening of both arteries.

Continued

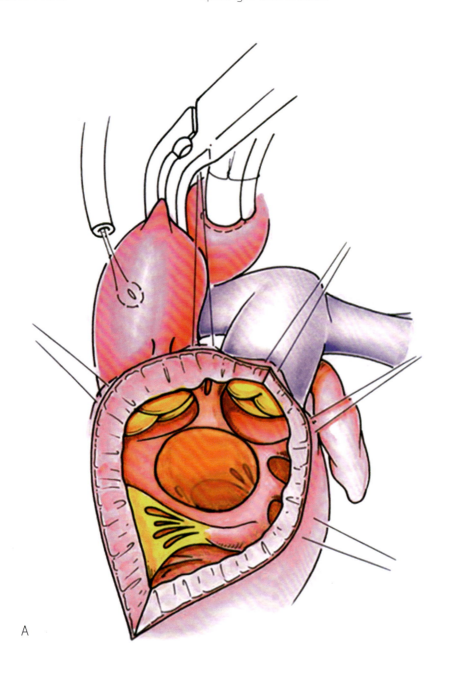

A

图 26-8（续）

B. 如双动脉下室间隔缺损的上缘距离主动脉瓣偏远，几乎横跨右心室流出道，为确保术后左心室流出道畅通，一般采用人工血管作补片，穹形补片的宽度至少是主动脉直径的 2/3。

Figure 26-8 cont'd

B. If the superior margin of the doubly committed VSD is distal to the aortic valve and almost spans the right ventricular outflow tract, in order to ensure the patency of the left ventricular outflow tract after the operation, an artificial vascular conduit is generally used as a patch, and the width of the dome-shaped patch is at least 2/3 of the diameter of the aorta.

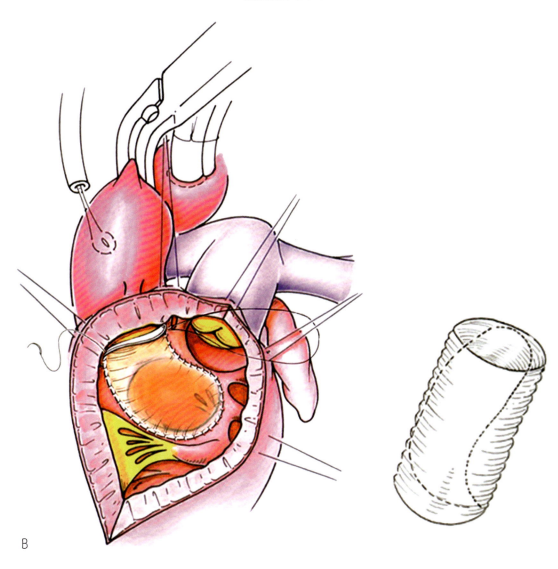

B

图 26-8（续）

C. 肺动脉没有狭窄，穹形补片修补室间隔缺损和重建左心室流出道后，如果右心室流出道还有足够空间，右心室流出道可直接用补片加宽重建。必要时可跨瓣把补片修补到主肺动脉。红色箭头所示动脉血由左心室经室间隔缺损、新建左心室流出道、主动脉瓣进入体循环。蓝色箭头的静脉血仍旧通过三尖瓣、右心室和新建流出道进入肺循环。

Figure 26-8 cont'd

C. After the repair of the VSD with a dome-shaped patch and reconstruction of the left ventricular outflow tract, if there is sufficient space in the right ventricular outflow tract without pulmonary stenosis, the right ventricular outflow tract can be directly widened with a patch. If necessary, the patch can be sutured to the main pulmonary artery across the valve. From the left ventricle, arterial blood, as indicated by the red arrow, travels through the VSD and the constructed left ventricular outflow tract and enters the systemic circulation via the aortic valve. Venous blood, indicated by the blue arrow, enters the pulmonary circulation through the tricuspid valve, the right ventricle, and the new outflow tract.

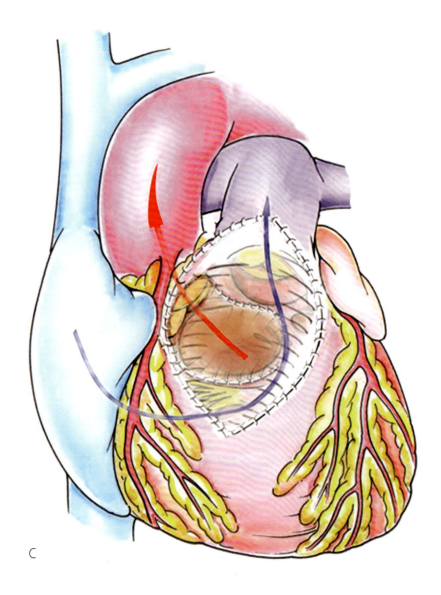

C

图 26-8（续）

D. 若有肺动脉瓣和肺动脉狭窄,特别是肺动脉瓣下有圆锥体或粗大异常肌束,则需要同时重建右心室与肺动脉连接。穹形补片修补室间隔缺损和重建左心室流出道后,按虚线横断主肺动脉。离断肺动脉的近端可以用连续缝合封闭。双动脉下室间隔缺损合并肺动脉狭窄多为婴幼儿。

Figure 26-8 cont'd

D. When the defect is complicated with pulmonary valve stenosis and pulmonary stenosis, especially with thick muscle bundle and the arterial cone under the pulmonary valve, it is necessary to simultaneously reconstruct the connection between the right ventricle and pulmonary artery and repair the defect. After the closure of the VSD and reconstruction of the left ventricular outflow tract with a dome patch, a transverse is performed in the main pulmonary artery as depicted by the dotted line. The proximal end of the transected pulmonary artery can be closed with a continuous suture. Doubly committed VSD combined with pulmonary stenosis mostly appears in infants and young children.

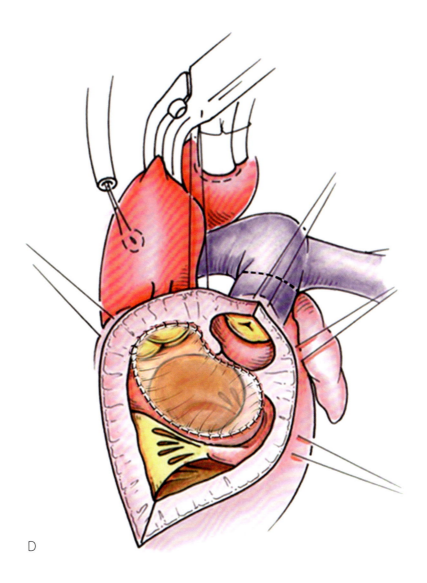

D

图 26-8（续）

E. 分叉部的肺动脉和右心室切口距离
较长，一般直接选用同种异体带瓣管道
（Homograft）或异种带瓣管道如牛颈静
脉，也可选用自制 ePTFE 带瓣管道，连
接肺动脉和右心室切口，新建右心室流
出道。

Figure 26-8 cont'd

E. The pulmonary artery at the bifurcation is distal to the right ventricle incision, so generally valved homograft or heterologous conduit such as bovine jugular vein, or self-made ePTFE valved conduit is taken to connect the pulmonary artery and right ventricle incision and reconstruct the right ventricular outflow tract.

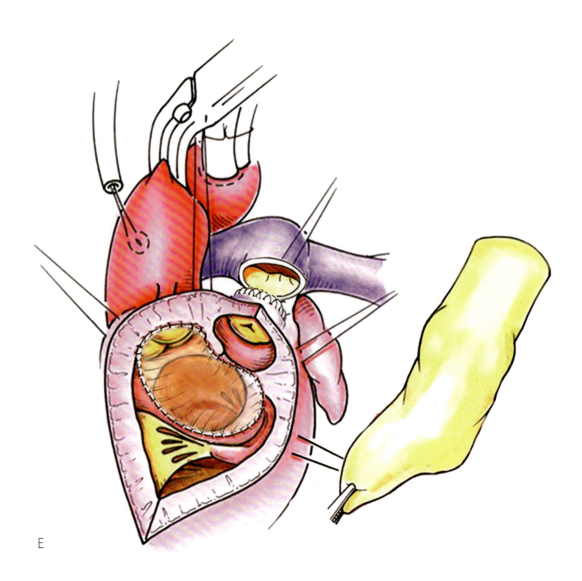

E

图 26-8（续）

F. 新建右心室流出道缝合完毕。红色箭头所示动脉血从左心室经室间隔缺损通过新建左心室流出道、主动脉瓣进入升主动脉。蓝色箭头所示静脉血从右心房经三尖瓣、新建右心室流出道进入肺动脉。

Figure 26-8 cont'd

F. The newly-built right ventricular outflow tract. Arterial blood (red arrows) originates in the left ventricle and passes through the new left ventricular outflow tract and the aortic valve into the ascending aorta. Venous blood (blue arrow) originates in the right atrium, and travels through the tricuspid valve and the established right ventricular outflow tract, and enters the pulmonary artery.

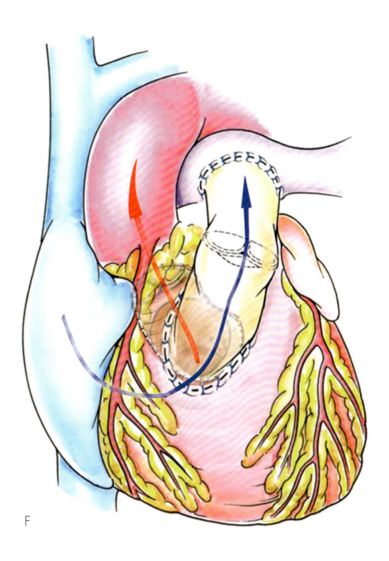

F

8. 远离两大动脉的不定性室间隔缺损：双心室矫治（内隧道 + Rastelli 手术） 右心室双出口合并远离两大动脉瓣的室间隔缺损靠近房室瓣，又称房室通道型室间隔缺损。这些患者的室间隔缺损可以做心室内隧道修补（图 26-9）。

图 26-9 **远离两大动脉的不定性室间隔缺损：双心室矫治（内隧道 +Rastelli 手术）**

A. 如果大动脉瓣下圆锥体或间隔圆锥体影响血流，需要向前上方扩大室间隔缺损以便建立内隧道。虚线显示扩大室间隔缺损切除圆锥体的部分。这部分操作是这一手术的关键也是难点。

8. Indefinite VSD remote from two large arteries: biventricular repair (baffle tunnel + the Rastelli procedure) A VSD in DORV which is far from both great arteries, is commonly near the atrioventricular valve, known as atrioventricular canal VSD. The patient can be treated with baffle tunnel repair (Figure 26-9).

Figure 26-9 Indefinite VSD remote from two large arteries: biventricular repair (baffle tunnel + the Rastelli procedure)

A. If the subaortic conus or septal cone interferes with blood flow, the VSD is to be enlarged anteriorly in order to establish an internal tunnel. The dotted line shows the portion to be widened and incised. This part of the operation is the key point and the difficulty of this procedure.

Continued

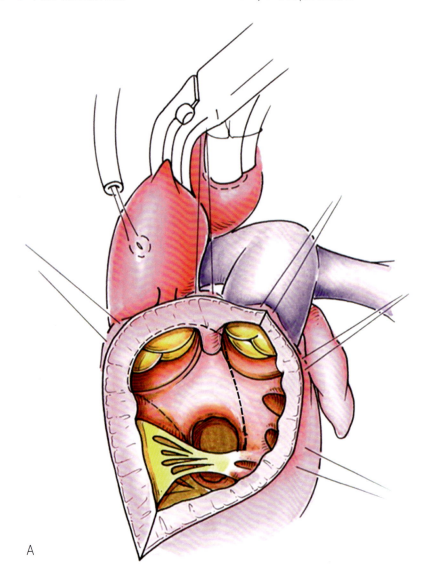

A

图 26-9（续）

B. 如果肺动脉瓣的圆锥体影响新建左心室流出道，必要时缝闭肺动脉瓣。横断肺动脉，近端缝闭，远端和带瓣管道重新建立右心室流出道。

Figure 26-9 cont'd

B. If the subpulmonary conus affects the new left ventricular outflow tract, close the pulmonary valve when necessary. Transect the pulmonary artery, close the proximal end of the artery, and use a valved conduit to reconstruct the right ventricular outflow tract at the distal end.

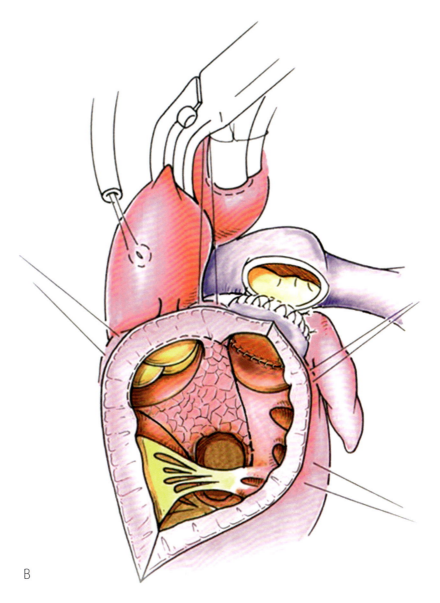

B

图 26-9（续）

Figure 26-9 cont'd

C. 和其他右心室双出口合并主动脉瓣下室间隔缺损一样使用穹形补片连接室间隔缺损和主动脉，也可采用双片法修补室间隔缺损。

C. The dome-shaped patch is used to connect the VSD to the aorta in the same way for DORV with subaortic VSD, or the two-patch technique can also be performed to repair the left ventricle.

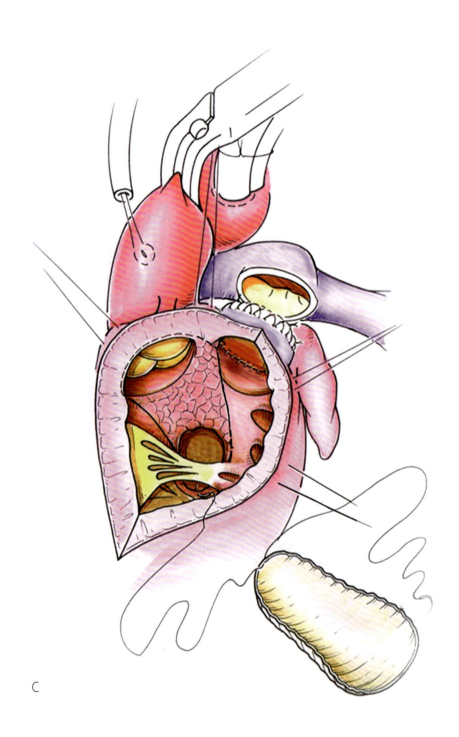

C

图 26-9（续）

D. 重新建立的左心室流出道,必须足够宽畅,确保动脉血直接从左心室经室间隔缺损流入主动脉。

Figure 26-9 cont'd

D. The reconstructed left ventricular outflow tract must be wide enough to ensure direct flow of arterial blood from the left ventricle into the aorta through the VSD.

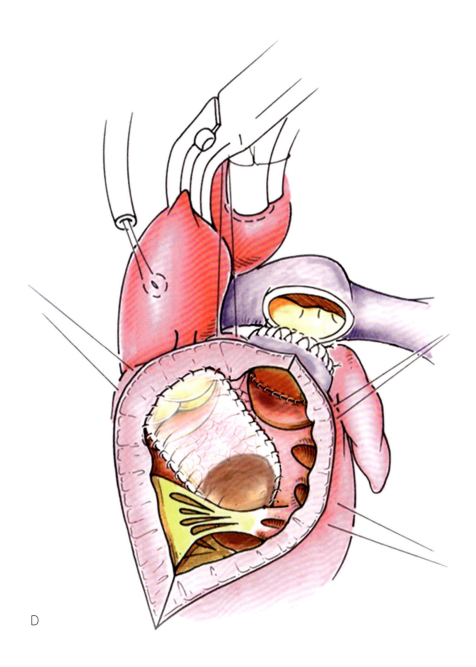

D

图 26-9（续）

Figure 26-9 cont'd

E. 植入同种或异种带瓣管道,用于右心室流出道重建。红色箭头示动脉血从左心室经室间隔缺损,新建流出道进入升主动脉。蓝色静脉血经带瓣管道进入肺动脉。

E. For right ventricular outflow tract reconstruction, valved homograft or heterologous conduits can be chosen for implantation. Red arrows indicate that arterial blood from the left ventricle travels through the VSD and a new outflow tract into the ascending aorta. Blue arrows show that the blue venous blood enters the pulmonary artery through the valved conduit.

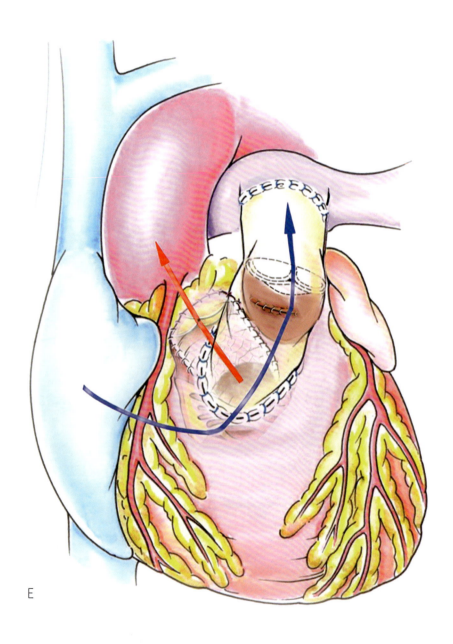

E

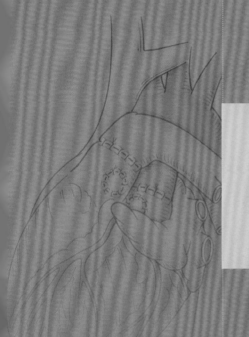

27 左心室双出口

27 Double Outlet Left Ventricle

左心室双出口（double outlet left ventricle, DOLV）是一种罕见的先天性心血管畸形，其心室动脉连接为两大动脉完全或大部分起源于形态学左心室。

1. 心室内补片修补 当肺动脉瓣环无梗阻、肺动脉瓣下梗阻为局限性，以及三尖瓣和右心室发育足够大时，可以考虑完全性心室内补片修补。一般采用经右心房、右心室或肺动脉切口来切除肺动脉下梗阻。使用内隧道技术将右心室与肺动脉相连（图 27-1）。

Double outlet left ventricle (DOLV) is a rare congenital cardiovascular malformation in which both great arteries originate entirely or predominantly from the morphologic left ventricle.

1. Intraventricular baffle repair Complete intraventricular baffle repair may be considered when the pulmonary annulus is not obstructed, the subvalvular pulmonary obstruction is limited, and the tricuspid valve and the right ventricle are sufficiently developed. A right atrium, right ventricle, or pulmonary artery incision is commonly used to relieve the subpulmonary artery obstruction, and an intraventricular tunnel repair is used to connect the right ventricle to the pulmonary artery (Figure 27-1).

图 27-1　心室内补片修补

A. 左心室双出口和右心室双出口一样，畸形的变异很多，手术方法的选择需依据两大动脉的左右前后位置不同，肺动脉是否有狭窄，室间隔缺损位置与大小。甚至有些病例会伴有心室发育不全。图示常见的左心室双出口，双大动脉前后位，肺动脉瓣下狭窄。

Figure 27-1　Intraventricular baffle repair

A. Like double outlet right ventricle (DORV), DOLV has many variants of the malformation, and the surgical approach depends on the different anterior and posterior positions of the two great arteries, the presence or absence of the stenosis in the pulmonary arteries, and the position and size of the VSD. In some cases, there may even be ventricular hypoplasia. The figure shows the common anatomical structure of DOLV, the anterior-posterior position of both great arteries and subpulmonary valve stenosis.

Continued

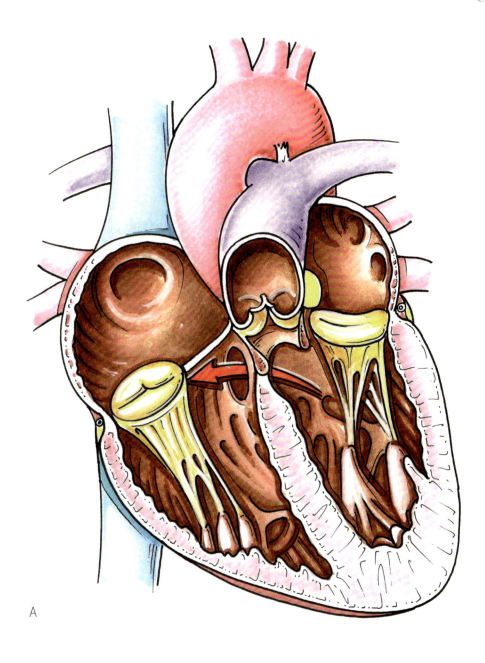

A

图 27-1 (续)

B. 这种病理类型可进行心内根治手术，经右心房三尖瓣或经右心室切除肺动脉瓣下造成瓣下梗阻的圆锥体。

Figure 27-1 cont'd

B. This type of pathology allows intracardiac radical surgery. The conus causing subvalvular obstruction under the pulmonary valve is excised through the right atrial tricuspid valve or via the right ventricle.

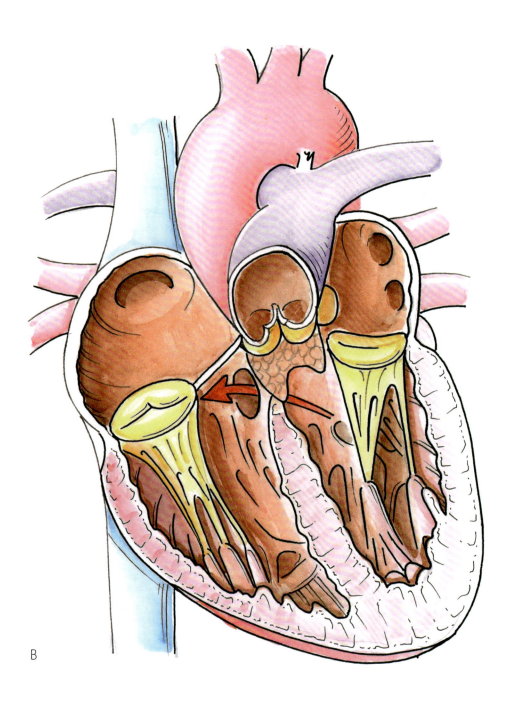

B

图 27-1（续）

C. 通过右心室切口建立从室间隔缺损到肺动脉的心内隧道。如果室间隔缺损太小，必须扩大室间隔缺损，保证右心室流出道的血流通畅。

Figure 27-1 cont'd

C. An intraventricular tunnel from the ventricular defect to the pulmonary artery is created through the right ventricular incision. If the VSD is too small, the defect must be enlarged to ensure unobstructed flow in the right ventricular outflow tract.

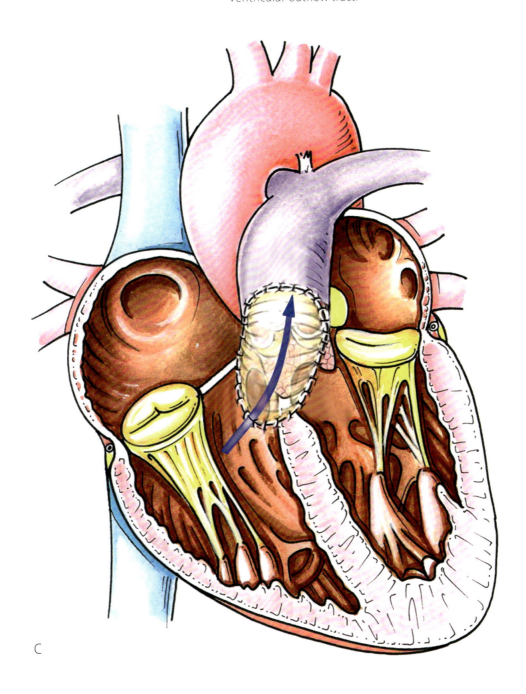

C

2. 肺动脉转位　左心室双出口患儿肺动脉瓣下圆锥梗阻且环绕肺动脉下很长，或者左冠状动脉紧靠肺动脉瓣环，无法进行心室内补片修补，可以进行肺动脉转位（图27-2）。

2. Pulmonary artery transposition　Pulmonary artery transposition could be performed in children with DOLV who have a subpulmonary conus obstruction with a long wrap around the inferior pulmonary artery or whose left coronary artery is close to the pulmonary annulus and cannot be repaired with an intraventricular baffle repair (Figure 27-2).

图 27-2　肺动脉转位
A. 右心室切口，避开冠状动脉，显露室间隔缺损。肺动脉瓣通常在左心室，室间隔缺损的背后。

Figure 27-2　Pulmonary artery transposition
A. A right ventricular incision is made, avoiding damaging the coronary arteries. Expose the septal defect. The pulmonary valve is usually in the left ventricle, behind the VSD.

Continued

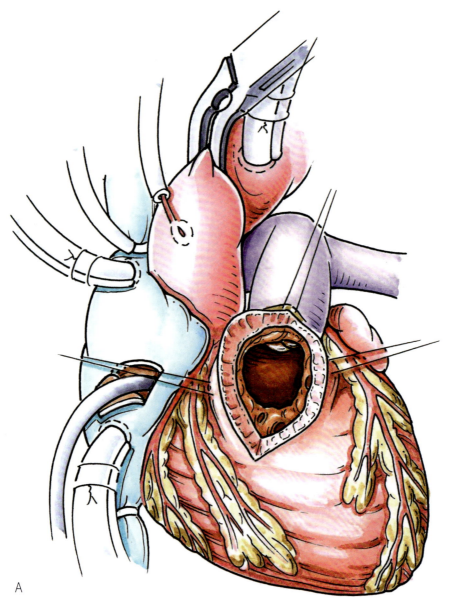

A

图 27-2（续）

B. 室间隔缺损补片修补，可以采用连续
缝合。

Figure 27-2 cont'd

B. Patch repair of VSD with running sutures.

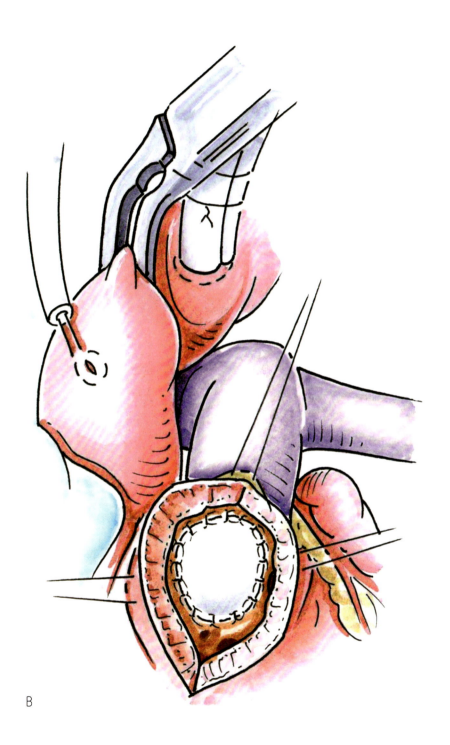

B

图 27-2（续）

C. 紧靠肺动脉瓣环，避开左冠状动脉，把肺动脉根部连同瓣膜从左心室切下，不要损伤瓣叶。左心室切口用 Prolene 缝线带垫片间断缝合。室间隔缺损补片的背面是左心室。

Figure 27-2 cont'd

C. The root of the pulmonary artery, along with the valve, are dissected right close to the pulmonary annulus from the left ventricle, avoiding damage to the left coronary artery and the leaflets. The left ventricular incision is closed with pledget-supported interrupted Prolene sutures. The dorsal aspect of the ventricular patch is the left ventricle.

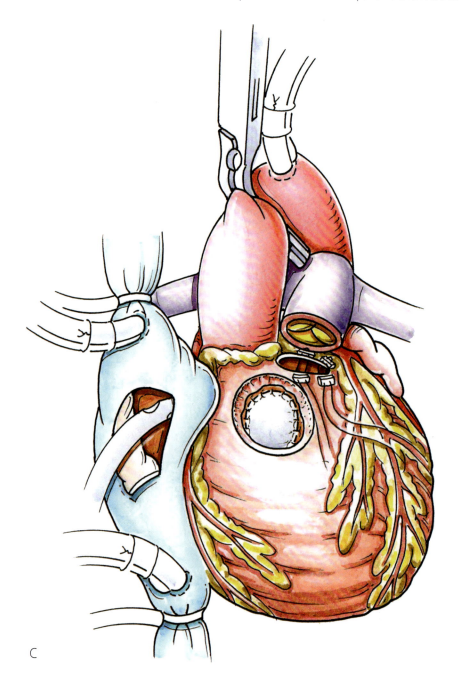

C

图 27-2（续）

Figure 27-2 cont'd

D. 切下的肺动脉根部后壁和右心室切口对合，连续缝合。

D. The posterior wall of the pulmonary artery root and the right ventricular incision are coapted and continuously sutured.

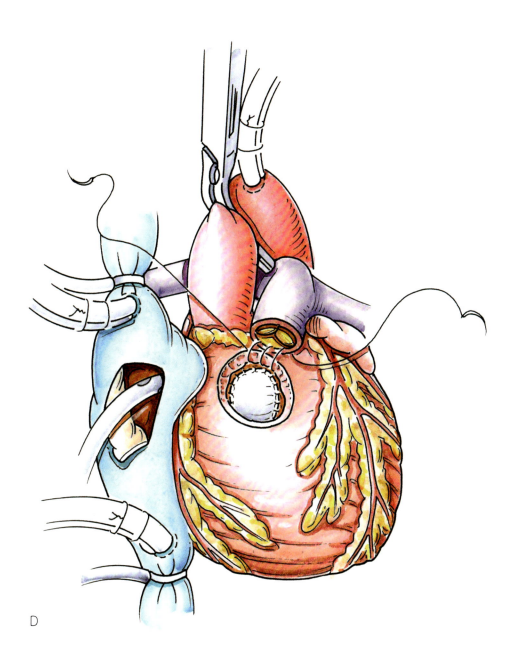

D

图 27-2（续）

E. 选择合适的补片,如自身心包、牛心包或 ePTFE 补片重建右心室流出道。

Figure 27-2 cont'd

E. Select an appropriate patch, such as autologous pericardial patch, bovine pericardial patch, or ePTFE patch, to reconstruct the RVOT.

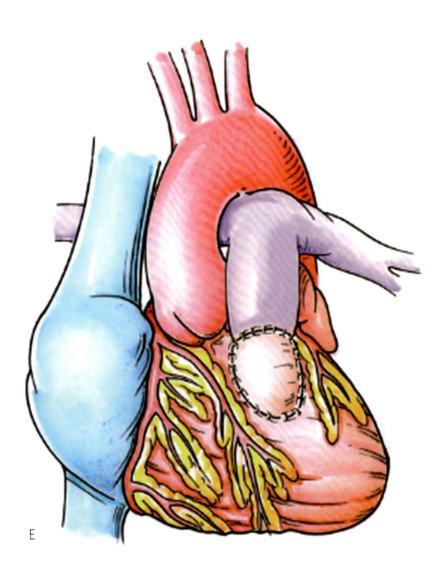

E

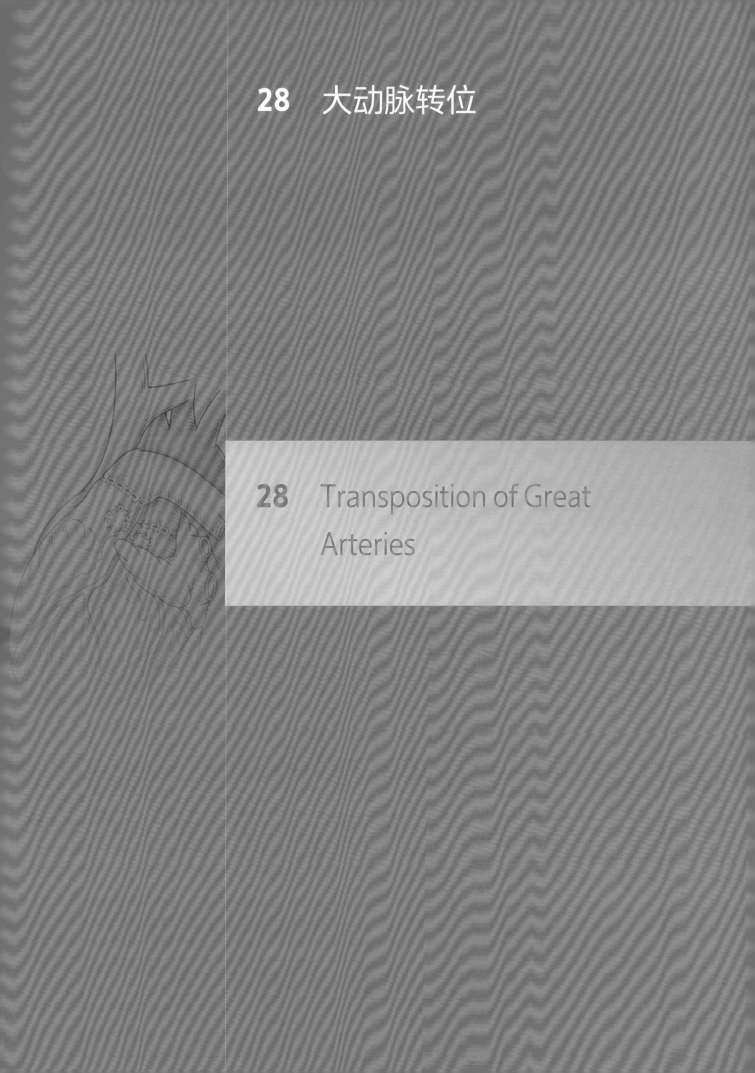

28 大动脉转位

28 Transposition of Great Arteries

大动脉转位(transposition of great arteries,TGA)是一种房室关系一致而心室大动脉关系不一致,形态学上主动脉起源于右心室而肺动脉起源于左心室的先天性心脏畸形。通常合并有动脉导管未闭和大小不等的房间隔缺损。如为室隔完整型的大动脉转位则必须在新生儿期就予以手术。常见合并畸形包括室间隔缺损、肺动脉狭窄等。冠状动脉的解剖学变异是这类畸形手术的最大挑战。

transposition of great arteries (TGA) is a congenital heart abnormality in which the atrioventricular connection is consistent, but the ventricular and aortic connections are reversed. Morphologically, the aorta originates from the right ventricle, and the pulmonary artery originates from the left ventricle. TGA is usually combined with patent ductus arteriosus (PDA) and atrial septal defect of varying sizes. TGA with intact ventricular septum must be operated in the neonatal period. Common malformations in combination with TGA include ventricular septal defect (VSD), pulmonary artery stenosis, etc. The anatomical deformity of the coronary arteries constitutes the biggest challenge for surgery.

一、解剖分型

I. Anatomical Typing

目前临床上最常用的是Yacoub 冠状动脉分支模式分类(图28-1)。

Currently, coronary artery branch typing proposed by Magdi Yacoub is mostly used in clinic (Figure 28-1).

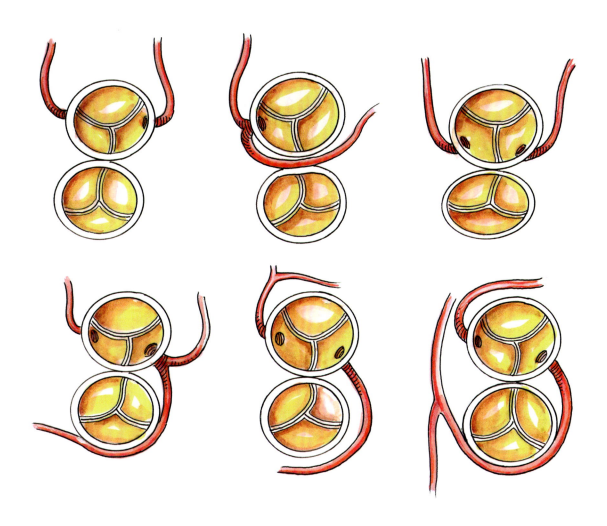

二、手术方法

Ⅱ. Surgical Methods

早年(20 世纪 70 年代前)使用心房内调转手术(Senning 或者 Mustard 手术)治疗大动脉转位。但是患者随访证明,担负体循环功能的右心室失代偿可引发心律不齐、心力衰竭,预后不佳。同时期成功开展的大动脉调转术,基本上取代了心房内调转手术。对于大多数新生儿或者婴幼儿患者,大动脉调转术已经成为常规的治疗。对极少

In the early years (before the 1970s), atrial switch operation (Senning procedure or Mustard procedure) was used to treat TGA. However, patients' follow-up studies proved that the decompensation of the right ventricle, which is responsible for systemic circulation, resulted in arrhythmia and heart failure with poor prognosis. The arterial switch operation, which was successfully carried out during the same period, basically has replaced the great atrial switch operation. For most neonates

数有其他合并症的病例,如肺动脉狭窄合并室间隔缺损,不可切除的左心室流出道梗阻,非典型的大动脉转位,或年龄已超出了做大动脉调转术的条件、冠状动脉异常等,也可选择心房内调转手术。

or infants, arterial switch operation has become routine management. In rare cases of other complications, such as pulmonary artery stenosis in combination with ventricular defect, unresectable left ventricular outflow tract obstruction, atypical TGA, or beyond the age for great arterial switch operation, coronary artery abnormalities, atrial switch operation is also an option.

1. 使用自身房间隔组织的心房内调转手(Senning 手术)(图28-2)

1. Intra-atrial switch operation using autologous atrial septal tissue (Senning procedure)(Figure 28-2)

图 28-2　使用自身房间隔组织的心房内调转手(Senning 手术)

A. Senning 手术一般采用心肺转流术,上下腔静脉插管,避免使用右心耳插管。由于需要部分右心房壁构成新房间隔,所以切口呈横 S 形。从右心耳起至下腔静脉心房连接部,并平行房间沟做左心房切口成为构成新的心房一部分(图中虚线所示)。

B. 切开右心房,注意右心房内结构。三条绿色虚线显示的是从窦房结到房室结的三条传导束支,术中避免损伤。黑色虚线是要切开的含缺损的房间隔。

Figure 28-2　Intra-atrial switch operation using autologous atrial septal tissue (Senning procedure)

A. Senning procedure generally requires cardiopulmonary bypass with cannulation in the superior and inferior vena cava, not cannulation in the right atrial appendage. The incision is transversely S-shaped because a portion of the right atrial wall is needed to create a new atrial septum. From the right atrial appendage to the atrial junction of the inferior vena cava. A left atriotomy is made in parallel with the atrial sulcus to form a portion of a new atrium (illustrated in the dotted line in the figure).

B. A right atriotomy is made, noting structures within the right atrium. The three green dotted lines illustrate the three conduction bundles from the sinoatrial node to the atrioventricular node, avoiding injury during the operation. The black dotted line illustrates the atrial septal defect that was incised.

Continued

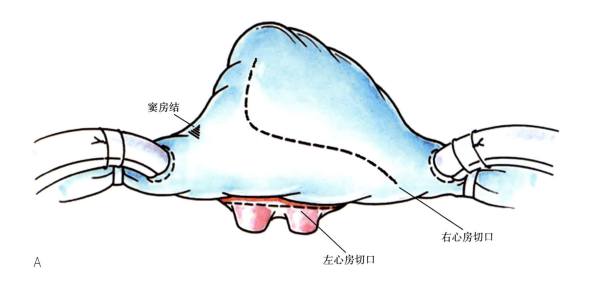

窦房结

右心房切口

左心房切口

A

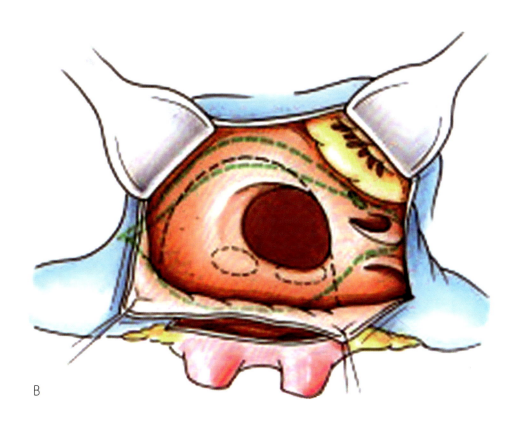

B

图 28-2（续）

C. 沿三尖瓣环上下切开房间隔,缺损的房间隔可用自身心包或者补片修补。

D. 房间隔缺损修补后三个边缘游离的房间隔将构成新的房间隔。把游离的房间隔板沿左右上下肺静脉开口连续缝合,成为新房间隔的一部分。

E. 将已经切开的右心房壁正中对着被切开房间隔的边缘,分别向上下腔静脉开口缝合、打结,构成新的右心房,上下腔静脉血由此进入二尖瓣到肺动脉。虚线所示是新房间隔。

Figure 28-2 cont'd

C. The atrial septum is incised from top to bottom along the tricuspid annulus, and the atrial septal defect may be repaired with its own pericardium or patch.

D. After the repair of the atrial septal defect, the atrial septal with three free edges would form a new atrial septum. The free septum is continuously sutured along the ostium of the left, right, superior, and inferior pulmonary veins as part of the new atrial septum.

E. The center of the incised right atrium wall is aligned with the edge of the incised atrial septum, and is sutured to the ostium of superior and inferior vena cava and knotted. A new right atrium is formed, from which blood in the superior and inferior vena cava enters the mitral valve, eventually to the pulmonary artery. The dotted line illustrates the new atrial septum.

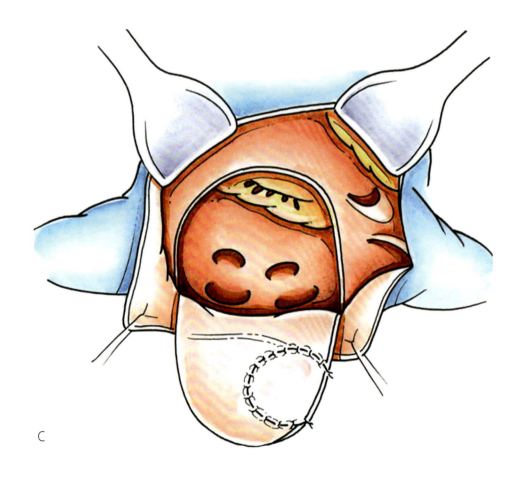

C

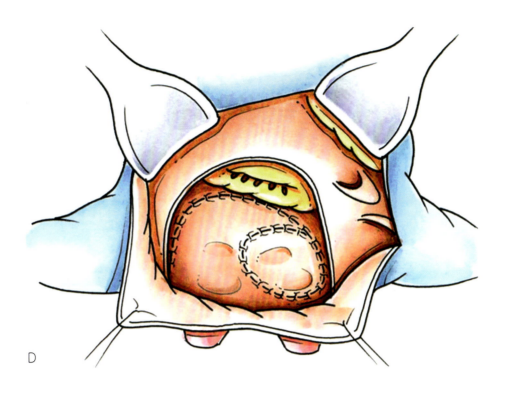

D

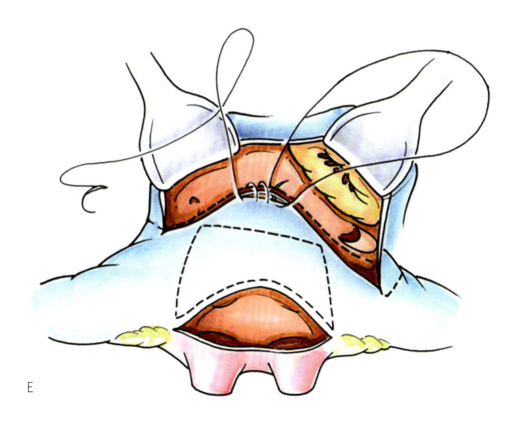

E

图 28-2 (续)

F. 把大部分右心房壁含整个右心耳缝于已经构成新右心房的房壁上。靠近上腔静脉处避免损伤窦房结,下缘覆盖部分下腔静脉。在左心房切口中部打结。

Figure 28-2 cont'd

F. Most of the right atrial wall containing the entire right atrial appendage is sutured to the atrial wall that has already formed the new right atrium. Avoid damage to the sinoatrial node near the superior vena cava, with the inferior border covering a portion of the inferior vena cava. The knot is tied in the middle of the left atrial incision.

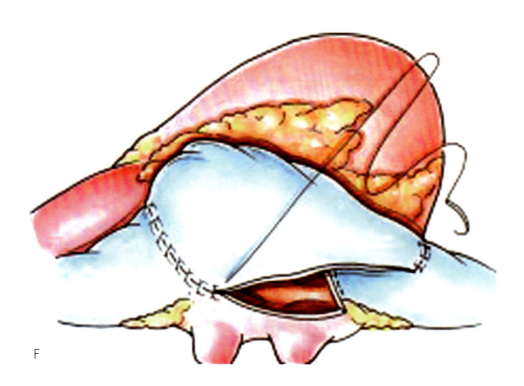

F

图 28-2（续）

G. 心脏背面观。动脉血从左右肺静脉通过被重新分隔后进入三尖瓣（心房内调转手术后）再进入和主动脉相连的体循环。上下腔静脉的静脉血被分隔后从二尖瓣进入和肺动脉连接的肺循环。

Figure 28-2 cont'd

G. Back view of the heart. Arterial blood passes from the left and right pulmonary veins to the tricuspid valve (after the atrial switch operation) through re-division, and then enters the systemic circulation connected to the aorta. The venous blood from the superior and inferior vena cava is separated and passes from the mitral valve into the pulmonary circulation connected to the pulmonary artery.

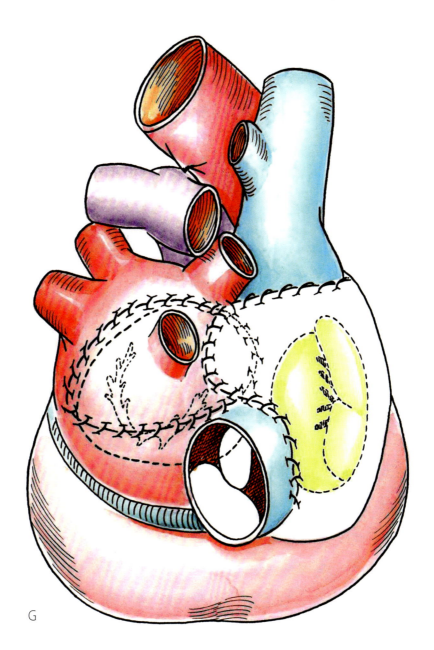

G

2. 应用补片做心房内调转手术（Mustard 手术）（图 28-3）

2. Intra-atrial switch operation with patch (Mustard procedure)(Figure 28-3)

图 28-3　应用补片做心房内调转手术（Mustard 手术）

A. 同 Senning 手术相同方法行心肺转流术。于右心房前壁中部平行房间隔做横行切口。在邻近上腔静脉右心房连接处，避免损伤窦房结。如果需要延长切口，可以向心耳方向伸展。

Figure 28-3　Intra-atrial switch operation with patch (Mustard procedure)

A. Cardiopulmonary bypass is established in the same manner as the Senning procedure. A transverse incision is made in the middle of the anterior wall of the right atrium parallel to the atrial septum. The incision is made near the right atrium junction of the superior vena cava, avoiding damage to the sinus node. If the incision needs to be extended, it can be extended toward the atrial appendage.

Continued

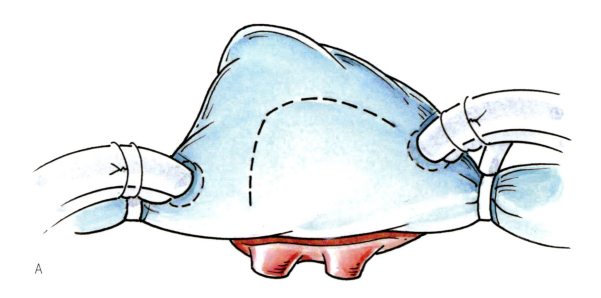

A

图 28-3（续）

B. 充分显露全部房间隔。虚线显示需扩大的房间隔。扩大切除可以直接从房间隔缺损开始,依次头侧、上腔静脉心房连接部、房间沟、下腔静脉心房连接部。房间隔上下腔静脉连接部和房间沟部,因为是双层组织叠折在一起,比较厚。切除时,要保留足够的组织(5mm 左右),避免心房壁穿孔。残留的房间隔虽然粗糙,但会很快内皮化,不必缝合。

Figure 28-3 cont'd

B. The entire atrial septum is adequately exposed. The dotted line illustrates the atrial septal defect to be enlarged. Resection can be performed directly from the ASD, followed by the head side, superior vena cava-atrial junction, the atrial sulcus, and inferior vena cava-atrial junction. The junctions of the superior and inferior vena cava with the atrial septum, together with the atrial sulcus, are thick because they are double-layered tissues. At the time of resection, it is necessary to preserve enough tissue (about 5mm) to avoid perforation of the atrial wall. The residual atrial septum, although rough, is rapidly endothelialized and does not need to be sutured.

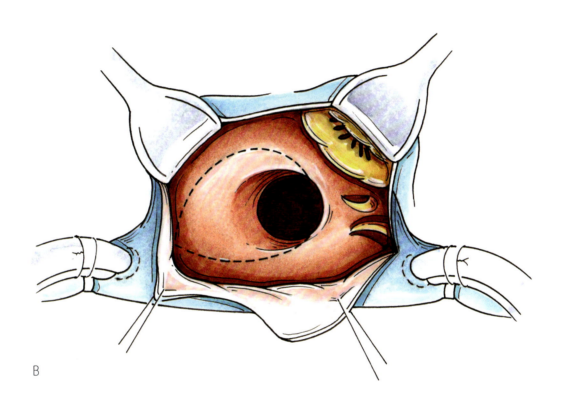

B

图 28-3（续）

Figure 28-3 cont'd

C. 按虚线选择补片剪成"裤样"重建房间隔。"裤管"分别和上下腔静脉右心房入口处缝合。"裤腰"正中对齐左心房后壁左上下肺静脉之间的组织。连续缝合从左心房后壁开始。

C. Select the appropriate patch according to the dotted line and cut it into a pants-like shape to reconstruct the atrial septum. The two "trousers" are sutured at the entrance to the right atrium of the superior and inferior vena cava, respectively. The "waistband" is medially aligned with the tissues between the left superior and inferior pulmonary veins on the posterior wall of the left atrium. The running suture starts from the posterior wall of the left atrium.

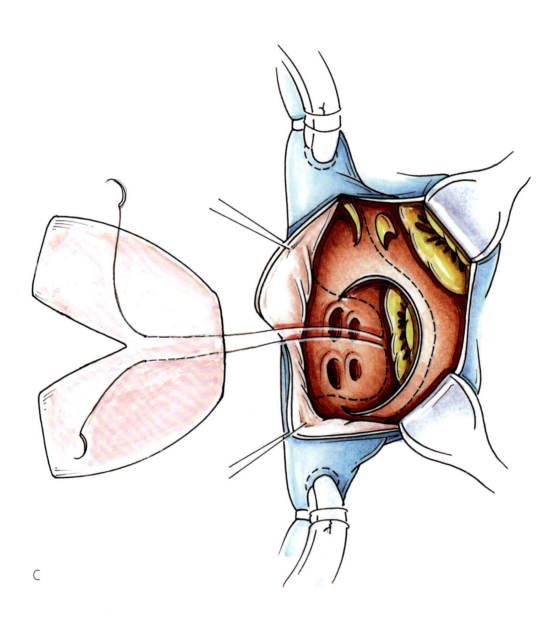

C

图 28-3（续）

D. 新建房间隔后壁完成缝合后，翻转补片，补片两头依次和上下腔静脉缝合。先缝合上腔静脉入口，注意吻合口要足够大，继续缝合二尖瓣和下腔静脉入口。二尖瓣入口处要同时接受上下腔静脉血流，此处开口必须足够大，避免补片狭窄。

Figure 28-3 cont'd

D. After completion of suturing the posterior wall of the newly created atrial septum, the patch is turned over, and both ends of the patch are sutured to the superior and inferior vena cava in turn. First, suture the entrance to the superior vena cava. The anastomosis should be large enough. Then, suture the mitral valve and the entrance to the inferior vena cava. Since the entrance to the mitral valve simultaneously receives blood flow from the superior and inferior vena cava, the opening here must be large enough to avoid stenosis of the patch.

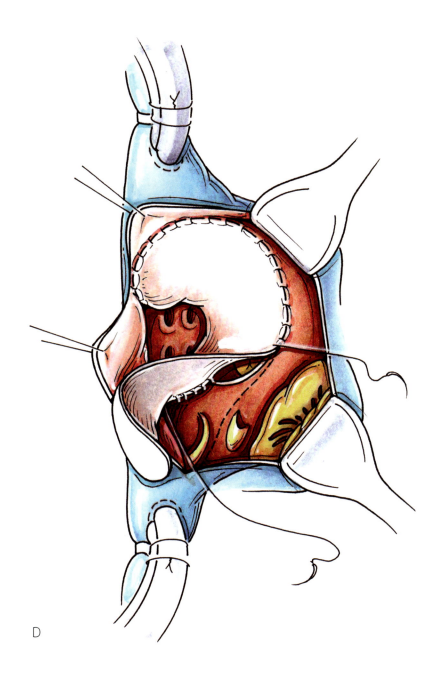

D

图 28-3（续）

Figure 28-3 cont'd

E. 将右心房切口缝合完毕。

E. Suturing right atrial incision is accomplished.

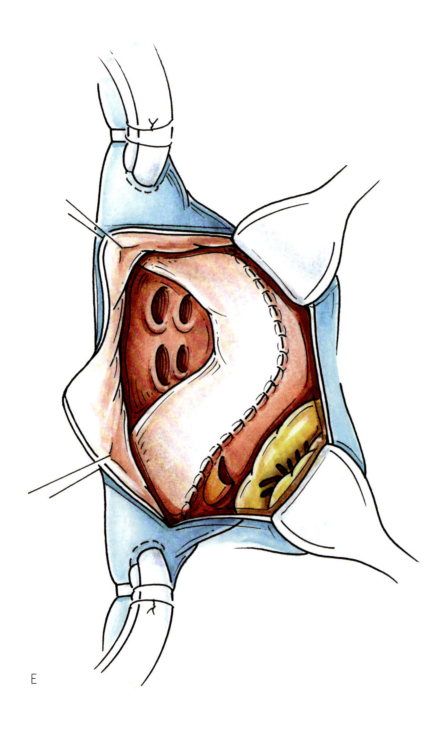

E

图 28-3（续）

F. 房间隔重建后，上下腔静脉血流二尖瓣进入肺循环，而肺静脉血流从留下的心房经三尖瓣到升主动脉进入体循环。

Figure 28-3 cont'd

F. After atrial septal reconstruction, the blood of the superior and inferior vena cava flows through the mitral valve and then enters the pulmonary circulation. The pulmonary venous blood flows from the remaining atrium through the tricuspid valve to the ascending aorta and finally enters the systemic circulation.

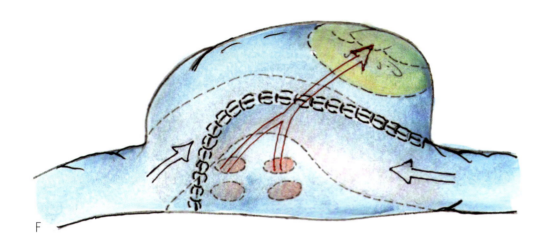

F

3. 大动脉调转术（Jatene 手术）

动脉调转手术常规应用于室间隔完整型的大动脉转位，最佳手术年龄为出生 1~2 周。此时，左心室尚未退化，仍能承受体循环压力，动脉调转手术成功性大。出生 3~4 周后的婴儿，如果左心室压力低于体循环压力的 60%，需要做左心室收缩功能训练，分期手术，先行肺动脉环束术，同时施行或不施行体循环至肺动脉的分流手术，根据左心收缩功能情况再进行动脉调转手术。仅合并小室间隔缺损的大动脉转位，左心室收缩功能减退较慢，可根据左心室收缩功能适当延长手术年龄（图 28-4）。

3. Great arterial switch operation (Jatene procedure)

Arterial switch operation is routinely applied to TGA with intact ventricular septum, and the optimal age for surgery is 1-2 weeks after birth. At this time, the left ventricle has not yet degenerated and can still withstand the systemic pressure, and the arterial switch operation has a high possibility of success. In infants of 3-4 weeks, if the left ventricular pressure is lower than 60% of the systemic circulation pressure, left ventricular systolic function training and staged surgery are required. Pulmonary artery banding is first performed, with or without systemic-pulmonary shunt. Whether to perform arterial switch operation is then decided by the left ventricular systolic function. In cases of the TGA with small VSD, the left ventricular systolic function declines more slowly than the one without VSD, and the operation age can be adjusted flexibly according to the left ventricular systolic function (Figure 28-4).

图 28-4　**大动脉调转术（Jatene 手术）**

A. 正中开胸，切除大部分或全部胸腺组织，打开心包，了解两大动脉位置和冠状动脉状况。

Figure 28-4　Arterial switch operation (Jatene procedure)

A. A median thoracotomy is performed, resect most or all the thymic tissue and open the pericardium, observe the location of both arteries and the condition of the coronary arteries.

Continued

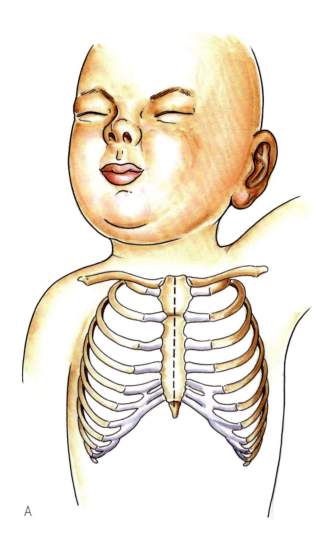

A

图 28-4（续）

B. 常规行心肺转流术。2kg 以上的新生儿可以升主动脉插管 10 Fr 和上下腔静脉插管 12 Fr。钝性分离动脉导管，穿结扎线。进行心肺转流术，同时缝扎切断动脉导管。通常主动脉插管的位置略高些，方便做两大血管的换位和吻合。中低温降温。

Figure 28-4 cont'd

B. Cardiopulmonary bypass is routinely established. The ascending aorta cannulation at 10 Fr and the superior and inferior vena cava cannulation at 12 Fr are performed for newborns over 2 kg. The ductus arteriosus is bluntly separated and ligated. Patients are placed on cardiopulmonary bypass and the ductus arteriosus is ligated and cut. Usually, the position of the aortic cannula is slightly higher to facilitate the transposition and anastomosis of the two major arteries. Moderate hypothermia is required.

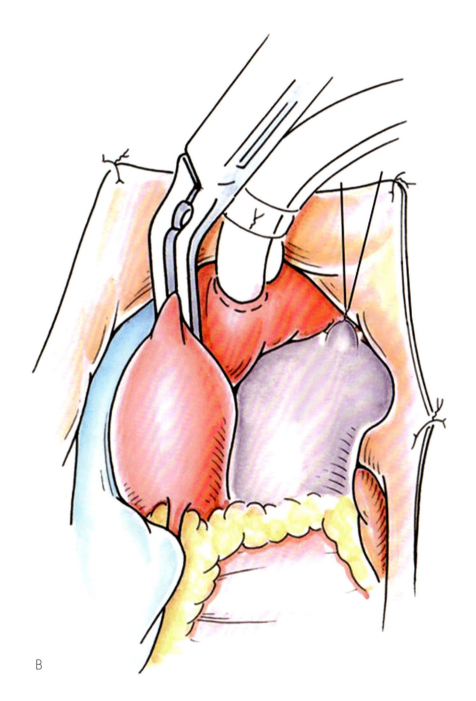

B

图 28-4（续）

C. 确定主动脉和肺动脉的横断切口。大动脉转位手术大多都要进行肺动脉换位到主动脉前的 Lecompte 步骤,所以肺动脉尽量靠近瓣膜处离断,而升主动脉离断位置可以高于肺动脉,使肺动脉在 Lecompte 操作后和主动脉根部吻合不会显得张力太大。右心房的切口通过房间隔缺损或未闭合的卵圆孔放置左心引流管。

Figure 28-4 cont'd

C. Determine the location of the transverse incision of the aorta and pulmonary artery. Most transposition operations of the great arteries require the Lecompte maneuver, so the pulmonary artery is transected as close to the valve as possible, and the ascending aorta can be transected at a higher position than the pulmonary artery. In this way, after the Lecompte maneuver, the anastomotic tension between the pulmonary artery and the aortic root will not be too great. A left heart drainage tube is placed through the atrial defect or a patent foramen ovale at the right atrium incision.

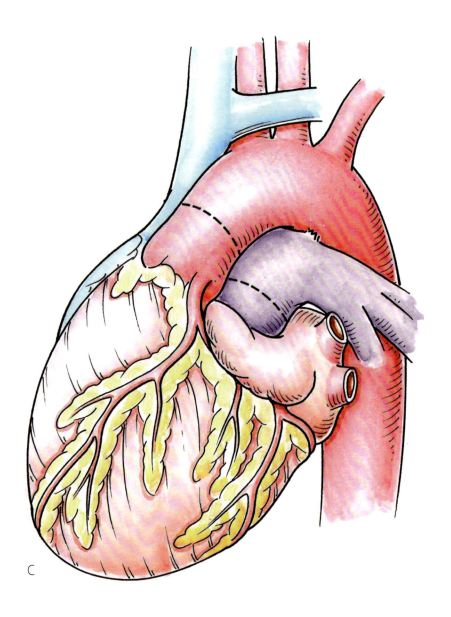

图 28-4（续）

D. 升主动脉横断后,显露左右冠状动脉窦。虚线示纽扣状取下冠状动脉开口的切口位置。一般主动脉和肺动脉直径差异不大,冠状动脉开口呈纽扣状切下,保留了两个大动脉根部的完整。心包补片缝闭两个缺口。

Figure 28-4 cont'd

D. The left and right coronary sinuses are exposed after the transection of the ascending aorta. The dotted liney represents the incision to take the coronary artery buttons. In general, the diameters of the aorta and pulmonary arteries are not much different. The coronary artery ostia are cut out in a button-like shape, leaving the roots of the two large arteries intact. The two defects are sutured and closed with pericardial patches.

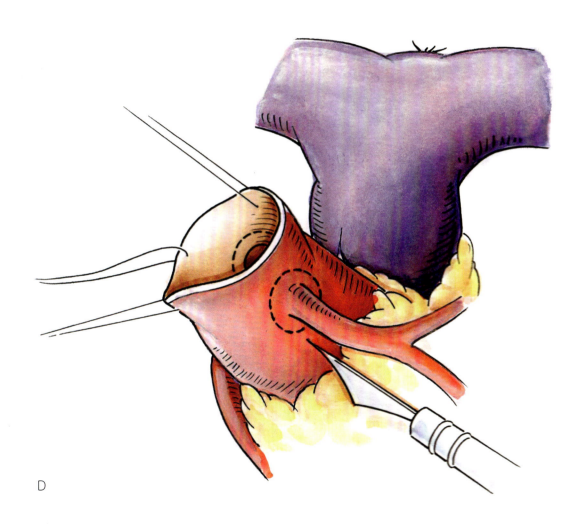

D

图 28-4（续）

E. 左右冠状动脉从冠状动脉窦被取下后,做充分游离,注意不要损伤冠状动脉分支。

Figure 28-4 cont'd

E. After the left and right coronary arteries are removed from the coronary sinuses, they are fully freed, taking care not to damage the branches of the coronary arteries.

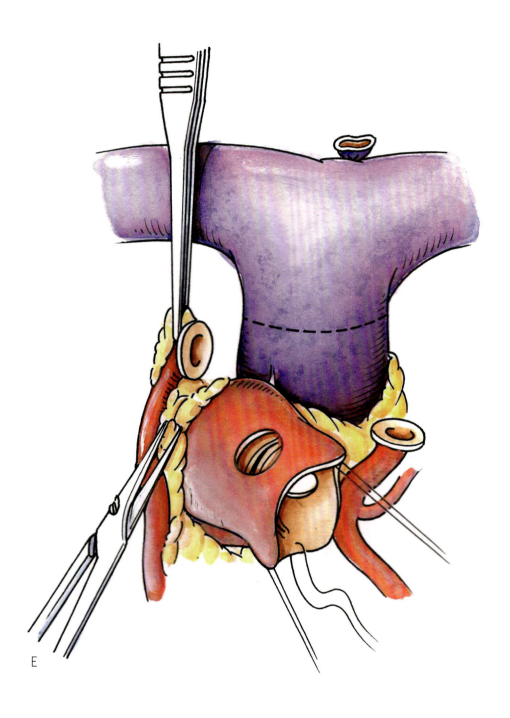

E

图 28-4（续）

Figure 28-4 cont'd

F. 在肺动脉根部相应的瓣膜窦做纽扣状切口，把充分游离的冠状动脉连续吻合在肺动脉根部。游离的冠状动脉要长度合适，太短使得冠状动脉张力太大，影响冠状动脉灌注。太长冠状动脉，扭曲也同样使心肌灌注不良。婴幼儿组织很脆弱，体重小于 3kg 的建议使用 7-0 的 Prolene 圆头针缝线。

F. A button-like incision is made in the corresponding valve sinus of the pulmonary artery root, and the fully freed coronary artery is continuously anastomosed to the pulmonary artery root. The freed coronary arteries should be of appropriate length since the too-short coronary arteries will cause high pressure and affect the perfusion of the coronary arteries, and the too-long coronary arteries will twist and cause poor myocardial perfusion. Infant tissues are very fragile, and a 7-0 Prolene suture with a round-headed needle is recommended for infants weighing less than 3kg.

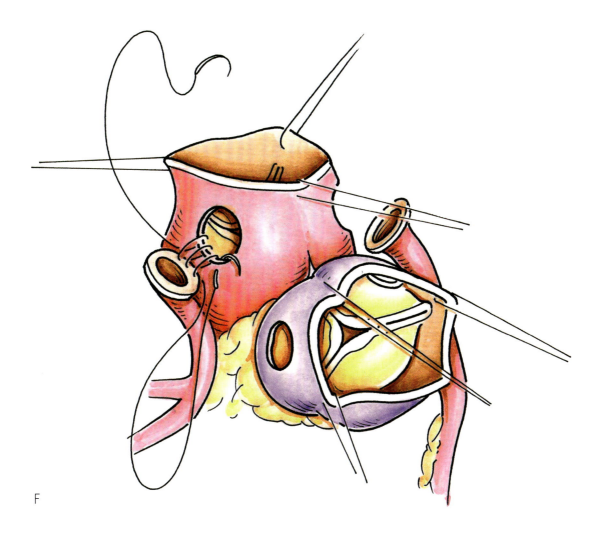

F

图 28-4（续）

Figure 28-4 cont'd

G. 充分游离左右肺动脉分别至它们的分叉,使骑跨在主动脉上的肺动脉在和起始于右心室的主动脉根吻合时能够无张力。降低主动脉灌注流量,交换升主动脉血流阻断钳把肺动脉提到升主动脉前方(Lecompte 操作),在主动脉切口远端重新上主动脉钳子。在肺动脉的下方进行新建主动脉吻合。视婴幼儿大小,使用 6-0 或者 7-0 的 Prolene 圆头针连续缝合。

G. Fully free the left and right pulmonary arteries to their bifurcations so that the pulmonary artery that overrides the aorta is tension-free when anastomosing to the aortic root starting from the right ventricle. Reduce perfusion flow, exchange the ascending aorta coarctation forceps and lift the pulmonary artery to the front of the ascending aorta (the Lecompte maneuver), and re-employ the aortic forceps at the distal end of the aortic incision. Make a new aortic anastomosis below the pulmonary artery. Depending on the weight and age of infants, use a 6-0 or 7-0 Prolene suture with a round-headed needle for running suture.

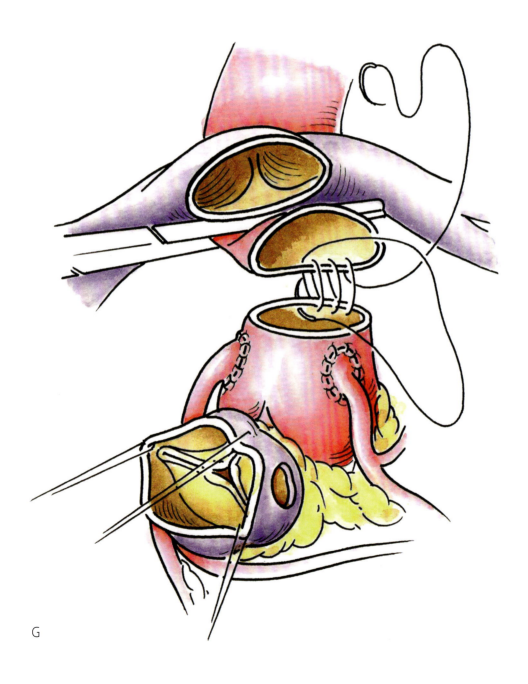

G

图 28-4（续）

H. 切除冠状动脉后的主动脉窦口，使用
7-0 的无创缝线，自身的没有处理过的
或 0.6% 戊二醛处理后的心包片缝闭。
在确定没有张力的情况下进行肺动脉
吻合。方法材料同升主动脉吻合。

Figure 28-4 cont'd

H. The aortic sinus ostium after coronary artery resection is closed with untreated or 0. 6% glutaraldehyde-fixed autologous pericardial patch by using 7-0 non-invasive sutures. The pulmonary artery anastomosis is performed under the condition that there is no tension, and the method and materials needed are the same as the ascending aorta anastomosis.

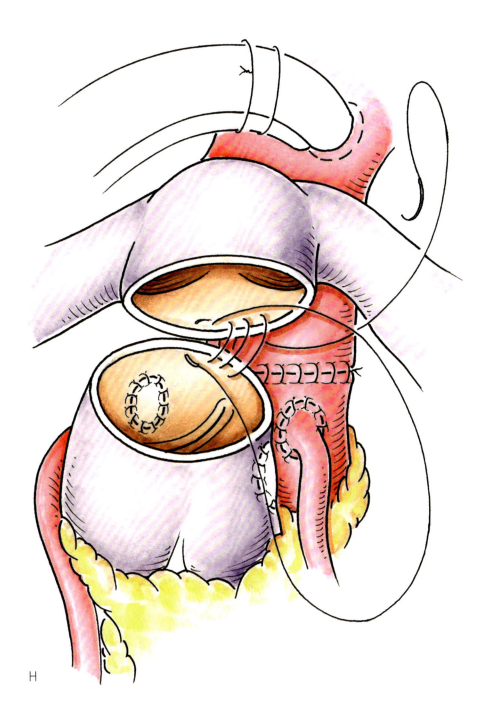

H

图 28-4（续）

Figure 28-4 cont'd

I. 大动脉转位矫正手术后,骑跨在主动脉上的肺动脉起始于右心室,肺动脉左侧后下的升主动脉起始于左心室。

I. After the operation for TGA, the pulmonary artery that overrides the aorta starts from the right ventricle, and the ascending aorta, at the posterioinferior portion on the left side of the pulmonary artery, starts from the left ventricle.

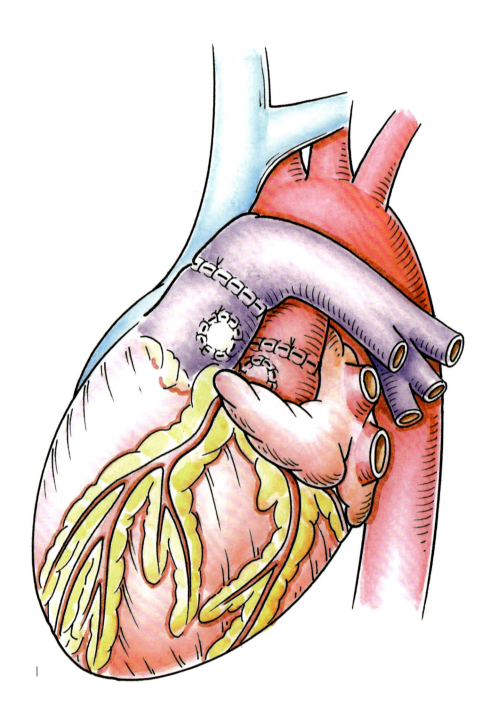

I

4. 大动脉转位合并室间隔缺损　大动脉转位合并室间隔缺损患者的大动脉调转术与前述动脉调转术相同,只需加做室间隔缺损修补术。建立主动脉、上下腔静脉插管以最大程度暴露右心房,室间隔缺损修补大多经右心房切口,也可经肺动脉或主动脉暴露室间隔缺损部位。一般在动脉调转术前关闭室间隔缺损,二次使用心肌保护液。但目前大多使用 HTK 心肌保护液,只需一次灌注(图 28-5)。

4. TGA associated with VSD　The arterial switch operation for patients with TGA associated with VSD is the same as the arterial switch operation aforementioned, but a repair of the ventricular defect is required. Cannulation in the aorta and superior and inferior vena cava are established to fully expose the right atrium. Most ventricular defect repairs are via the right atrium incision, and the VSD can also be exposed through the pulmonary artery or aorta. Generally, the ventricular defect is closed before arterial switch procedure, and the second dose of cardioplegic solution is used. But at present, HTK solution is mostly used, and only one perfusion is required (Figure 28-5).

图 28-5　室间隔缺损大动脉调转术

图 28-5　室间隔缺损大动脉调转术
A. 经右心房修补室间隔缺损,切开右心房,牵开三尖瓣组织,暴露室间隔缺损的位置。

Figure 28-5　Surgical management for TGA associated with VSD

A. The VSD is repaired through the right atrium. The right atrium is incised, and the tricuspid valve tissue is retracted to expose the position of the VSD.

Continued

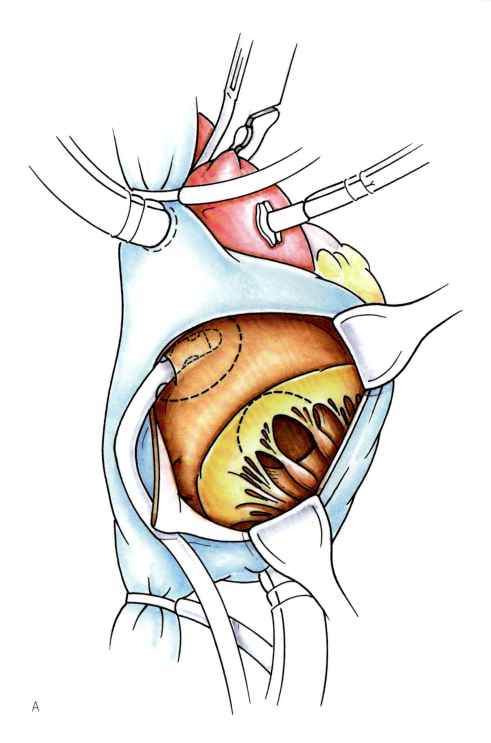

A

图 28-5（续）

B. 一般采用自身心包补片，5-0 Prolene 缝线连续缝合。图示补片修补室间隔缺损后。

Figure 28-5 cont'd

B. Autologous pericardial patch is generally employed using running sutures of 5-0 Prolene. The figure shows the completion of repairing VSD with a patch.

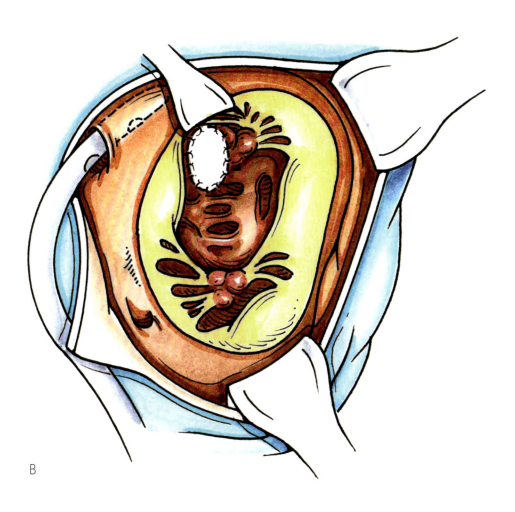

B

图 28-5（续）

C. 大部分病例，在横断大动脉后，小室间隔缺损显示得很清楚，也可以经肺动脉或经主动脉修补。大动脉调转术方法同前。

Figure 28-5 cont'd

C. In most cases, the VSD is clearly displayed after the aorta is transected, and it can also be repaired via the pulmonary artery or via the aorta. The surgical method of aortic switch operation is the same as before.

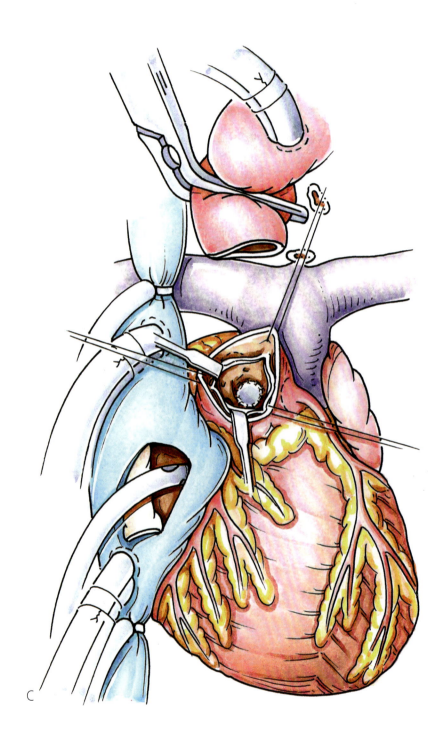

图 28-6 大动脉转位合并冠状动脉异常

A. 在大动脉转位患者中，主动脉最常转向肺动脉的前方，少数情况下，大血管并行排列，且主动脉位于肺动脉的右侧。冠状动脉通常起源于朝向肺动脉的主动脉窦中。这样，不朝向肺动脉的主动脉窦最常位于前方。

Figure 28-6   TGA associated with coronary artery abnormalities

A. In patients with TGA, the aorta most often turns to the front of the pulmonary artery. In a few cases, the great arteries are arranged in parallel, and the aorta is located on the right side of the pulmonary artery. Coronary arteries usually originate in the aortic sinus towards the pulmonary artery. In this way, the aortic sinus that does not face the pulmonary artery is most often anteriorly located.

Continued

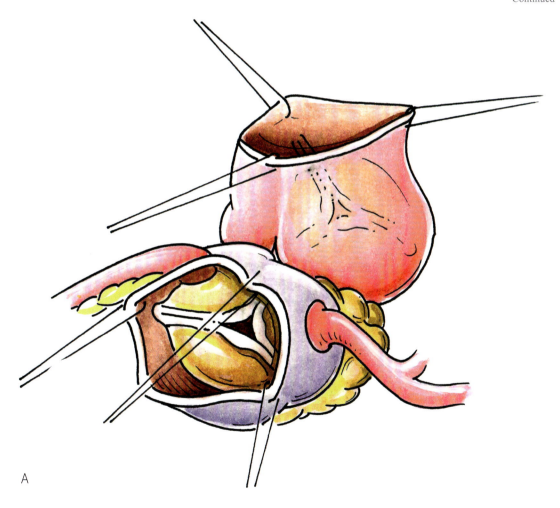

A

图 28-6（续）

B. 按照 Leiden 规则，从不朝向肺动脉的无冠状窦来看，1 号主动脉窦位于右手侧，2 号主动脉窦为 1 号主动脉窦的逆时针方向的下一个瓣窦。约 70% 的患者左前降支和回旋支冠状动脉作为单独的动脉干起自 1 号主动脉窦，而右冠状动脉起自 2 号主动脉窦。

Figure 28-6 cont'd

B. According to the Leiden convention, from the perspective of the non-coronary sinus that does not face the pulmonary artery, the valve sinus 1 is located on the right-hand side, and the valve sinus 2 is the next valve sinus of the valve sinus 1 in the counterclockwise direction. In about 70% of patients, the left anterior descending and circumflex coronary arteries originate from sinus 1 as a separate trunk, while the right coronary artery originates from sinus 2.

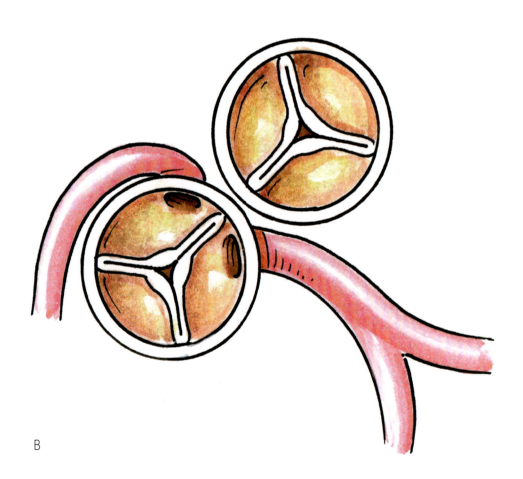

B

图 28-6(续)

C. 在约 15% 的患者中，左前降支动脉起自 1 号主动脉窦，而右冠状动脉和回旋支一起起自 2 号主动脉窦。

Figure 28-6 cont'd

C. In approximately 15% of patients, the left anterior descending artery originates from sinus 1, while the right coronary artery and the circumflex artery originate from sinus 2.

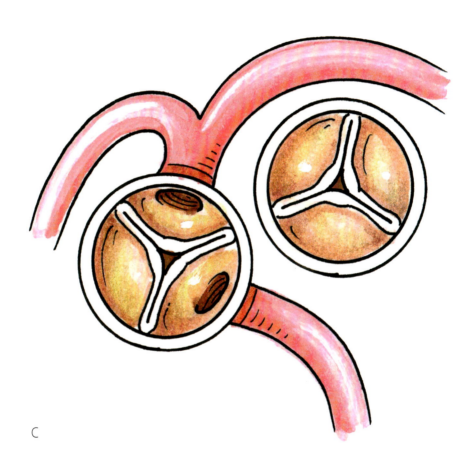

C

图 28-6（续）

D. 极少的情况下，所有三支主要的冠状动脉起自单个瓣窦，最常见的为 2 号主动脉窦。在有些病例中，左前降支或左主冠状动脉可为壁内型。

Figure 28-6 cont'd

D. In rare cases, all three major coronary arteries originate from a single valve sinus, the most common being the valve sinus 2. In some cases, the left anterior descending artery or left main coronary artery may be intramural.

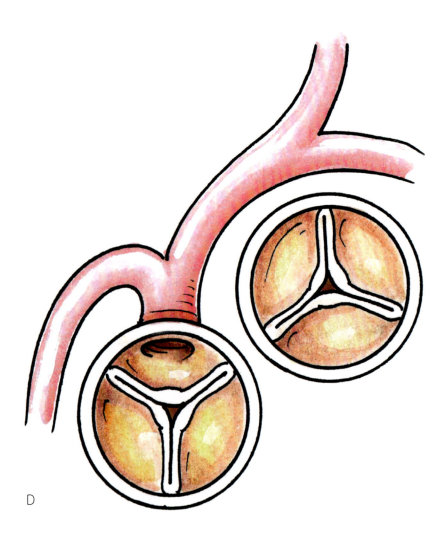

D

6. 壁内走行冠状动脉的移植

大动脉转位合并冠状动脉异常,特别是壁内走行冠状动脉是手术的高危因素(图 28-7)。

6. Intramural coronary artery transplantation

TGA with coronary artery abnormalities, especially intramural coronary artery transplantation, remain high-risk factors for surgery (Figure 28-7).

图 28-7 壁内走行冠状动脉的移植
A. 冠状动脉异常走行于主动脉壁内,两个冠状动脉开口距离很近。

Figure 28-7 Intramural coronary artery transplantation
A. The coronary arteries travel abnormally in the aortic wall, and the openings of the two coronary arteries are very close.

Continued

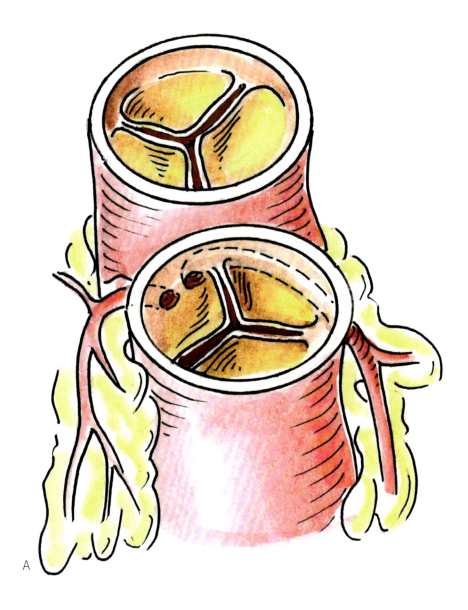

A

图 28-7（续）

B. 冠状动脉开口若靠近主动脉瓣交界，先将瓣叶交界从主动脉壁上剥离下来。注意避免损伤瓣叶。

Figure 28-7 cont'd

B. If the coronary ostium is close to the aortic valve commissure, the leaflet commissure is first freed off the aortic wall. Take care to avoid damaging the valve leaflets.

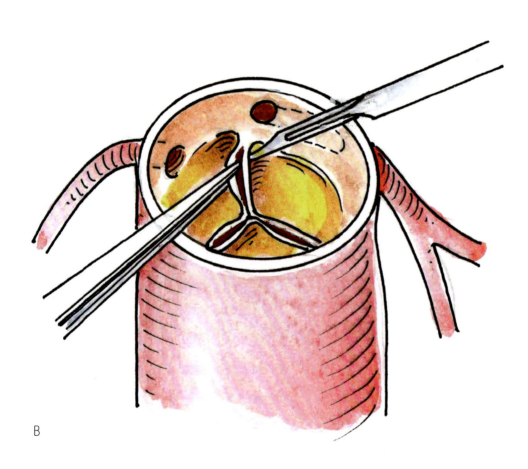

B

图 28-7（续）

Figure 28-7 cont'd

C. 用冠状动脉探条探查壁内走行冠状动脉的长度，然后剪除冠状动脉开口后的主动脉壁组织壁内走行部分。

C. The length of the intramurally coursing coronary artery is explored with a coronary probe, and then the intramural aortic wall tissue following the coronary ostium is excised.

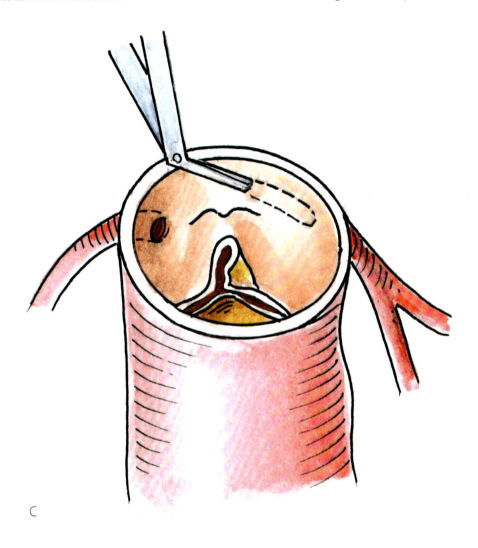

C

图 28-7（续）

D. 将左、右冠状动脉开口分别取下，用自身心包和补片修补缺损的主动脉壁。

Figure 28-7 cont'd

D. The left and right coronary ostium are removed separately, and the defective aortic wall is repaired with autogenous pericardium and patch.

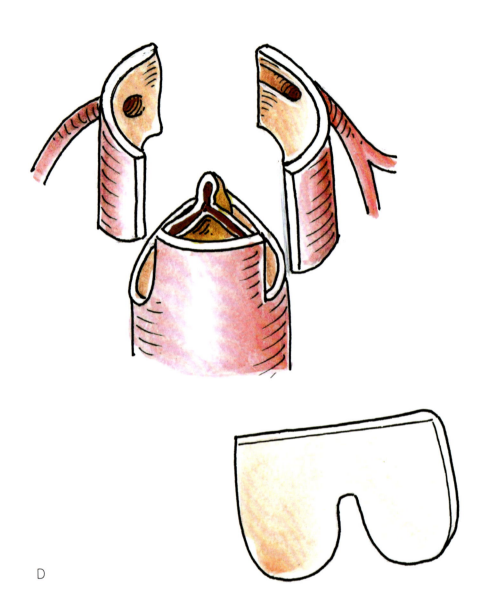

D

图 28-7(续)

Figure 28-7 cont'd

E. 将游离下来的主动脉瓣叶交界重新固定在补片上,以后的步骤与普通 TGA 手术相同。所有的缝合大多采用 7-0 Prolene 缝线。移植后的右冠状动脉位置要比左冠状动脉开口稍高些,避免右冠状动脉的扭曲。

E. Re-fix the freed aortic valve leaflet junction to the patch. The subsequent procedures are the same as ordinary TGA surgery. All sutures generally use 7-0 Prolene sutures. The position of the right coronary artery after transplantation is slightly higher than the opening of the left coronary artery to avoid distortion of the right coronary artery.

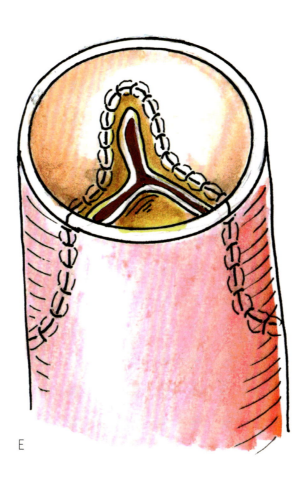

E

7. 左右冠状动脉同时起始于一个瓣窦（图 28-8）

7. The right and left coronary sinuses simultaneously originating from one sinus (Figure 28-8)

图 28-8　左右冠状动脉同时起始于一个瓣窦

A. 左右冠状动脉同时起始于一个瓣窦的窦往往大于另外两个。为了保证冠状动脉开口的再吻合，尽量多地切下主动脉壁组织。

B. 虚线显示一个瓣窦同时含有左右冠状动脉窦时的切割位置。

Figure 28-8　The right and left coronary sinuses simultaneously originating from one sinus

A. The left and right coronary arteries originate from one sinus at the same time, which is often larger than the other two sinuses. In order to ensure the re-anastomosis of the coronary ostium, large aortic wall tissue is removed as much as possible.

B. The dotted liney indicates the removal position when one sinus contains both left and right coronary sinuses.

Continued

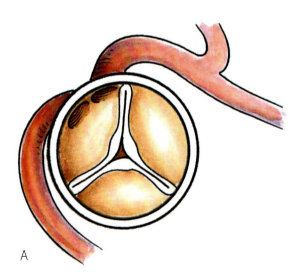

A

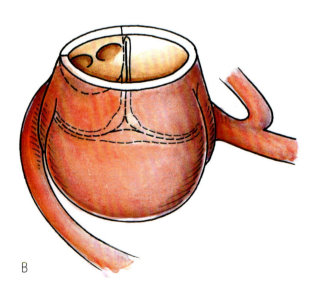

B

图 28-8(续)

C. 缺损的瓣窦可以用自身心包补片修补。一般尽可能将左右冠状动脉平均分开。

Figure 28-8 cont'd

C. Valvular sinuses with defect can be repaired with an autogenous pericardial patch. Typically, the left and right coronary arteries should be divided equally.

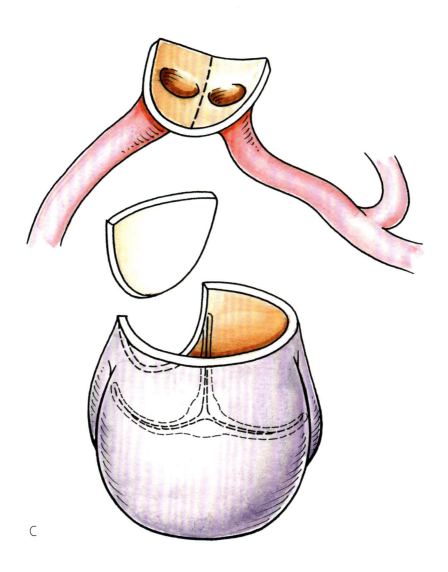

C

图 28-8（续）

Figure 28-8 cont'd

D. 在左右冠状动脉没有张力的情况下，可以分别单独和肺动脉瓣窦吻合。

D. In the absence of tension in the left and right coronary arteries, they can be anastomosed separately to the pulmonary sinus.

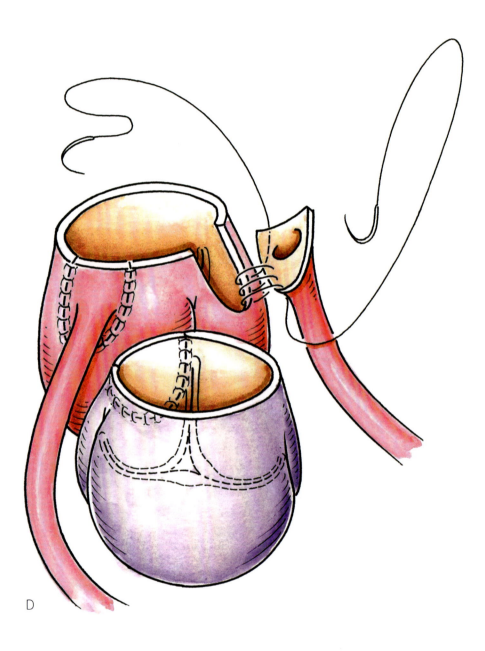

D

图 28-8（续）

E. 如果两个冠状动脉靠得很近，剪开会损伤冠状动脉的开口，可将两个冠状动脉开口一并取下，纽片翻转 90° 与相邻的新的主动脉窦做吻合。

Figure 28-8 cont'd

E. If the two coronary arteries are very close, cutting them will damage the opening of the coronary arteries. The two coronary artery openings can be removed together, and the button can be turned 90° to make an anastomosis to the adjacent new aortic sinus.

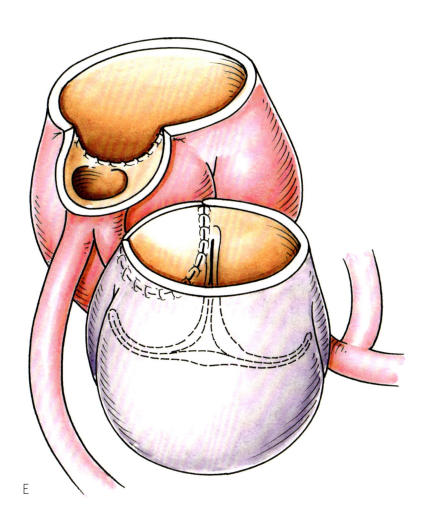

E

图 28-8（续）

Figure 28-8 cont'd

F. 然后再用自身心包补片构建前壁顶部，重要的是确保吻合后左、右冠状动脉不能张力过大或扭曲。

F. Then the roof of the anterior wall is constructed with an autologous pericardial patch. It is important to ensure that the left and right coronary arteries should not be over-tensioned or twisted after the anastomosis.

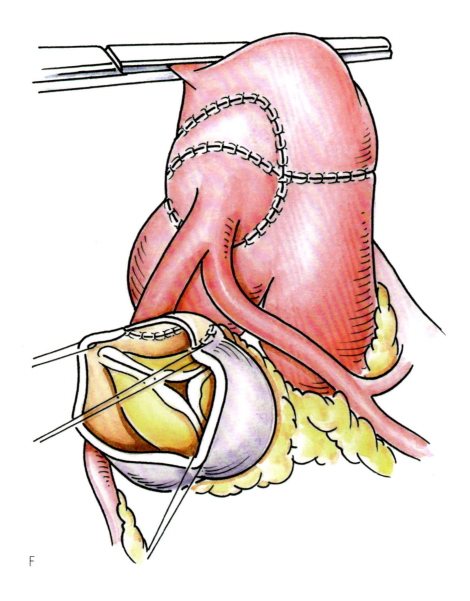

F

8. 单支冠状动脉（图 28-9）

8. Single coronary artery (Figure 28-9)

图 28-9 单支冠状动脉

A. 有些病例只有一支冠状动脉，再分叉成左右支、回旋支，几乎都在 2 号主动脉窦，而且靠近交界，极少数也可能有一支是壁内型走向。

B. 虚线显示单个冠状动脉窦的切除范围。近交界处动脉窦壁少，切开时小心不要损伤瓣膜。

Figure 28-9 Single coronary artery

A. In some cases, there is only one coronary artery, which bifurcates into left and right branches and circumflex branches, almost in sinus 2 and close to the commissure. In rare cases, there may also be an intramural coronary artery.

B. The dotted line shows the resection range of a single coronary sinus. Since there are few arterial sinus walls near the commissure, be careful not to damage the valve during incision.

Continued

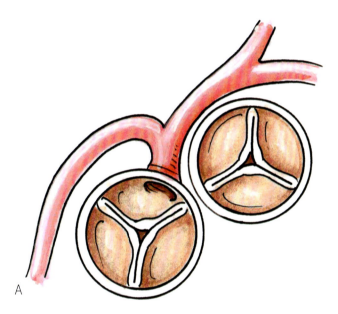

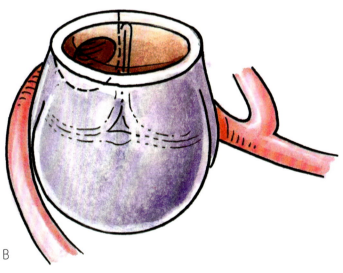

图 28-9（续）

Figure 28-9 cont'd

C. 将冠状动脉小心取下,注意不要损伤细小分支,缺损的瓣窦用自身心包修补。

C. Carefully remove the coronary artery, taking care not to damage the small branches, and repair the defective sinus with autologous pericardium.

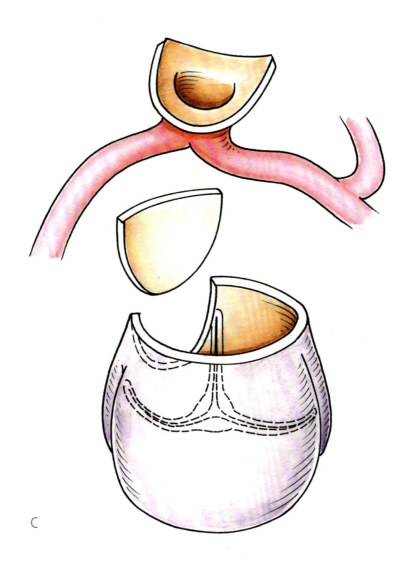

C

图 28-9（续）

D. 选择肺动脉邻近的瓣窦在相应位置
做吻合。融合在一起的冠状动脉窦往
往很大，相对地，大动脉根部较小。

Figure 28-9 cont'd

D. The valve sinus adjacent to the pulmonary artery is selected for anastomosis at the corresponding position. Coronary sinuses fused together tend to be large, with relatively small aortic roots.

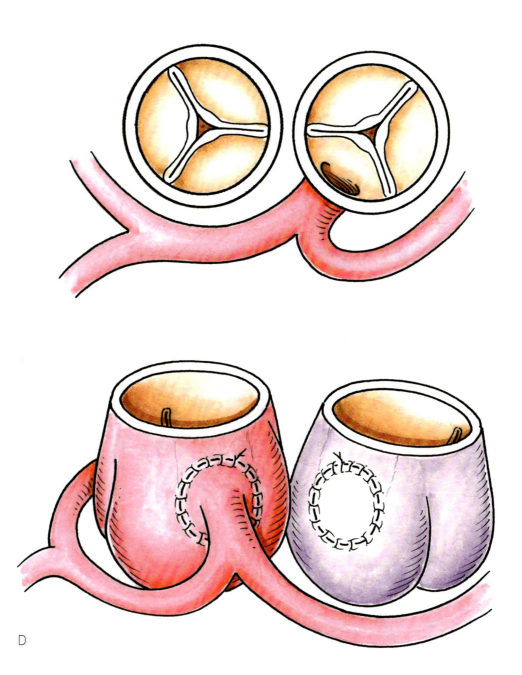

D

图 28-9（续）

E. 如果单支冠状动脉开口在一个冠状动脉窦的位置合适,也可以把冠状动脉开口纽扣状取下。原来的冠状动脉窦缺口可以用圆形心包补片关闭。原主动脉根部和肺动脉端端吻合,这样吻合口合适,一般不会引起肺动脉吻合口远期狭窄。

Figure 28-9 cont'd

E. If a single coronary artery opens in a coronary sinus, and the coronary ostium is appropriately positioned in the sinus, the coronary ostium can also be resected in a button shape. The original coronary sinus defect can be closed with a round pericardial patch. The aortic root and the pulmonary artery are end-to-end anastomosed so the anastomosis is suitable and generally will not cause long-term stenosis of the pulmonary artery anastomosis.

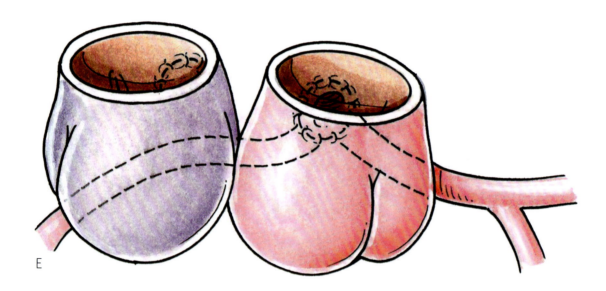

E

9. 大动脉转位合并主动脉弓发育不良

这类手术的心肺转流术大多采用深低温低流量脑灌注或深低温停循环方法（图 28-10）。

9. TGA complicated with dysplasia of aortic arch

Deep hypothermic low-flow cerebral perfusion or deep hypothermic circulatory arrest is usually employed in the cardiopulmonary bypass techniques in these procedures (Figure 28-10).

图 28-10　大动脉转位合并主动脉弓发育不良

A. 升主动脉和主动脉弓发育不良，升主动脉直径通常为肺动脉直径的 1/3~1/2。

Figure 28-10　TGA complicated with dysplasia of aortic arch

A. The ascending aorta and aortic arch are dysplastic. The diameter of the ascending aorta is usually about 1/3-1/2 of the diameter of the pulmonary artery.

Continued

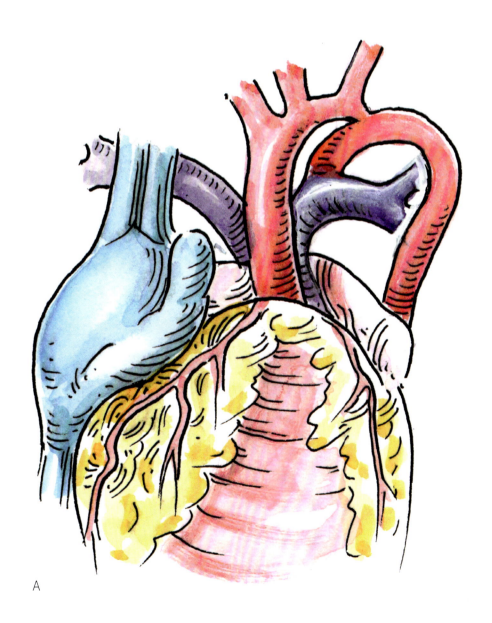

A

图 28-10（续）

B. 主动脉瓣上横断升主动脉，纵行剪开远端发育不良的升主动脉和主动脉弓，用自身心包或牛心包补片扩大成形。

Figure 28-10 cont'd

B. The ascending aorta above the aortic valve is transected, the dysplastic ascending aorta and dysplastic aortic arch at the distal end are incised longitudinally, and autologous pericardium or bovine pericardial patch is employed for enlargement.

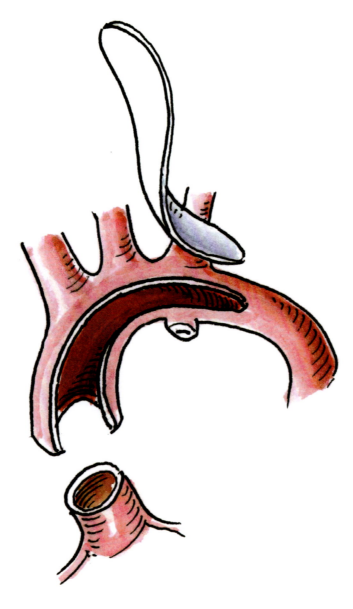

B

图 28-10（续）

C. 横断主肺动脉（虚线处），完成 Lecompt 转位。常规取下左右冠状动脉开口并分别移植，缺损的新的主动脉壁用裤片状心包补片修复。

Figure 28-10 cont'd

C. Transect the main pulmonary artery (refer to the dotted line) and perform the Lecompte maneuver to accomplish transposition. The left and right coronary artery openings are routinely removed and transplanted separately, and the new aortic wall defect is repaired with a pant-shaped pericardial patch.

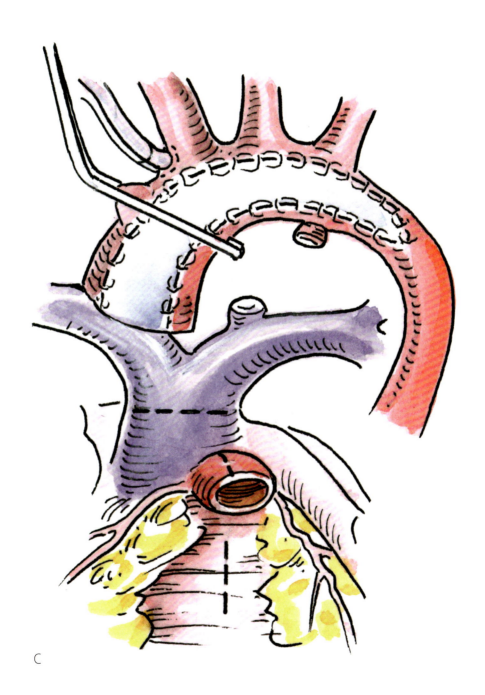

C

图 28-10（续）

D. 主动脉弓发育不良通常会合并右室漏斗部发育不良。取漏斗部纵行切口，离断部分漏斗部肌束，并用心包补片扩大右心室流出道。

Figure 28-10 cont'd

D. Dysplasia of the aortic arch is usually associated with dysplasia of the right infundibulum. A longitudinal incision is made at the infundibulum, a portion of the infundibular muscle bundle is dissociated and the right ventricular outflow tract is enlarged with a pericardial patch.

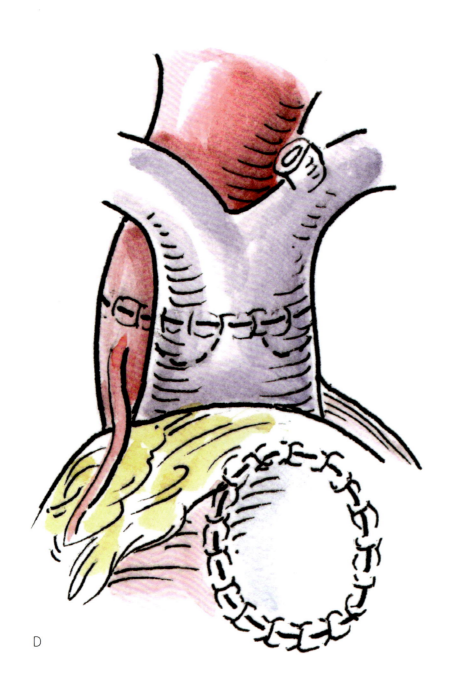

D

图 28-10（续）

E. 大动脉调转，主动脉弓扩大和右心室流出道扩大完成。

Figure 28-10 cont'd

E. After switching the great arteries, and the enlargement of the aortic arch, and enlargement of the right ventricular outflow tract are accomplished.

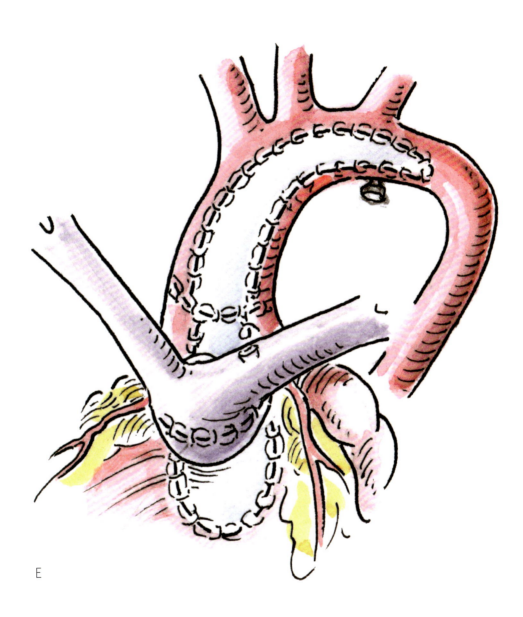

E

10. 大动脉转位的分期手术

大动脉转位合并室间隔完整的分期矫治用于已错过最佳手术时机的大动脉转位婴幼儿。这主要是因为新生儿生理性肺动脉高压已下降，导致左心室心肌逐渐退化，收缩压力也下降，心肌收缩功能不能承受体循环负荷。这种情况下分期矫治对于锻炼左心室，使其左心室心肌增厚以适应术后足够的体循环支持是十分必要的。分期矫治包括第一期肺动脉环束术和主动脉肺动脉分流和第二期大动脉转位手术。

新生儿的肺动脉环束术，可以在主肺动脉使用薄型的 ePTFE 系带，环束时逐步收紧，直至理想的程度，再用 Prolene 线缝合固定防止环束带松弛或移位。主动脉肺动脉分流一般建立在无名动脉近端和右肺动脉处。再手术时主动脉端直接缝闭，肺动脉侧可以用心包片修补。结扎动脉导管。肺动脉环缩的程度以保持动脉血氧饱和度在 80% 左右为宜，同时观察心脏窘迫程度，若心动过速（超过环束前的 30%）则提示环束过紧。同时也可测肺动脉和左心室压力阶差，一般控制在 50~60mmHg，对于房间隔缺损过小的患者，还需同时扩大房间隔缺损。

10. Staged procedure for TGA

The staged repair of TGA with intact ventricular septum is used for infants who have missed the optimal surgical timing for TGA. This is mainly because the physiological pulmonary hypertension of the newborn has decreased, leading to the gradual degeneration of the left ventricular myocardium and the decrease of systolic pressure, and myocardial systolic function cannot bear the load of the systemic circulation. In this case, staging repair is necessary to exercise the left ventricle and thicken the left ventricular myocardium to accommodate adequate systemic circulation support after surgery. Staged repair includes pulmonary artery banding and aortic-pulmonary shunt in the first stage, and aortic switch operation in the second stage.

For neonatal pulmonary artery banding, a thin ePTFE band can be employed on the main pulmonary artery, which is progressively tightened until the desired level, and then a Prolene suture is used to fix it to prevent the band from loosening or shifting. The aortic-pulmonary shunt is generally established at the proximal end of the innominate artery and the right pulmonary artery. During the second stage operation, the aortic end is directly sutured, and the pulmonary artery side can be repaired with a pericardial patch. The ductus arteriosus is ligated. The degree of pulmonary artery banding should maintain arterial oxygen saturation at approximately 80%, while the degree of cardiac distress should be observed, and tachycardia (more than 30% before banding) indicates that the banding is too tight. At the same time, the pressure gradient between the pulmonary artery and the left ventricle can also be measured, which is generally controlled at 50-60mmHg. For patients with a small atrial septal defect, the atrial septal defect needs to be enlarged at the same time.

通常取 4mm 直径的 ePTFE 管道,在无名动脉和右肺动脉之间做主动脉肺动脉分流手术,同时结扎动脉导管。主肺动脉上环束带并测压,观察环束后的压力变化(图28-11)。

Usually, an ePTFE conduit with a diameter of 4 mm is used to perform a systemic-pulmonary shunt operation between the innominate artery and the right pulmonary artery, and the ductus arterious is ligated at the same time. The main pulmonary artery is banded, and the pressure is measured. Observe the pressure change after banding (Figure 28-11).

术后主要依靠超声心动图评估左心室壁厚度和收缩功能、射血分数及左心室肌质量,再决定是否行动脉调转术。进行动脉调转术的条件是:①左心室与右心室压力比大于 70%;②左心室容量和心肌重量达到或接近该年龄的正常值。

Postoperatively, echocardiography is mainly employed to evaluate left ventricular wall thickness and systolic function, ejection fraction (EF) and left ventricular muscle mass, and then decide whether to perform arterial switch operation. The conditions for arterial switch operation are: ① The ratio of left ventricular to right ventricular pressure is greater than 70%; ② Left ventricular volume and myocardial weight reach or approach the normal value of this age.

图 28-11　TGA 分期手术　　　　　　　　Figure 28-11　Staged procedure for TGA

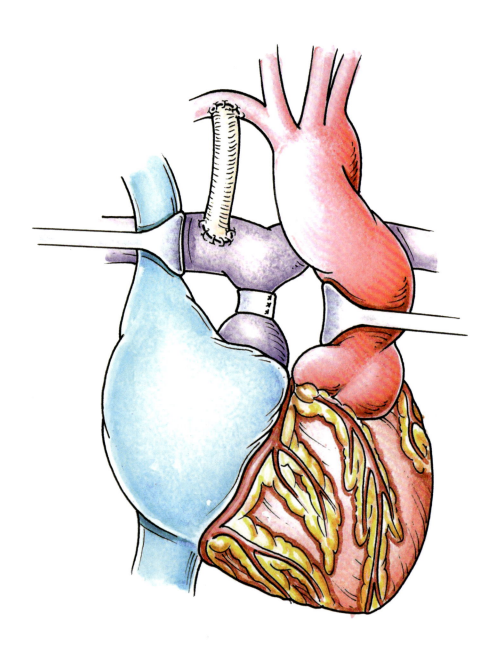

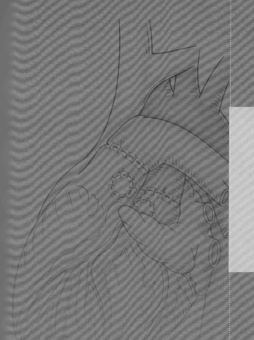

29 大动脉转位合并室间隔缺损和肺动脉狭窄

29 Transposition of Great Arteries Complicated with Ventricular Septal Defect and Pulmonary Stenosis

大动脉转位合并室间隔缺损和肺动脉狭窄的患者治疗方法取决于肺动脉狭窄的程度和室间隔缺损的位置和大小。手术年龄大多在 1 岁以后。

The treatment of patients with transposition of great arteries (TGA), ventricular septal defect (VSD), and pulmonary stenosis (PS) depends on the severity of the PS and the location and size of the VSD. Surgery is mostly performed after the age of one year old.

1. 升主动脉根部移位，室间隔缺损修补并扩大流出道，肺动脉半移位（Nikaidoh 手术） 对于大动脉转位合并室间隔缺损和左心室流出道狭窄，Nikaidoh 手术采用了整个升主动脉连同左右冠状动脉移位到左心室，同时进行室间隔缺损修补和双心室流出道重建。出于左右冠状动脉位置原因，此手术很合适于主动脉肺动脉前后位的患者。该手术和大动脉调转术一样，采用心肺转流术、中低温（图 29-1）。

1. Translocation of the aortic root, closure of VSD and enlargement of the outflow tract, semi-displacement of the pulmonary artery (Nikaidoh procedure) For TGA with VSD and stenosis of the left ventricular outflow tract, the entire ascending aorta and the left and right coronary arteries are translocated to the left ventricle, the VSD is closed, and the biventricular outflow tract is reconstructed in Nikaidoh procedure. Due to the location of the left and right coronary arteries, this procedure is appropriate for patients with anterior-to-posterior relation of the aorta and the pulmonary artery. Like arterial switch operation, the Nikaidoh procedure is also performed under cardiopulmonary bypass and moderate hypothermia (Figure 29-1).

图 29-1　Nikaidoh **手术**

A. 结扎并离断动脉导管，阻断升主动脉，灌注心肌停搏液。
B. 如果双大动脉位置有偏移，左右冠状动脉在升主动脉移位后不合适，可以进行冠状动脉再移植术。

Figure 29-1　Nikaidoh procedure

A. Ligate and transect the ductus arteriosus, block the ascending aorta, and then perfuse with the cardioplegic solution.
B. If the two great arteries are transposed from the common position and the left and right coronary arteries are not appropriate on completion of the ascending aorta translocation, coronary re-transplantation can be performed.

Continued

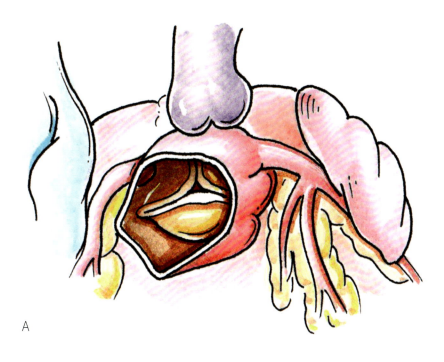

A

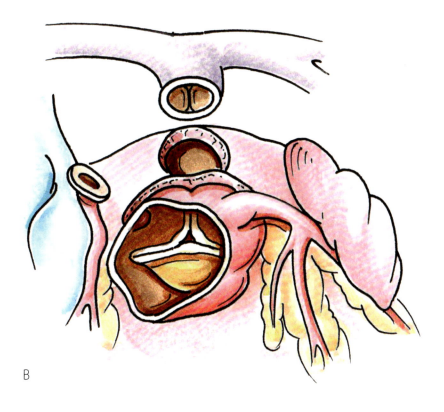

B

图 29-1（续）

C. 从主动脉根部离瓣环 5mm 左右游离升主动脉和紧邻升主动脉的肺动脉根部，避免损伤主动脉瓣。游离后的心室流出道显示左心室流出道狭小、室间隔缺损，室间隔缺损上的虚线显示要扩大的室间隔缺损。

Figure 29-1 cont'd

C. The ascending aorta and the pulmonary artery root adjacent to the ascending aorta are dissociated from the aortic root (approximately 5mm below the annulus), avoiding injuries to the aortic valve. After the ventricular outflow tract is freed, the left ventricular outflow tract stenosis and VSD can be exposed. The dotted line on the VSD indicates the defect is to be enlarged.

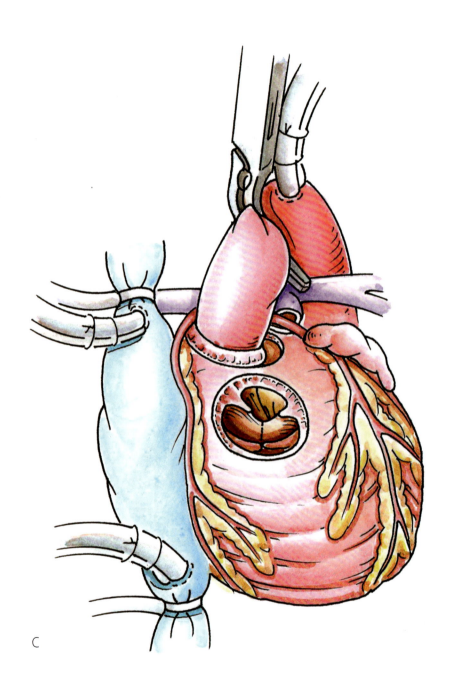

C

图 29-1（续）

Figure 29-1 cont'd

D. 沿室间隔缺损上的虚线切口扩大室间隔缺损，以便使用补片扩大左心室流出道。带冠状动脉的主动脉根部准备向左心室移位。移位时注意避免冠状动脉扭曲，过长或过短。必要时要进行单个或左右冠状动脉移植。本图显示的是右冠状动脉取下后再移植。如果左右冠状动脉在升主动脉移位时长度合适，没有扭曲，可以不移植。

D. Make an incision on the defect and enlarge the VSD along the dotted line to augment the left ventricular outflow tract with a patch. The aortic root with the coronary artery is to be displaced to the left ventricle. Care should be taken to avoid contorting the coronary artery or making it too long or too short during translocation. Single or left and right coronary artery grafts should be performed as necessary. This image shows the right coronary artery is removed and re-grafted. If the length of the left and right coronary arteries is appropriate without tortuosity during translocation of the ascending aorta, the arteries may not be grafted.

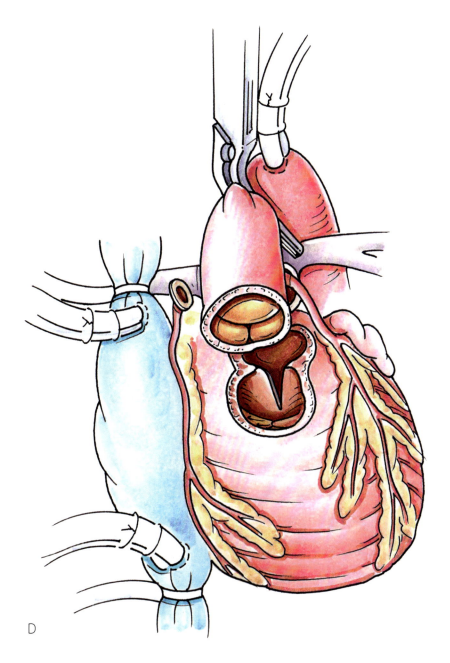

D

图 29-1 (续)

Figure 29-1 cont'd

E. 移位到左心室流出道的升主动脉。在确定升主动脉和左心室流出道一致时先进行后壁吻合。视婴儿大小使用5-0 或 6-0 的 Prolene 线连续缝合。扩大的室间隔缺损可使用心包片或人工补片闭合。

E. The ascending aorta is translocated to the left ventricular outflow tract. When the consistency between the ascending aorta and left ventricular outflow tract is confirmed, posterior wall anastomosis is performed at first with running sutures of 5-0 or 6-0 Prolene, depending on the baby's weight. The enlarged ventricle can be closed with a pericardial patch or prosthetic patch.

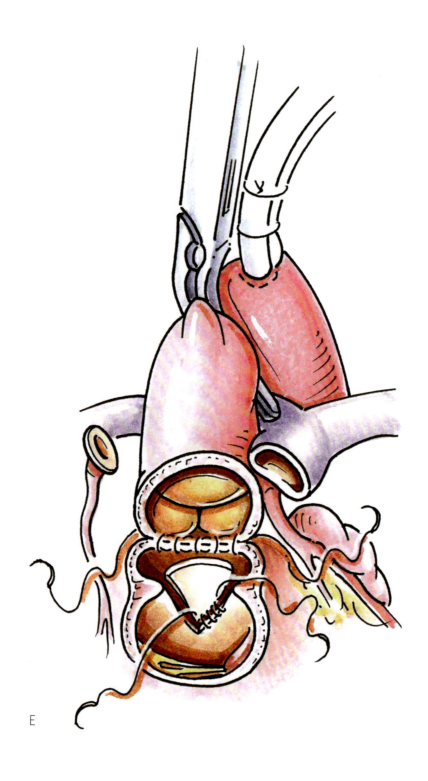

E

图 29-1（续）

F. 升主动脉移位完毕后可见新建的左心室流出道因为室间隔缺损的补片而扩大,此时可以进行冠状动脉移植。横断的肺动脉依靠邻近升主动脉侧壁进行右心室流出道再建。

Figure 29-1 cont'd

F. The newly constructed left ventricular outflow tract is augmented with the patch on the VSD after the displacement of the ascending aorta. Then, coronary artery transplantation can be performed. The transected pulmonary artery lies adjacent to the lateral wall of the ascending aorta for right ventricular outflow tract reconstruction.

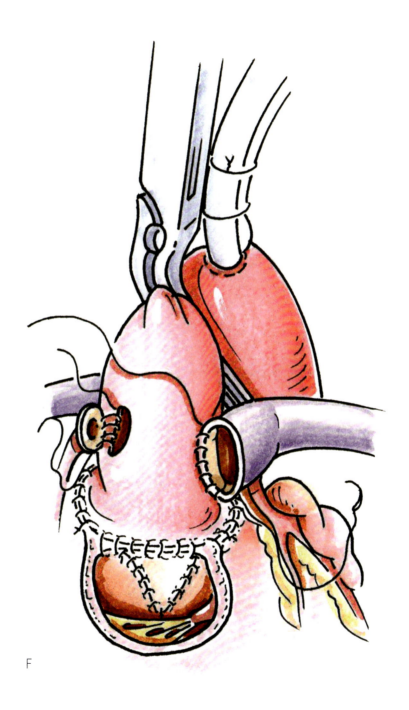

F

图 29-1（续）

G. 如果肺动脉比较狭小,可以在主肺动脉前壁纵行切开扩大,留在肺动脉根部的瓣膜可以部分减少肺动脉反流。选择合适的补片修剪成葫芦形状缝合扩大右心室流出道。

Figure 29-1 cont'd

G. If the pulmonary artery is relatively narrowed, a longitudinal incision can be made in the anterior wall of the main pulmonary artery for widening, as the remaining valves at the root of the pulmonary artery can partially decrease pulmonary regurgitation. An appropriate patch trimmed into a gourd shape is used to widen the right ventricular outflow tract.

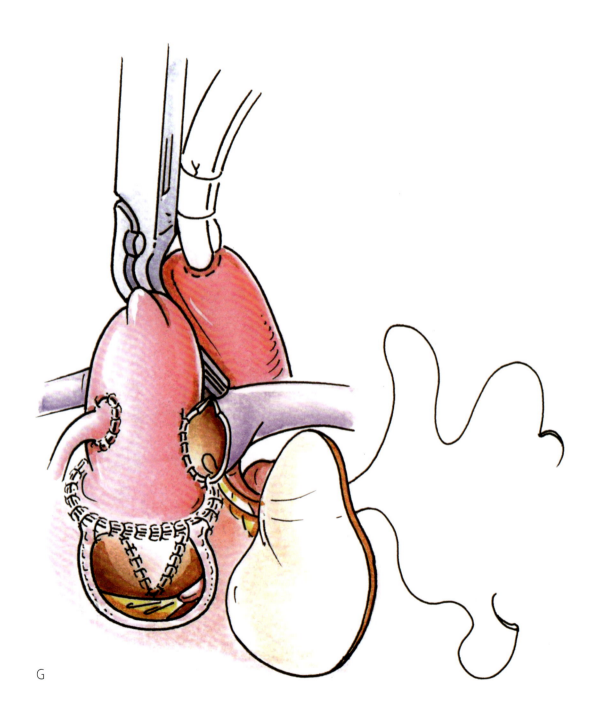

G

图 29-1（续）

Figure 29-1 cont'd

H. 经典的 Nikaidoh 手术包括升主动脉连同冠状动脉移位，室间隔缺损扩大并修补，左心室流出道和右心室流出道扩大成形。

H. The classic Nikaidoh procedure consists of displacement of the ascending aorta with the coronary artery, VSD enlargement and repair, and left ventricular outflow tract and right ventricular outflow tract enlargement.

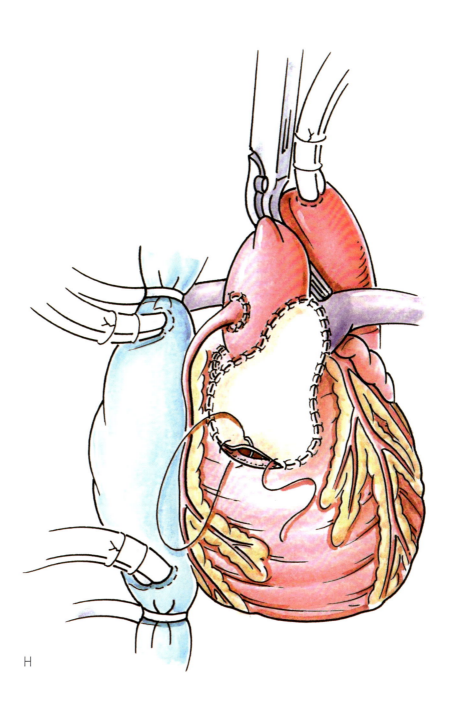

H

2. 大动脉根部整块旋转移植 对于大动脉转位合并室间隔缺损和左心室流出道狭窄，可以把左右冠状动脉从主动窦处切下，把整个大动脉根部进行180°旋转，使得肺动脉可以和右心室相连、主动脉和左心室连接。将左右冠状动脉移植到主动脉窦，同时进行室间隔缺损修补和双心室流出道重建。手术方法和大动脉转位相似（图29-2）。

2. En-block transposition of pulmonary and aortic root For TGA with VSD and stenosis of the left ventricular outflow tract, the left and right coronary arteries can also be dissected from the active sinus and the entire root of the great arteries is rotated 180°. The pulmonary artery is connected to the right ventricle, the aorta is connected to the left ventricle, and then the right and left coronary arteries are grafted to the aortic sinus when performing VSD repair and biventricular outflow tract reconstruction. The surgical approach of this procedure is like TGA surgery (Figure 29-2).

图 29-2　**大动脉根部整块旋转移植**

A. 横断双大动脉，切下左右冠状动脉。

Figure 29-2　En-block transposition of pulmonary and aortic root

A. Both great arteries are transected, and the left and right coronary arteries are excised.

Continued

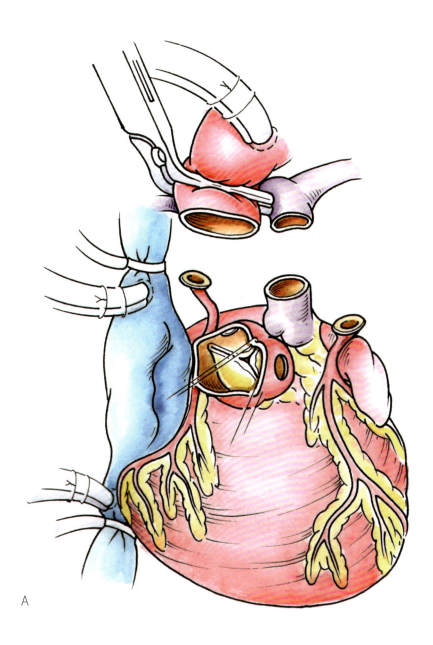

A

图 29-2（续）

B. 从主动脉根部离瓣环 5mm 左右游离升主动脉和紧邻升主动脉的肺动脉根部，整块切下，避免损伤主动脉瓣。游离后的心室流出道显示左心室流出道狭小（1），整块切下大动脉根部，左右冠状动脉已经从主动脉根部切下（2），大动脉根部 180°旋转后，肺动脉位于升主动脉前（3）。

Figure 29-2 cont'd

B. Free the ascending aorta at approximately 5mm from the annulus and dissect the pulmonary root adjacent to the ascending aorta, avoid injury to the aortic valve. After the ventricular outflow tract is freed, the left ventricular outflow tract stenosis and VSD are exposed (1). The excised en-block root, and the left and right coronary artery have been excised from the aortic root (2). After a 180° rotation of the great artery, the pulmonary artery is located anterior to the ascending aorta (3).

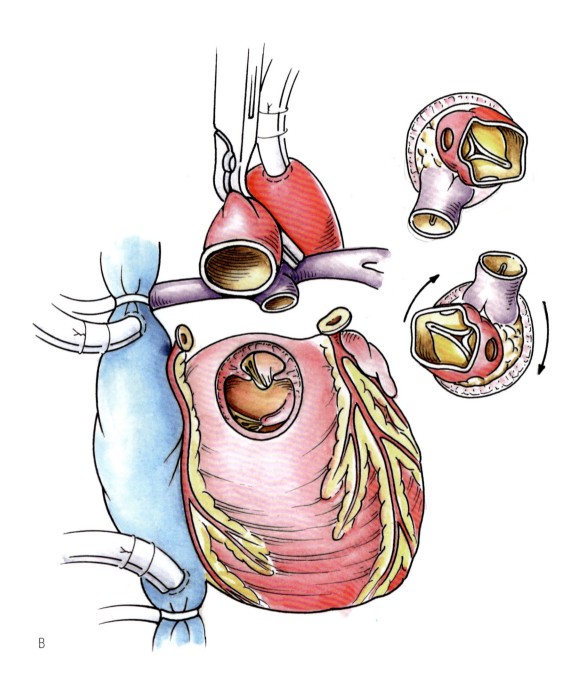

B

图 29-2（续）

C. 将旋转后的大动脉根部移位到左右心室流出道正确的位置，细小的肺动脉在前，正对右心室流出道，在确定升主动脉和左心室流出道一致时先进行后壁吻合。视婴儿大小使用 5-0 或 6-0 的 Prolene 线连续缝合。室间隔缺损上的虚线显示要扩大的室间隔缺损，肺动脉根部正中虚线处准备切开，扩大右心室流出道。

Figure 29-2 cont'd

C. Displacement of the rotated great artery roots into the correct position of the left and right ventricular outflow tracts. As the small pulmonary artery lies in front of the right ventricular outflow tract, the posterior wall is sutured first with continuous sutures using 5-0 or 6-0 Prolene based on the baby's weight after confirming the consistency between the ascending aorta and left ventricular outflow tract. The dotted line on the VSD shows the defect to be enlarged, and an incision is to be made in the middle of the pulmonary artery root along the dotted line, followed by enlargement of the right ventricular outflow tract.

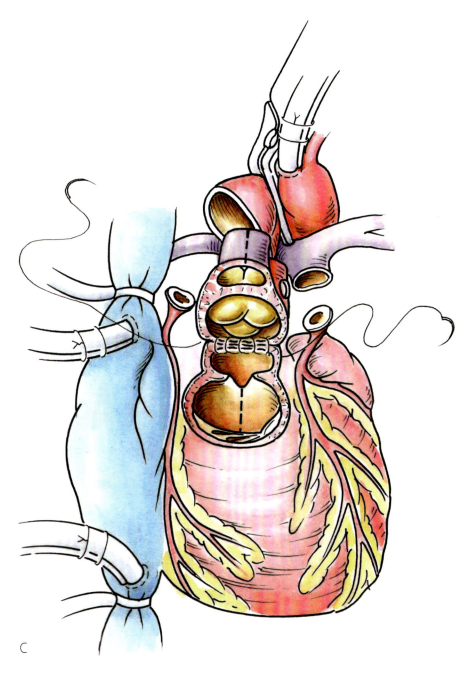

C

图 29-2（续）

D. 切断双动脉下的漏斗隔组织,使之与室间隔缺损相通,扩大的室间隔缺损可使用心包片或人工补片闭合。狭小的肺动脉经常只有两个瓣叶,要尽量保证瓣叶的完整性。

Figure 29-2 cont'd

D. The infundibular septum tissue under the great arteries is dissected and connected to the VSD, which can be closed with a pericardial patch or prosthetic patch. Narrowed pulmonary arteries often only have two leaflets, and the integrity of the leaflets should be ensured as much as possible.

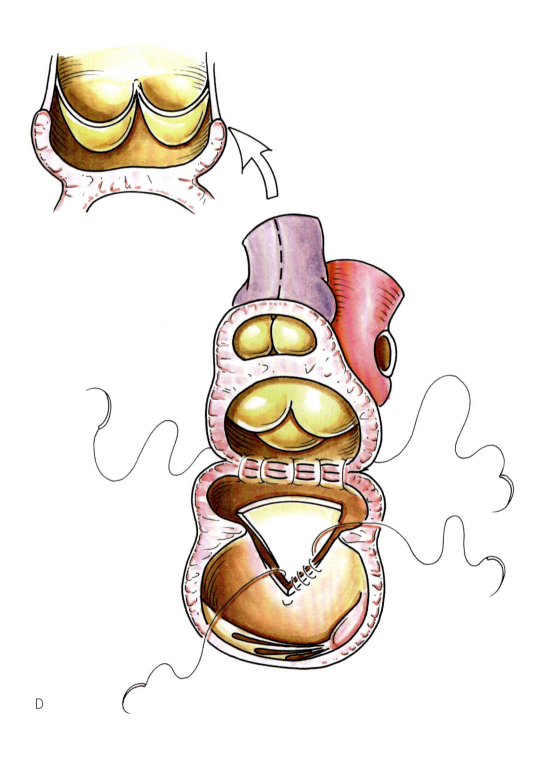

D

图 29-2 (续)

Figure 29-2 cont'd

E. 大多数情况切下的左右冠状动脉长度位置适合原有的冠状动脉窦，只是左右方向对调而已。冠状动脉再吻合，大多使用 7-0 的 Prolene 线。扩大的室间隔缺损应用补片修补。

E. In most cases, the position and length of the left and right coronary arteries fit the original coronary sinus, and displacements only need to swap the left and right directions of the sinus. The coronary artery is then re-anastomosed, mostly using 7-0 Prolene sutures. An enlarged VSD is repaired with a patch.

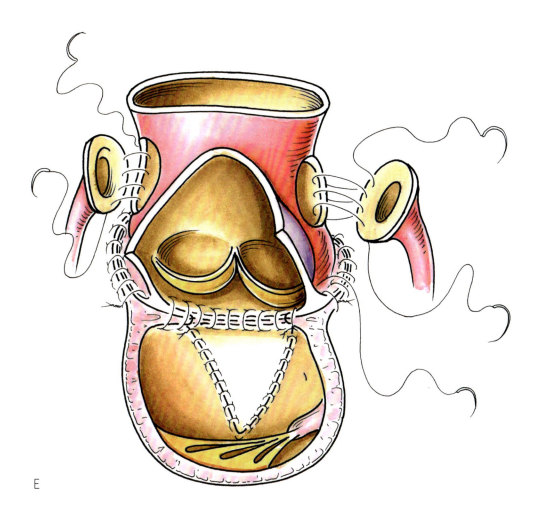

E

图 29-2（续）

F. 进行 Lecompte 操作，把充分游离好的肺动脉提到升主动脉前，做升主动脉和左心室流出道后壁连续吻合。

Figure 29-2 cont'd

F. The Lecompte maneuver is performed to advance the dissociated pulmonary artery to the ascending aorta, followed by a running suture of the ascending aorta and the posterior wall of the left ventricular outflow tract.

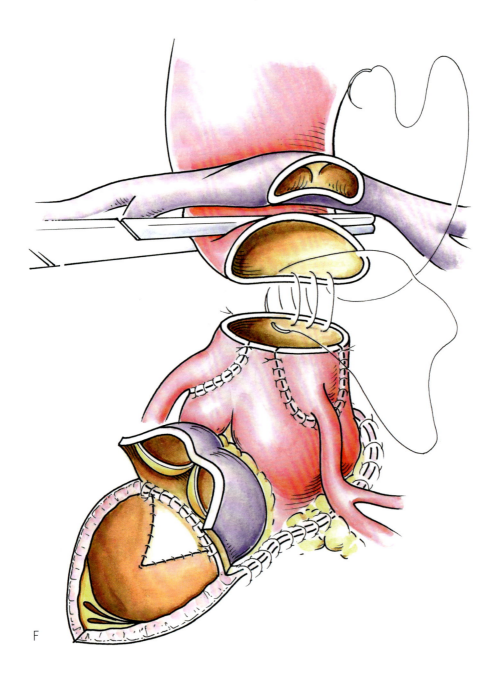

图 29-2（续）

Figure 29-2 cont'd

G. 肺动脉和被切开的肺动脉根部进行后壁吻合。

G. Anastomosis of the posterior wall between the pulmonary artery and the incised pulmonary root.

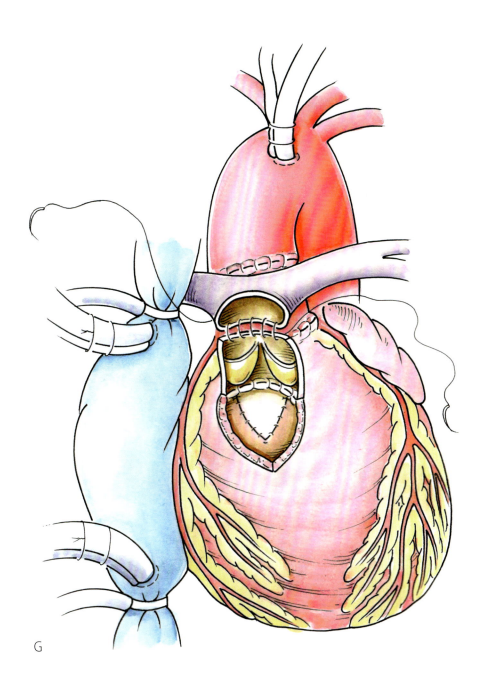

G

图 29-2（续）

H. 用自制的带瓣叶心包补片（最好不要经过固定处理）关闭右心室流出道。

Figure 29-2 cont'd

H. Close the right ventricular outflow tract with a homemade valvular pericardial patch (preferably without fixation).

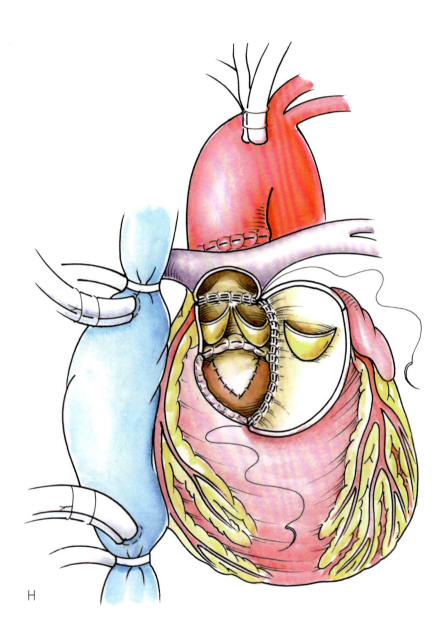

H

3. 大动脉双根调转术（改良 Nikaidoh 手术） 大动脉转位合并室间隔缺损和肺动脉狭窄，矫正手术除了 Nikaidoh 手术、大动脉根部旋转手术方法外，大动脉双根调转术也可以治疗这类畸形（图 29-3）。

3. Double-root transposition (modified Nikaidoh procedure) For TGA with a VSD and PS, in addition to the Nikaidoh procedure and transposition of great arteries, the double-root transposition is available for this malformation (Figure 29-3).

图 29-3　**大动脉双根调转术（改良 Nikaidoh 手术）**

A. 大动脉转位合并室间隔缺损和肺动脉狭窄。

Figure 29-3　Double-root transposition (modified Nikaidoh procedure)

A. TGA with a VSD and PS.

Continued

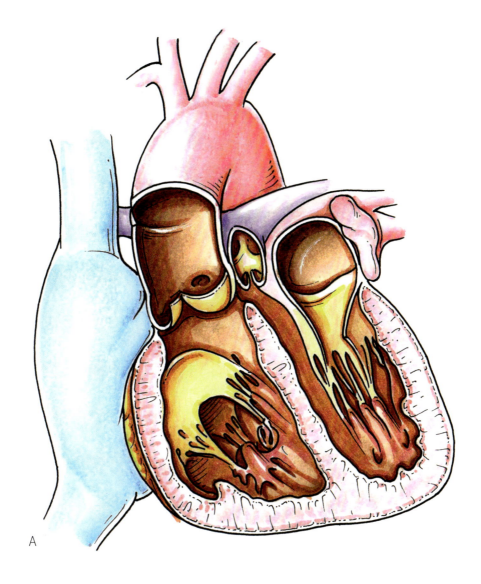

A

图 29-3（续）

B. 手术在心肺转流术下进行,基本方法和 Nikaidoh 手术、主动脉根部旋转手术一样。在升主动脉根部,瓣上 1 cm 左右横断升主动脉。离瓣环 5mm 处切下主动脉根部,避免损伤瓣叶和冠状动脉。

Figure 29-3 cont'd

B. This operation is performed under cardiopulmonary bypass with the same basic methods as those of the Nikaidoh procedure and transposition of great arteries. At the root of the ascending aorta, a transverse incision is made in the ascending aorta about 1 cm above the valve. The aortic root is resected at 5 mm below the annulus, while avoiding damage to the leaflets and coronary arteries.

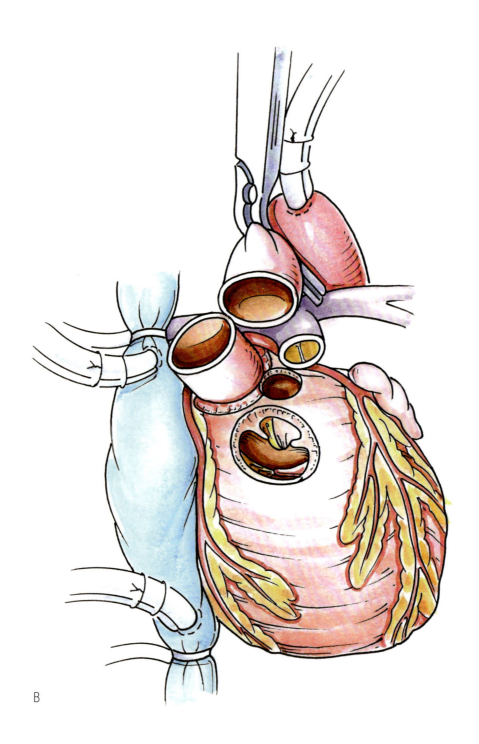

B

C. 和主动脉根部切除方法一样,从左心室切下整个带瓣的肺动脉。切断双动脉下的漏斗隔组织,与室间隔缺损相通。扩大左心室流出道。虚线显示室间隔缺损纵向切开准备补片扩大左心室流出道。

C. Like the aortic root resection method, the entire pulmonary artery with the valve is excised from the left ventricle. The infundibular septum tissue under both great arteries is cut and linked to the VSD. The left ventricular outflow tract is to be enlarged by patches through a longitudinal incision, as revealed by the dotted line.

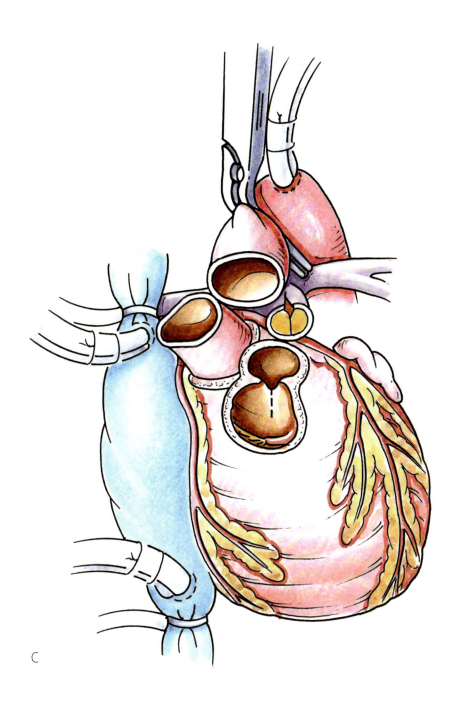

C

图 29-3（续）

D. 使用自身心包或者人工补片修补室间隔缺损同时扩大左心室流出道。

Figure 29-3 cont'd

D. Repair the VSD with an autologous pericardial patch or prosthetic patch while extending the left ventricular outflow tract.

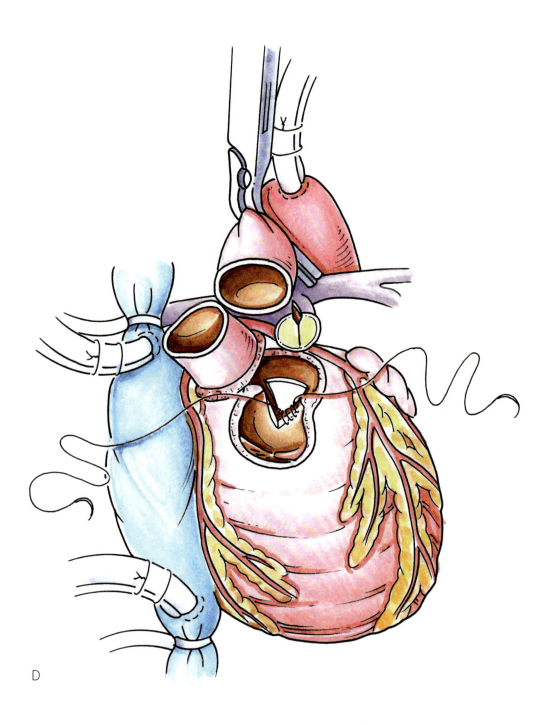

D

图 29-3（续）

E. 大多数患儿的左右冠状动脉适合 Leiden 规则,左冠状动脉(左前降支和回旋支)位于冠状动脉窦 1,右冠状动脉位于冠状动脉窦 2。在升主动脉根部向左心室移位后,视冠状动脉的位置和长度决定接下来的操作,如左右冠状动脉的长度不够,造成冠状动脉牵拉过紧或扭曲,则必须把一根或两根冠状动脉从根部切下。把主动脉根部后壁连续缝合在左心室后壁,前壁与扩大的室间隔缺损补片缝合。

Figure 29-3 cont'd

E. The Leiden convention is available for the left and right coronary arteries of most children with their left coronary artery (left anterior descending and circumflex) located in the coronary sinus 1 and the right coronary sinus in the sinus 2. After migration of the ascending aortic root to the left ventricle, one or both coronary arteries must be excised from the root if the left and right coronary arteries are not long enough to cause the tightness or tortuosity of the coronary artery, which depends on the position and length of the coronary artery. The posterior wall of the aortic root is sutured continuously to the posterior wall of the left ventricle, and the anterior wall is sewed with an enlarged ventricular patch.

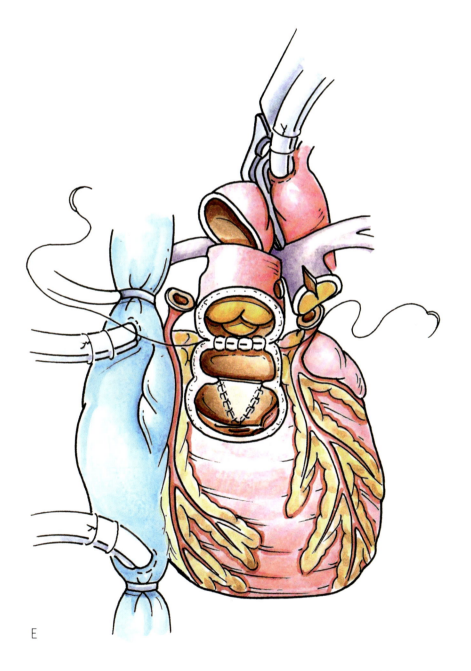

E

图 29-3（续）

Figure 29-3 cont'd

F. 主动脉根部移植到左心室后,右心室流出道后壁显示的是室间隔缺损使用补片后加宽的室间隔。左右冠状动脉分别被移植到升主动脉前壁。

F. After the aortic root is grafted to the left ventricle, the right ventricular outflow tract posterior wall is the interventricular septum widened by patches. The left and right coronary arteries are grafted to the anterior wall of the ascending aorta, respectively.

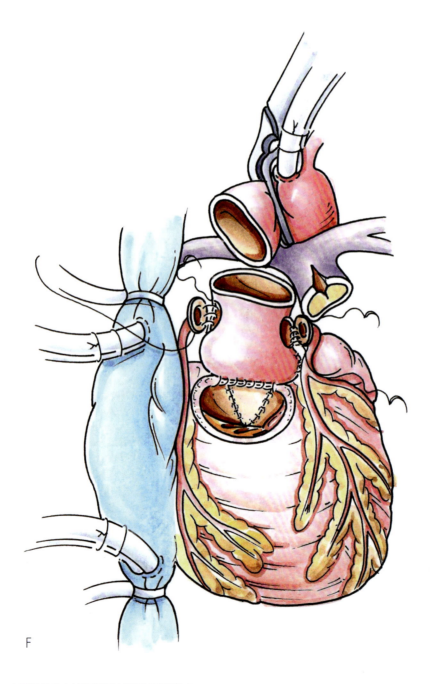

F

图 29-3（续）

G. 进行 Lecompte 换位操作,把肺动脉提到升主动脉前。升主动脉和主动脉根部连续缝合。

Figure 29-3 cont'd

G. The Lecompte maneuver is conducted to advance the pulmonary artery to the anterior aspect of the ascending aorta, with running suturing of the ascending aorta and aortic root.

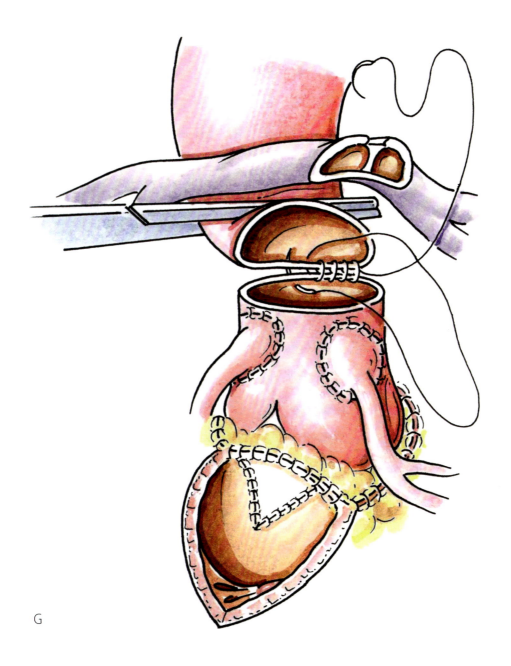

G

图 29-3（续）

Figure 29-3 cont'd

H. 接下来的步骤视肺动脉发育情况而定，如肺动脉发育好则尽量保留肺动脉瓣，下缘用一块心包补片扩大右心室流出道，反之则纵向切开狭窄肺动脉至分叉处，肺动脉后壁正好和补片修补后的室间隔连续缝合。

H. The following step depends on the development of the pulmonary artery. If the pulmonary artery is well developed, the pulmonary valve should be preserved as much as possible. On the lower edge, a pericardial patch is used to expand the right ventricular outflow tract. On the contrary, a longitudinal incision is made to the bifurcation of the narrowed pulmonary artery, and the posterior wall of the pulmonary artery and the VSD repaired by patches are closed with a running suture.

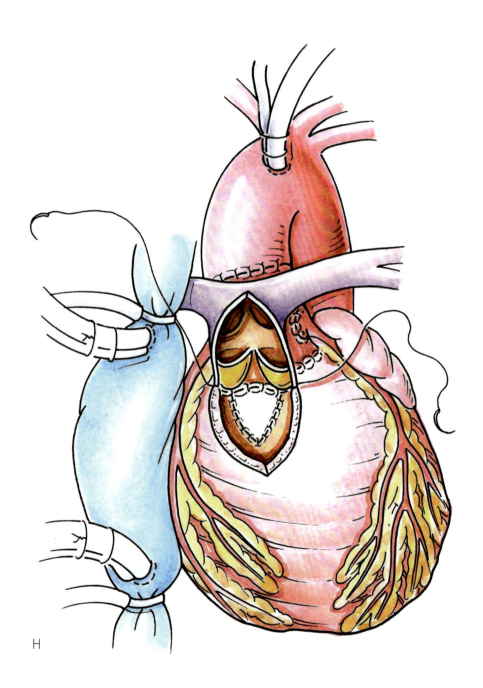

图 29-3（续）

I. 使用自制带瓣叶的补片关闭右心室流出道。根据法洛四联症矫治经验，这种方法可以有效防止肺动脉反流，保护右心室功能。

Figure 29-3 cont'd

I. Close the right ventricular outflow tract using a homemade valvular patch. According to the evidence on tetralogy of Fallot treatment, this procedure can effectively prevent pulmonary regurgitation and protect right ventricular function.

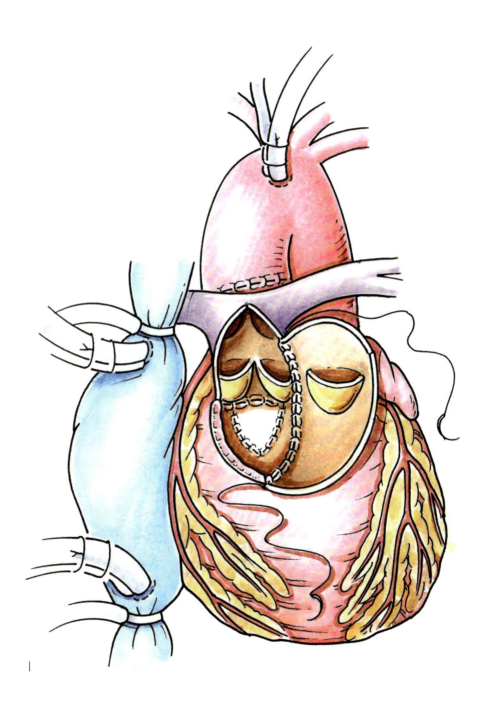

图 29-3（续）

J. 大动脉转位合并室间隔缺损和肺动脉狭窄调转术后的主动脉、肺动脉根部。

Figure 29-3 cont'd

J. Aortic and pulmonary artery root in the cases of TGA with VSD and PS can be inversed after the transposition surgery.

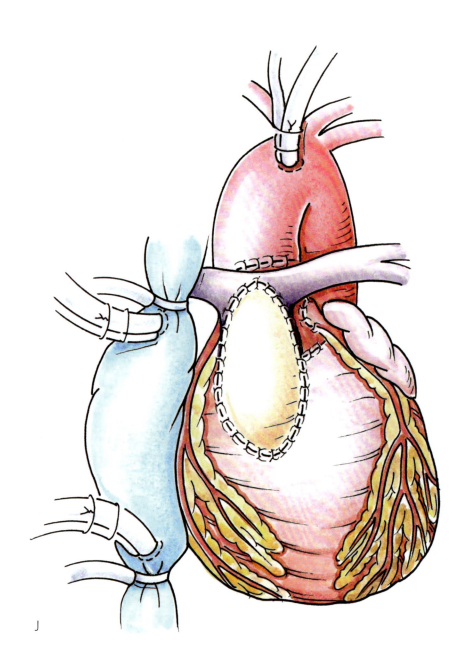

J

图 29-4　大动脉转位的冠状动脉再移植

A. 大动脉转位的大血管所占空间位置大，转位的变异性也大。一般情况下主动脉在肺动脉的右前方（1）。事实上每一病例主动脉窦和冠状动脉开口均面对相应的肺动脉的动脉窦（2），这样有利于冠状动脉的转移和大动脉调转术。仅一小部分冠状动脉调转困难。

Figure 29-4　Retransplantation of coronary artery after arterial switch operation

A. In TGA, the great arteries take up large space, and the variability of transposition is high, and the aorta usually lies anterior to the right of the pulmonary artery (1). In fact, the aortic sinus and coronary ostium, in each case, face the corresponding arterial sinus of the pulmonary artery (2), which facilitates coronary artery transfer and arterial switch operation. Only a small proportion of coronary transfer is difficult.

Continued

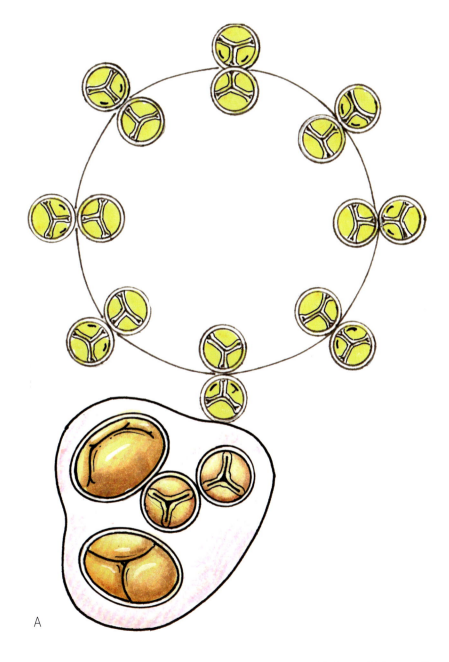

A

图 29-4（续）

Figure 29-4 cont'd

B. 大多数病例左冠状动脉位于冠状动脉窦 1，右冠状动脉在冠状动脉窦 2 (1)，为了使主动脉在移位到左心室流出道时避免产生冠状动脉张力，切下左右冠状动脉后，使主动脉根部进行 180° 转位，以便左右冠状动脉共同移植到无冠状动脉窦的瓣窦上 (2)。

B. In most cases, the left coronary artery is located in the coronary sinus 1 and the right coronary artery in the coronary sinus 2 (1). In order to avoid coronary tension when migrating the aorta to the left ventricular outflow tract, the aortic root is transposed 180° after the left and right coronary arteries are excised so that the left and right coronary arteries are co-grafted to the valve sinus with noncoronary sinus (2).

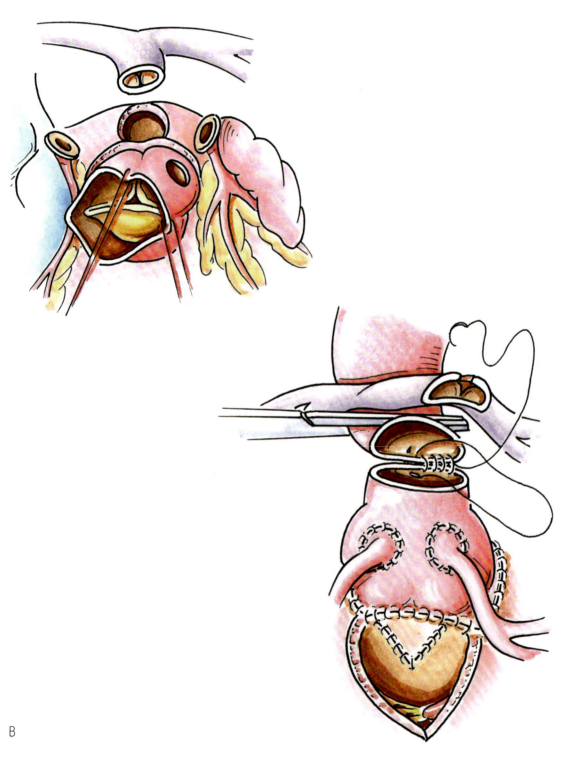

B

图 29-4（续）

Figure 29-4 cont'd

C. 如果左心室流出道上的肺动脉在升主动脉根部左后侧(1)，左冠状动脉在升主动脉移植后不会有张力，而右冠状动脉在升主动脉移植后因为长度不够，需要再移植(2)。

C. If the pulmonary artery of the left ventricular outflow tract lies left and posterior to the ascending aortic root (1), the left coronary artery does not have tension after ascending aortic grafting, while the right coronary artery needs to be re-grafted because it is not long enough (2).

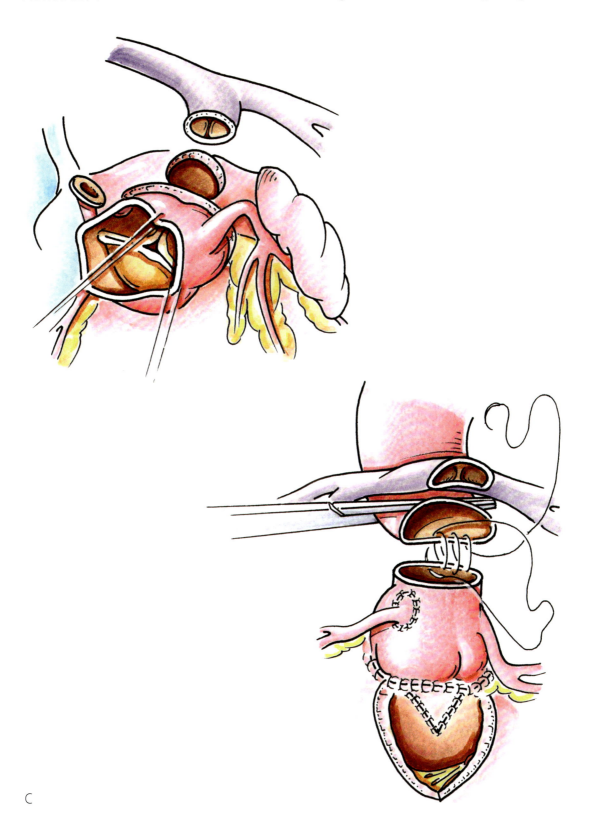

C

图 29-4（续）

Figure 29-4 cont'd

D. 肺动脉在升主动脉根部的右后侧
(1)，升主动脉根部在移位到左心室流出
道时，右冠状动脉不太会有张力，而左
冠状动脉必须要再移植(2)。

D. Pulmonary arteries lie right and posterior to the
ascending aortic root (1). When the ascending aortic root is
displaced into the left ventricular outflow tract, there is little
tension in the right coronary artery, while the left coronary
artery must be re-grafted (2).

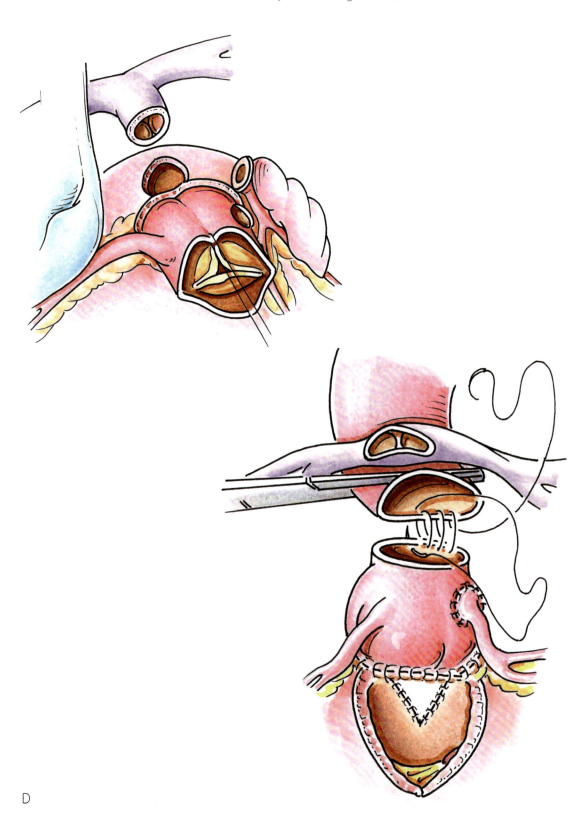

D

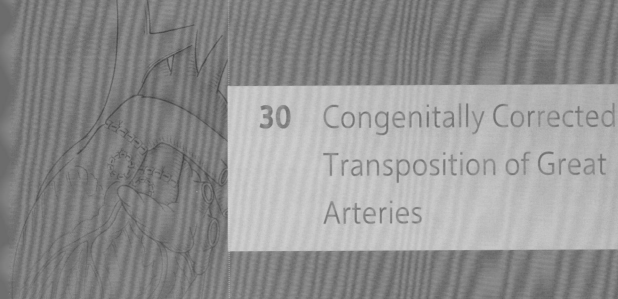

30 矫正型大动脉转位

30 Congenitally Corrected Transposition of Great Arteries

一、解剖分型

矫正型大动脉转位（congenitally corrected transposition of great arteries，ccTGA）是一组心房和心室连接不一致、心室和大动脉连接不一致的复杂型先天性心脏病。主动脉起始于和左心房相连的右心室，肺动脉起始于和右心房连接的左心室。生理学上血流动力学与正常循环一致，但是解剖学上结构不一致。由于其功能上已得到矫正，主动脉仍然接受肺静脉血，肺动脉仍然接受体静脉血，临床上并无重要的病理意义。但是，在有其他心内畸形并存而需要手术时，则必须充分了解矫正型大动脉转位的解剖学特征。其常见伴有的心脏畸形有室间隔缺损、肺动脉瓣狭窄等。下面以常见的 S.L.L 矫正型大动脉转位为例加以说明（图 30-1）。

左右心房位置正常，左右心室并排于两侧，室间隔近于矢状位，前室间沟也比正常心脏靠近中线，升主动脉在左前方，主肺动脉在右后方，冠状动脉发自左、右冠状动脉窦内而无冠状动脉窦被移至前方，前降支发自右侧冠状动脉主干。

I. Anatomical Typing

Congenitally corrected transposition of great arteries (ccTGA) is a complex congenital heart defect with inconsistent atrial and ventricular connections and inconsistent ventricular and aortic connections. The aorta arises from the right ventricle connected to the left atrium, and the pulmonary artery from the left ventricle connected to the right atrium. Physiologically, the hemodynamics are consistent with normal circulation but anatomically inconsistent. Since the heart actually "corrects" the abnormal development, the aorta still receives pulmonary venous blood, and the pulmonary artery still receives systemic venous blood, which has no important pathological significance in clinical practice. However, if other intracardiac malformations co-exist and surgery is required, the anatomic characteristics of the corrected transposition of great arteries must be well understood. Common associated cardiac malformations include ventricular septal defect (VSD), pulmonary valve stenosis, etc. The common ccTGA (S, L, L) is illustrated below (Figure 30-1).

The left and right atria are normal. The left and right ventricles are juxtaposed on both sides. The interventricular septum is close to the sagittal position, and the anterior interventricular sulcus is also closer to the midline than the normal heart. The ascending aorta is in the left anterior, and the main pulmonary artery is in the right rear. The coronary artery arises from the left and right sinuses, the noncoronary sinus is moved to the front, and the anterior descending artery arises from the right main coronary artery.

S.L.L 矫正型大动脉转位的心房位置正常，但右侧心室腔为二尖瓣心室腔，二尖瓣环在室间隔的附着缘仍然高于对侧的三尖瓣隔瓣附着缘，膜样间隔位于二尖瓣环之下。因此，在切开心室腔后可以发现膜样间隔位于右侧房室环（二尖瓣环）的下方。这和正常心脏的右心室所见恰恰相反，因为正常情况下膜样间隔位于右侧房室环（三尖瓣环）的上方。

The atrial position of ccTGA (S, L, L) is normal, but the right ventricular chamber is the mitral valve ventricular chamber. The attachment margin of the mitral annulus in the interventricular septum is still higher than that of the tricuspid valve on the opposite side. The membranous septum is located below the mitral annulus. Thus, the membranous septum can be found below the right atrioventricular ring (mitral annulus) after incision of the ventricular chamber. This is quite the opposite of what is seen in the right ventricle of a normal heart, where the membranous septum is normally located above the right atrioventricular ring (tricuspid annulus).

矫正型大动脉转位的肺动脉流出道是一个斜行管道，深嵌于逆位的二尖瓣环和三尖瓣环之间。肺动脉瓣环与后方的中心纤维体相接，右侧与二尖瓣环呈纤维性连续，左侧为膜样间隔，前方以圆锥间隔和主动脉瓣环相邻，肺动脉瓣环骑跨于肌性室间隔之上。矫正型大动脉转位并发肺动脉流出道梗阻的原因包括肺动脉瓣狭窄、瓣下肌肉肥厚性狭窄以及膜样间隔突向流出道的组织团块等所致的梗阻。

The pulmonary outflow tract for ccTGA is an oblique conduit embedded deeply between the mitral annulus and the tricuspid annulus in the reverse position. The pulmonary annulus is connected to the posterior central fibrous body, and the right side is fibrously continuous with the mitral annulus, the left side is the membranous septum, the anterior side is adjacent with a conic septum and an aortic annulus, and the pulmonary annulus rides over the muscular septum. The causes of ccTGA complicated by pulmonary outflow tract obstruction include pulmonary valve stenosis, hypertrophic stenosis of the subvalvular muscles, and obstruction caused by tissue masses protruding from the membranous septum into the outflow tract.

ccTGA 的传导束起于前房室结，该房室结位于肺动脉瓣和二尖瓣的连接处相当于房间隔和右心耳的延续部位。传导束沿肺动脉瓣环

The conduction bundle of ccTGA arises from the anterior atrioventricular node, which is located at the junction of the pulmonary valve and mitral valve, corresponding to the continuity of the

的前缘绕行至肌部室间隔的上方后分成左、右束支。左束支分布于解剖左心室，右束支下行至解剖右心室，如果有膜部室间隔缺损，则传导束走行于缺损的前缘。

atrial septum and right atrial appendage. The conduction bundle travels along the anterior border of the pulmonary annulus to the superior portion of the muscular septum and then divides into left and right bundle branches. The left bundle branch is distributed in the anatomical left ventricle, the right bundle branch goes down to the anatomical right ventricle, and if there is a membranous VSD, the conduction bundle goes up to the anterior edge of the defect.

图 30-1　S.L.L 矫正型大动脉转位

A. 心脏外观。

Figure 30-1　S. L. L congenitally corrected transposition of great arteries

A. The appearance of the heart.

Continued

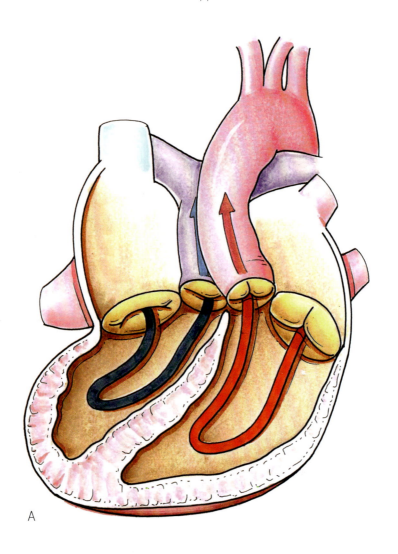

A

图 30-1（续）

B. 冠状动脉解剖。

Figure 30-1 cont'd

B. The anatomy of the coronary arteries.

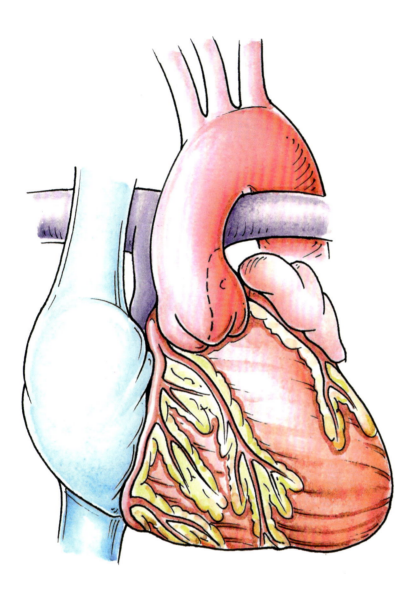

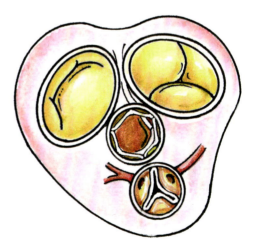

B

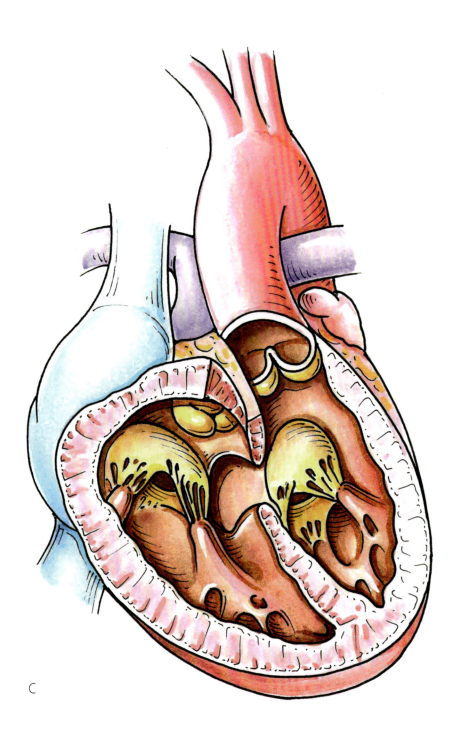

C

图 30-1（续）

Figure 30-1 cont'd

D. 传导束走行。

D. The conduction bundle of corrected transposition of great arteries.

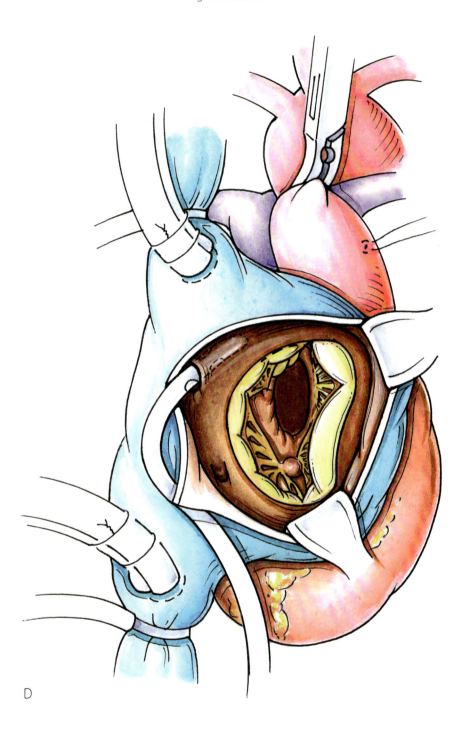

D

二、手术方法

II. Surgical Methods

1. 单纯合并室间隔缺损的外科修补 矫正型大动脉转位的室间隔缺损可以通过右心房切口经二尖瓣修补（图 30-2）。

1. Surgical repair of the associated VSD The ventricular defect of ccTGA can be repaired via mitral valve repair through an incision in the right atrium (Figure 30-2).

图 30-2　**单纯合并室间隔缺损的外科修补**

A. 切开右心房牵开二尖瓣暴露室间隔缺损。矫正型大动脉转位的房室结位于肺动脉瓣和二尖瓣的连接处相当于房间隔和右心耳的延续部位。

Figure 30-2　Surgical repair of the associated VSD
A. The right atrium is dissected to retract the mitral valve to expose the VSD. The atrioventricular node of the ccTGA is located at the junction of the pulmonary valve and the mitral valve, which corresponds to the continuation of the atrial septum and the right atrial appendage.

Continued

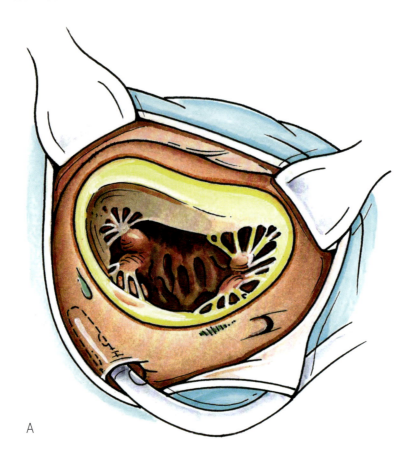

A

图 30-2 (续)

B. 传导束沿肺动脉瓣环的前缘绕行至肌部室间隔的上方。因此,室间隔缺损前缘用间断缝合,小垫片置于室间隔缺损背面(右心室缘)。其余部分可以连续缝合。

Figure 30-2 cont'd

B. The conduction bundle runs along the leading edge of the pulmonary annulus to the superior aspect of the muscular septum. Therefore, interrupted sutures are made to the anterior edge of the VSD, and a small pledget is placed in the dorsal surface of the VSD (right ventricular margin). The rest can be sutured continuously.

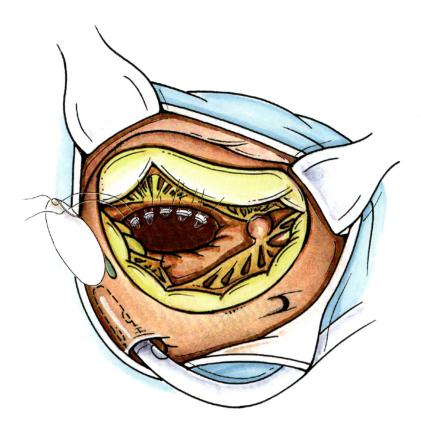

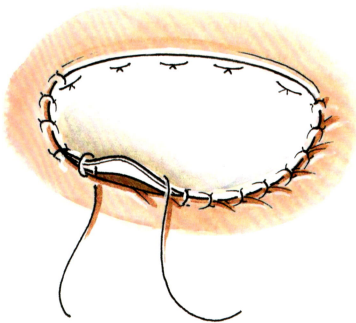

B

2. 矫正型大动脉转位合并室间隔缺损、形态学右心室流出道狭窄的手术 包括室间隔缺损修补，心房内调转手术（Senning 或者 Mustard 手术）联合带瓣管道连接功能性左心室和肺动脉（Rastelli 手术）（图 30-3）。

2. Surgery for ccTGA with VSD and snatomical right ventricular outflow tract stenosis It includes repair of the VSD, atrial switch procedure (Senning or Mustard procedure) with valved conduit connecting functional left ventricle to pulmonary artery (Rastelli procedure)(Figure 30-3).

图 30-3 矫正型大动脉转位合并室间隔缺损、形态学右心室流出道狭窄的手术
A. 先做心房内调转，可选择 Mustard 或 Senning 手术。

Figure 30-3 Surgery for ccTGA with VSD and anatomical right ventricular outflow tract stenosis
A. Atrial switch procedure can be performed firstly with the option of a Mustard or Senning procedure.

Continued

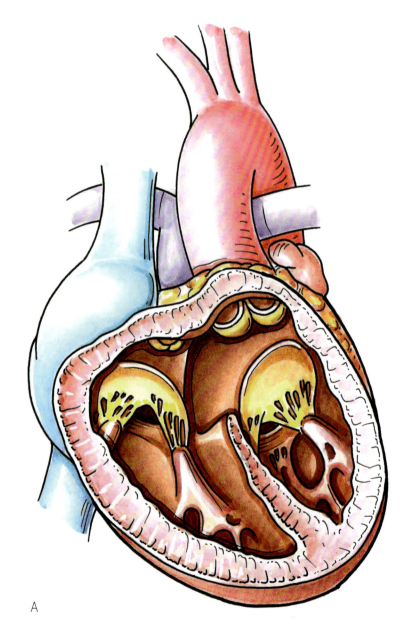

A

图 30-3（续）

Figure 30-3 cont'd

B. Mustard 手术（详见第二十八章）。
C. Senning 手术（详见第二十八章）。

B. Mustard procedure (see Chapter 28 for details).
C. Senning procedure (see Chapter 28 for details).

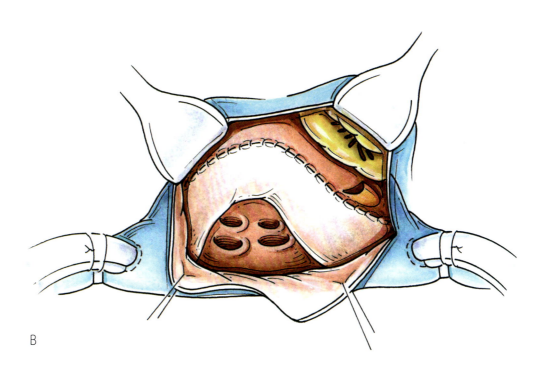

B

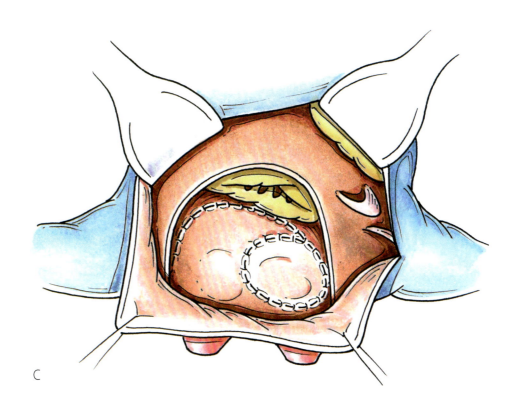

C

图 30-3（续）

D. 形态学右心室切口，计划建立从形态学左心室经室间隔缺损到主动脉的内隧道，以减少损伤传导束的危险，因为室间隔缺损缝合在形态学右心室侧。

Figure 30-3 cont'd

D. Morphologic right ventricular incision is performed, planning to create an internal tunnel from the morphologic left ventricle through the VSD to the aorta, reducing the risk of injury to the conduction bundle as the VSD suture is on the morphologic right ventricular side.

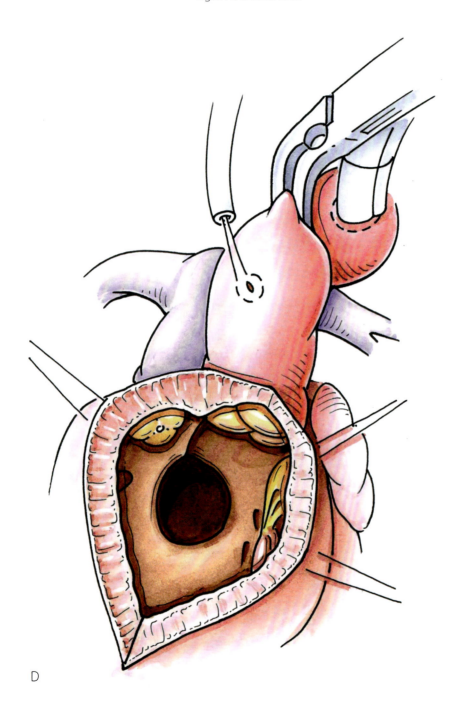

D

图 30-3（续）

E. 在狭窄肺动脉的根部横断肺动脉，近端连续缝合关闭。虚线显示的是室间隔缺损主动脉瓣补片缝合线，靠近传导束处要采用间断缝合，其余可采用连续缝合。使升主动脉通过室间隔缺损和已经左右心房调转过的心房（形态学右心房）相连，在三尖瓣右侧。垫片放在形态学右心室面。避开室间隔缺损前上方靠近形态学左心室的传导束。

Figure 30-3 cont'd

E. Transect the pulmonary artery at the root of a stenotic pulmonary artery. The proximal end is closed by running sutures. The dotted line shows the suture line of the aortic ventricular valve patch. An interrupted suture should be used near the conduction bundle, and a running suture could be used for the rest. The ascending aorta is connected to the corrected atria (morphologic right atrium) through the VSD at the right side of the tricuspid valve, and the pledget is placed on the morphologic right ventricular surface. Conduction bundles in the anterior superior aspect of the VSD close to the morphometric left ventricle should be avoided.

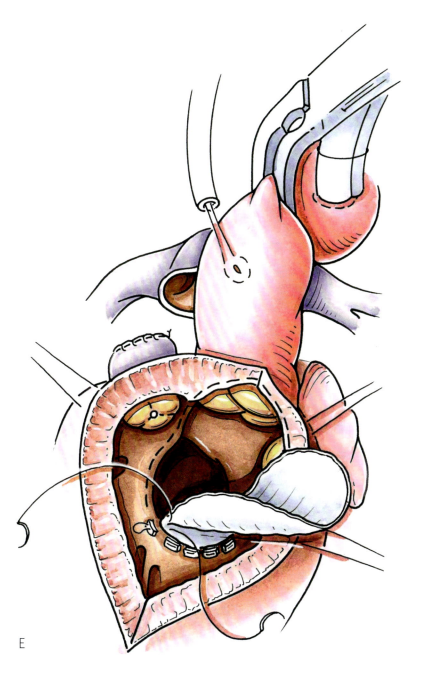

E

图 30-3(续)

Figure 30-3 cont'd

F. 补片下面是重建的左心室流出道。

F. The reconstructed left ventricular outflow tract under the patch.

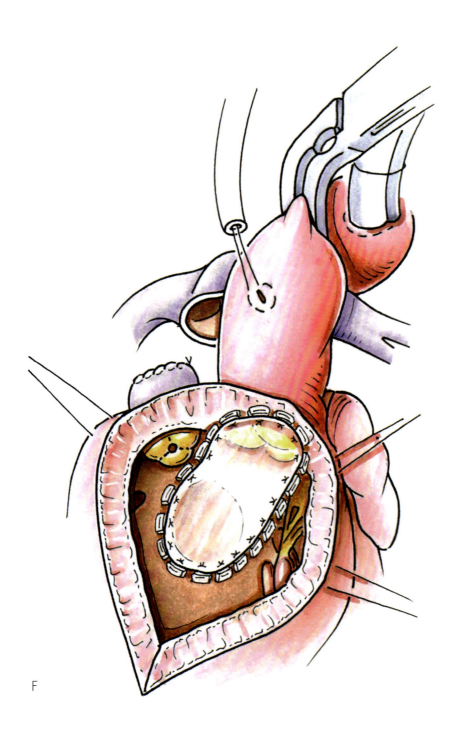

F

图 30-3（续）

G. 同种或者异种带瓣管道建立形态学右心室到肺动脉的通道,带瓣管道最好放在主动脉的左侧,避免关胸时直接挤压外管道。

Figure 30-3 cont'd

G. The valved homograft or heterologous conduits establish a pathway from morphometric right ventricular to the pulmonary artery, with the valved conduit preferably placed on the left side of the aorta. Avoid direct compression of the extracardiac conduit while closing the chest.

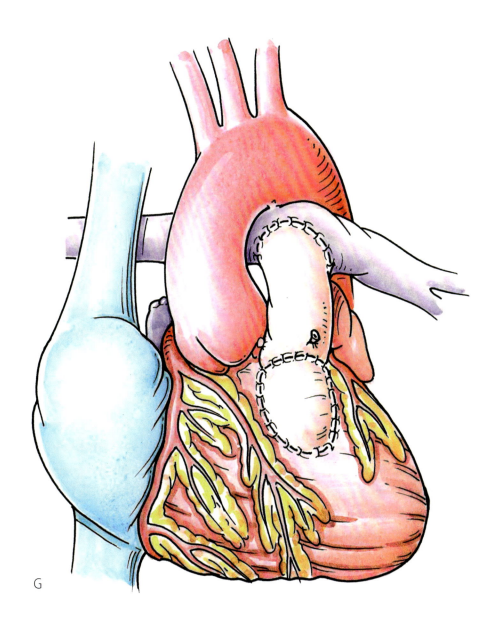

G

图 30-3（续）

Figure 30-3 cont'd

H. 心房调转联合 Rastelli 手术治疗矫正型大动脉转位合并室间隔缺损和左心室流出道狭窄手术后的血流示意图。红色箭头示动脉血流由左右肺静脉直接通过二尖瓣、室间隔缺损 - 主动脉补片隧道进入升主动脉。蓝色箭头示上下腔静脉血流在心房转流板障引导下通过三尖瓣和带瓣管道进入肺动脉。

H. Blood flow diagram after atrial transposition combined with the Rastelli procedure for the treatment of ccTGA with VSD and left ventricular outflow tract stenosis. Red arrows show the arterial blood flow enters the ascending aorta from the right and left pulmonary veins directly through the mitral valve, and VSD-aortic patch tunnel. Blue arrows indicate superior and inferior vena cava blood flow enters the pulmonary artery through the tricuspid valve and valved conduit under the guidance of the intraventricular baffle.

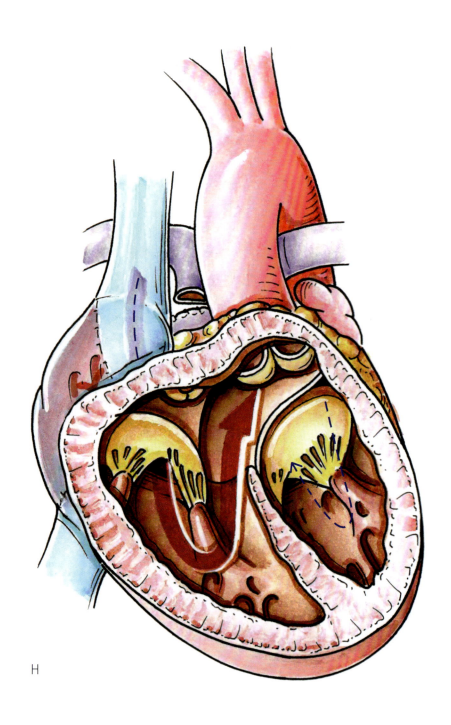

H

3. 矫正型大动脉转位合并室间隔缺损、形态学左心室流出道狭窄的手术 矫正型大动脉转位的左心室流出道狭窄部位和程度变化很多。左心室流出道靠后侧并嵌在两个房室瓣之间。此外，需要切除狭窄的部位有传导束经过。除非不计较传导束损伤或者只是瓣膜狭窄，且瓣下为膜性组织，可以考虑本手术，因为形态学左心室的解剖结构在生理上可以较好地耐受心室压力的上升。部分性解除左心室流出道梗阻时，术后左心室压力适度上升比放置心外管道效果好（图 30-4）。

3. Surgery for ccTGA combined with VSD and anatomical left ventricular outflow tract stenosis There are great variations in the location and extent of left ventricular outflow tract stenosis with ccTGA. The left ventricular outflow tract usually lies posterior and is embedded between the two atrioventricular valves. In addition, the conduction bundle passes through the site where the stenosis needs to be excised. If the damage to the conduction bundle is not considered or there is only valve stenosis, and the subvalvular is membranous tissue, the surgery can be considered, because the morphologic left ventricle can physiologically tolerate the rise in ventricular pressure. When left ventricular outflow tract obstruction is partly relieved, moderate postoperative pressure increase in the left ventricle is more effective than placement of an extracardiac conduit (Figure 30-4).

A. 左心室流出道狭窄。

A. Left ventricular outflow tract stenosis.

Continued

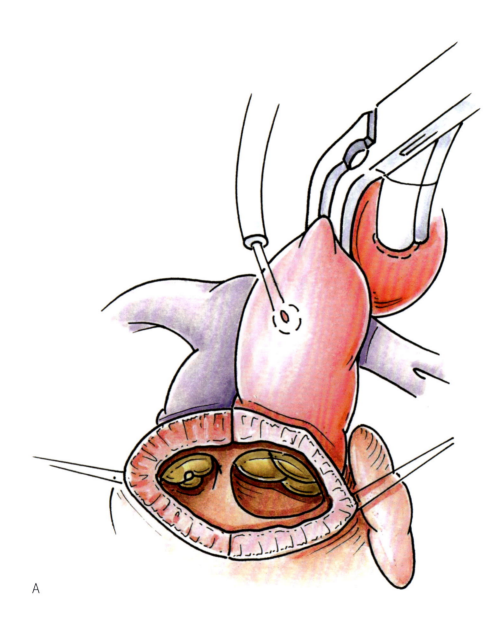

A

图 30-4（续）

B. 通过形态学左心室切口修补室间隔缺损,用补片把两组半月瓣隔置在形态学右心室侧。

Figure 30-4 cont'd

B. Repair of the ventricular defect via the morphologic left ventricular incision. The patch separates the two semilunar valves into the morphologic right ventricle.

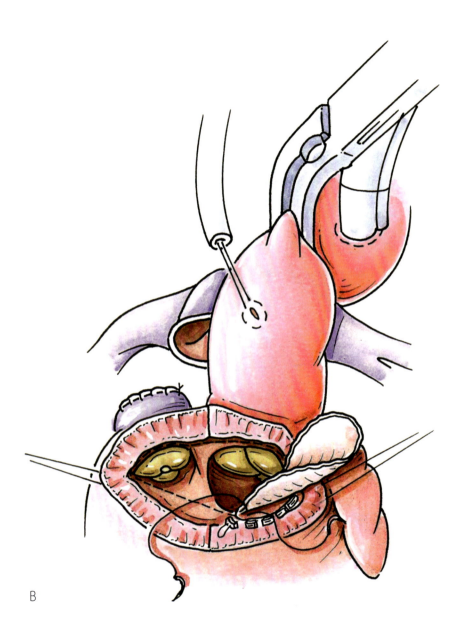

B

图 30-4（续）

C. 室间隔缺损还可以通过二尖瓣修补。室间隔缺损补片垫片通过室间隔缺损置于形态学右心室面，避免损伤形态学左心室前上方的传导束。

Figure 30-4 cont'd

C. VSD can also be repaired by the mitral valve. The ventricular septal patch pledget is placed in the morphologic right ventricular plane through the VSD to avoid damage to the morphologic left ventricular anterosuperior conduction bundle.

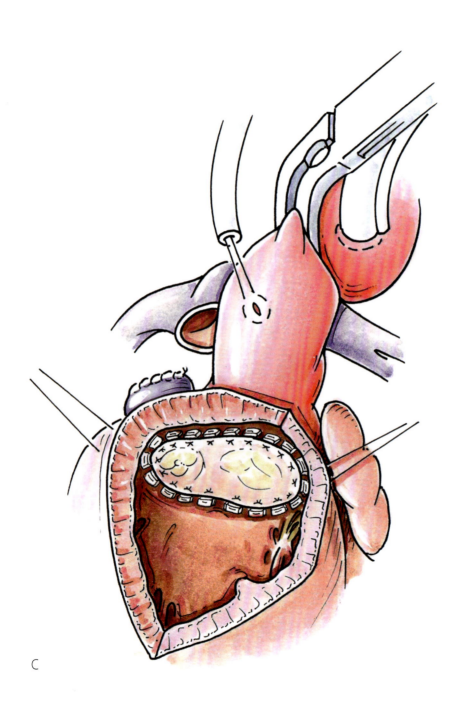

C

图 30-4（续）

D. 与经典的 Rastelli 右心室肺动脉外管道比较，矫正型大动脉转位的形态学左心室肺动脉外管道位置比较低，并且因为冠状动脉左前降支经常起始于右冠状动脉窦，吻合口靠近形态学左心室的心尖。吻合口位置受到乳头肌和冠状动脉的影响，管道在纵隔的右侧方，在主动脉右侧连接肺动脉。避免关胸时外管道紧贴在胸骨后。同种异体带瓣管道可选择升主动脉或者人工血管带生物瓣。图示为同种异体带瓣管道建立形态学左心室肺动脉的连接。

Figure 30-4 cont'd

D. Compared with the classic Rastelli right ventricular extrapulmonary artery duct, the position of the morphologic left ventricular extrapulmonary artery duct in ccTGA is lower, and the anastomosis is close to the apex of the morphologic left ventricle because the left anterior descending coronary artery often begins at the right coronary sinus. The location of the anastomosis is affected by the papillary muscle and coronary artery, with the duct on the right side of the mediastinum and the pulmonary artery connected to the right side of the aorta. Avoid closing the chest with the extracardiac conduit clinging to the back of the sternum. For valved homograft conduits, it is feasible to select ascending aorta or prosthetic valve. This is an illustration of a valved homograft conduit establishing a morphologic left ventriculopulmonary connection.

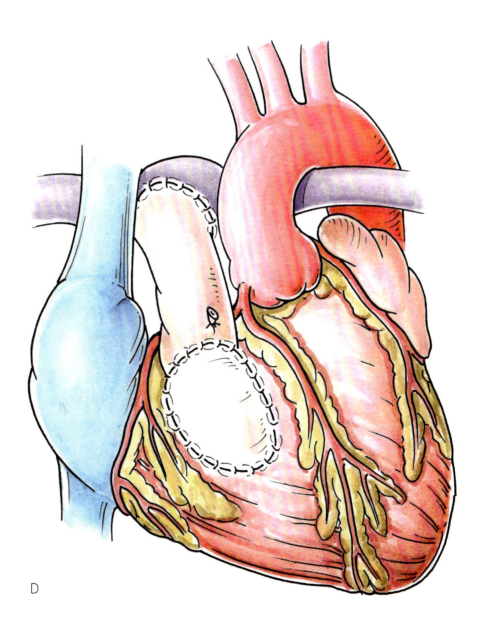

D

4. 心房和大动脉双调转手术 目前,这种手术方法在临床上较普遍,即所谓双调转(double switch)手术(图30-5)。

4. Double switch for the corrected atrium and great artery At present, this surgical procedure is commonly used in clinical practice, that is, so-called double switch surgery (Figure 30-5).

图30-5 **心房和大动脉双调转手术**

A. 升主动脉插管,在上下腔静脉直接静脉插管,中深低温心肺转流术,是否停循环视术者手术经验。右心房虚线是心房内调转手术切口。

Figure 30-5 Double switch for the corrected atrium and great artery

A. Ascending aorta cannulation and superior and inferior vena cava cannulation are performed under moderate and deep hypothermic cardiopulmonary bypass. Whether to terminate the bypass or not depends on the operator's surgical experience. The right atrial dotted line is the atrial switch surgical incision.

Continued

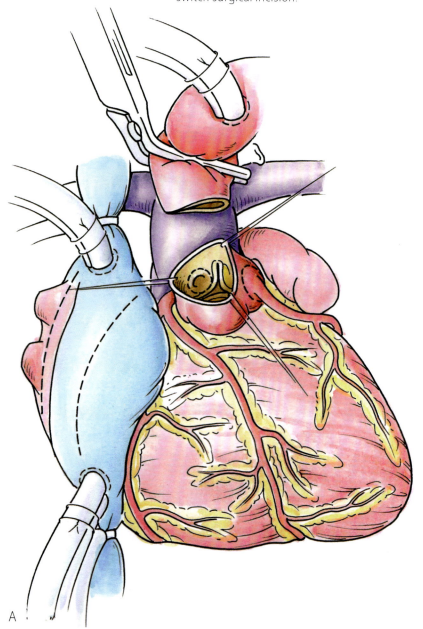

A

图 30-5（续）

B. 矫正型大动脉转位的双调转手术基本上是转位的心房和大动脉一次性手术调转。心房调转大多采用 Senning 手术,因为心房调转隔板采用的是自身的房间隔组织,有生长可能。图示房间隔部位切口。

Figure 30-5 cont'd

B. The double switch procedure for ccTGA is a one-time surgical switch of the transposed atria and great arteries essentially. The Senning procedure is mostly used for the atrial switch because the atrial switch septum uses its own atrial septal tissue and thus has growth potential. The incision at the atrial septal site is illustrated.

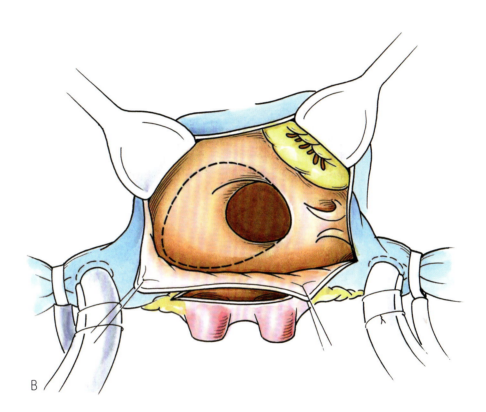

B

图 30-5(续)

C. Senning 手术的新房间隔。

D. 在心房内调转手术后腔静脉血通过三尖瓣进入形态学右心室。

Figure 30-5 cont'd

C. New atrial septal after Senning procedure.

D. The caval venous blood passes through the tricuspid valve and enters the morphologic right ventricle after the atrial switch procedure.

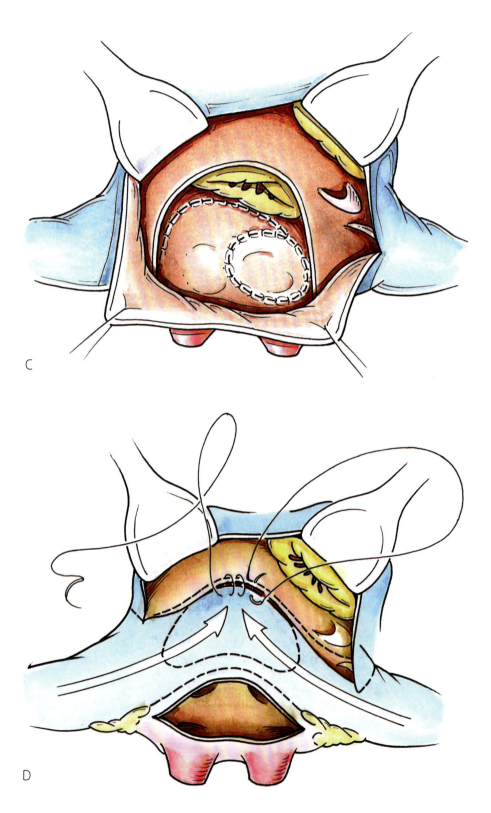

C

D

图 30-5（续）
E. 冠状动脉解剖位置和获取冠状动脉
纽扣状血管（同 TGA 手术相同）。

Figure 30-5 cont'd
E. Coronary artery anatomical location and access to a coronary button vessel (same as the TGA procedure).

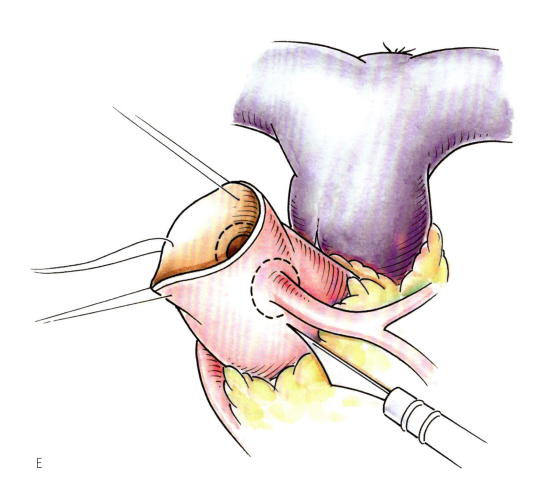

E

图 30-5（续）

Figure 30-5 cont'd

H. 图示矫正型大动脉转位双调转手术后的血流动力学。心房内调转手术采用的是 Mustard 手术。腔静脉血（蓝色）经调转后通过三尖瓣进入形态学右心室再到肺动脉。动脉血（红色）经由肺静脉 - 二尖瓣 - 形态学左心室 - 主动脉进入体循环。

H. This is an illustration of the hemodynamics after double-switch surgery for ccTGA. The atrial switch procedure is performed using the Mustard technique. After the switch, the caval vein blood (in blue) passes through the tricuspid valve to enter the morphologic right ventricle and then to the pulmonary artery. The arterial blood (in red) enters the systemic circulation via the pulmonary vein-mitral valve-morphologic left ventricle-aorta.

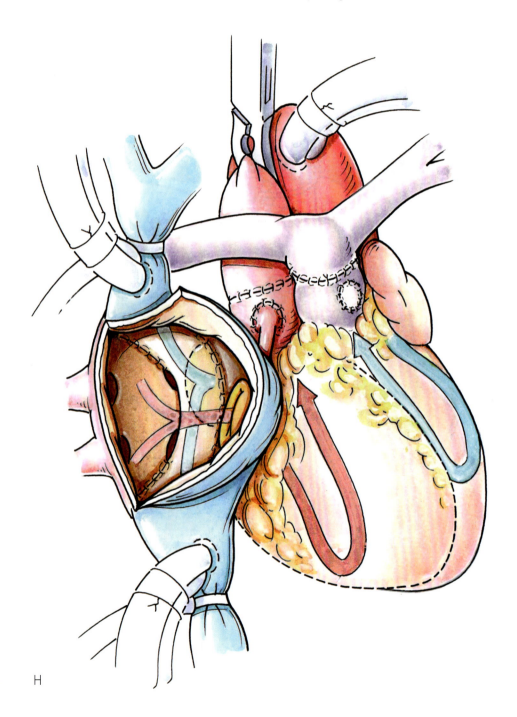

H

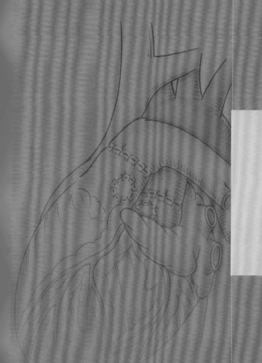

31 儿童机械辅助循环

31 Pediatric Mechanical
Circulatory Support

儿童体外生命支持主要有两个目的。

1. 临时性机械辅助循环 主要用于急性心肌炎或复杂型先天性心脏病手术后心功能障碍。通常使用的支持模式为短期心室辅助装置（ventricular assist device，VAD）或体外膜肺氧合（extracorporeal membrane oxygenation，ECMO）。待到患者心功能恢复便可中断辅助。

2. 长期机械辅助循环 通常用在患者自身心脏功能不可逆性障碍时，需长期机械辅助循环。一般使用长期 VAD 或人工心脏装置（Berlin Heart EXCOR）直至患者接受心脏移植。

一、儿童常用的机械辅助循环装置

1. 心室辅助装置 可作为短期心室辅助装置，最常用的为左心室辅助装置（left ventricular assist device，LVAD）。该装置主要应用于先天性心脏病术后左心室功能不全的患儿，如冠状动脉起源于肺动脉矫治术后，以及年长儿童大动脉转位术后左心室功能低下。LVAD 通常用离心泵，动脉插管置于升主动脉上。若先天性心脏病术后即需安

There are primarily two main purposes for pediatric mechanical circulatory support.

1. Temporary mechanical circulatory support Mainly used for cardiac dysfunction after acute myocarditis or complicated congenital heart disease surgery. Generally, the support mode is short-term ventricular assist device (VAD) or extracorporeal membrane oxygenation (ECMO). The assistance could be stopped after the patient's heart function recovers.

2. Long-term mechanical circulatory support It is usually employed in patients with irreversible heart dysfunction who require long-term mechanical circulatory support. A long-term VAD or artificial heart device (Berlin Heart EXCOR) is generally used until the patient receives a heart transplant.

I. Available Devices Commonly Used for Pediatric Mechanical Circulatory Support

1. VAD VAD can be used as a short-term ventricular assist device, and the left ventricular assist device (LVAD) is the most common one. The device is mainly used in children with left ventricular dysfunction after congenital heart surgery, such as the repair of coronary arteries originating from the pulmonary artery, and elderly children with left ventricular dysfunction after the transposition of great arteries. LVAD is

装,则可应用心肺转流术时的主动脉插管。静脉回流可置于右上肺静脉开口处。插管可选用普通上腔静脉插管(图 31-1)。

usually based on the centrifugal pump, and the arterial cannulation is placed on the ascending aorta. If it is necessary to place LVAD immediately after the congenital heart surgery, the aortic cannula during cardiopulmonary bypass may be used. A venous cannula can be placed at the ostium of the right superior pulmonary vein. The common superior vena cava cannulation may be employed (Figure 31-1).

图 31-1　LVAD 循环示意图

Figure 31-1　Schematic representation of LVAD circulation

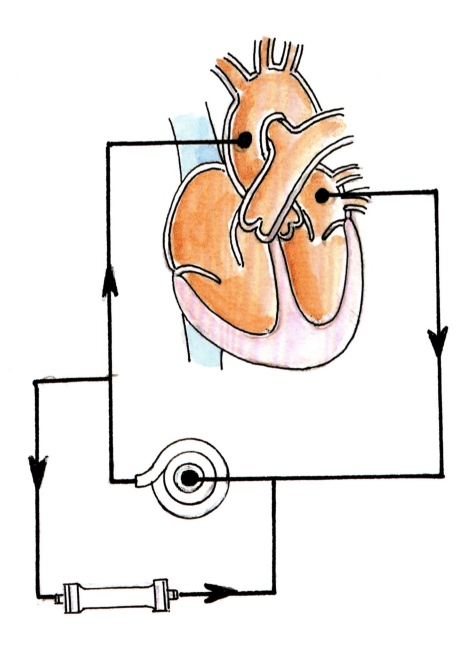

2. ECMO ECMO 是儿童机械辅助循环的最常用方法,最早用于治疗新生儿呼吸衰竭(先天性膈疝等),目前也常用于先天性心脏病术后心功能不全的患儿。其插管方法包括两种:静脉 - 静脉 ECMO(veno-venous ECMO,VV-ECMO)和静脉 - 动脉 ECMO(veno-arterial ECMO,VA-ECMO)。前者主要用于儿童肺部疾病治疗,而心血管疾病患者主要应用 VA-ECMO,可增加组织灌注,改善循环。特别是对于心脏,可减轻其工作负荷,减少强心药的使用,让心脏得到休息恢复。目前,对于复杂危重先天性心脏病术后心肺转流术撤机困难的儿童,首选保留主动脉和上腔静脉插管,右上肺静脉处放置左心房引流管。这类患者术后通常采用延迟关胸。所有引出的管道必须在胸壁上予以固定,避免滑脱(图 31-2)。

2. ECMO ECMO is the most common method for mechanical circulatory support in children. ECMO was first used to treat neonates with respiratory failure (such as congenital diaphragmatic hernia). ECMO is also currently used in children with cardiac insufficiency after congenital heart surgery. There are two types of cannulations: veno-venous ECMO (VV-ECMO) and veno-arterial ECMO (VA-ECMO). VV-ECMO is mainly employed in the treatment of lung diseases in children, while VA-ECMO is mainly used in patients with cardiovascular diseases, which can increase tissue perfusion and improve circulation. In particular, it can reduce the workload of the heart, reduce the use of cardiotonic, and allow the heart to rest and recover. At present, for children who can not be weaned from the device during cardiopulmonary bypass after complicated and critical congenital cardiac surgery, preserving cannula in the aorta and superior vena is the first choice, and the left atrium drainage tube is placed in the right superior pulmonary vein. Postoperatively, delayed closure of the chest is often employed in such patients. All outflow cannulae must be secured to the chest wall to avoid slipping (Figure 31-2).

图 31-2　ECMO 循环示意图　　　　Figure 31-2　Schematic representation of ECMO circulation

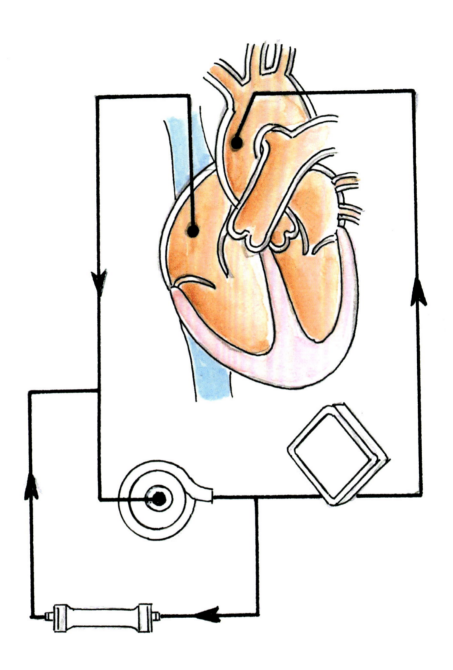

3. 柏林心泵 "柏林心泵" 是最常用于儿童长期心脏机械辅助循环的装置,已通过美国食品药品监督管理局(Food and Drug Administration,FDA) 批准。 其基本设备包括一个体外气动驱动型血泵和将血泵与心房或心室、大动脉相连的各类插管(图 31-3)。血泵分为气体腔室和血液腔室,可按患者体重选择不同大小。插管方法: 左心室辅助最常选用方法是升主动脉(输入)和左心室心尖部插管(引出)。因人工心脏都为相对长期的辅助循环,插管选择好合理的进出管道皮下隧道是十分重要的。儿童皮下隧道出口大多在上腹部,但须注意不要穿入腹腔。

3. Berlin Heart EXCOR The Berlin Heart EXCOR is mostly used for long-term cardiac mechanical circulatory support in children and has been approved by the U. S. Food and Drug Administration (FDA). The Berlin Heart EXCOR includes an extracorporeal pneumatically driven blood pump and a variety of cannula connecting the blood pump to the atrium or ventricle and aorta (Figure 31-3). The blood pump is divided into a gas chamber and a blood chamber, and blood pumps of different sizes can be selected according to the patient's weight. Cannulation method: The most employed method for left ventricular assistance is ascending aorta (input) and left ventricular apical cannulation (extraction). Because the artificial heart supports a relatively long-term auxiliary circulation, it is very important to reasonably choose the subcutaneous tunnel for the inflow cannula and outflow cannula. The exit of children's subcutaneous tunnel is mostly located in the upper abdomen, without penetrating the abdominal cavity.

图 31-3　柏林心泵　　　　　　　Figure 31-3　Berlin Heart EXCOR

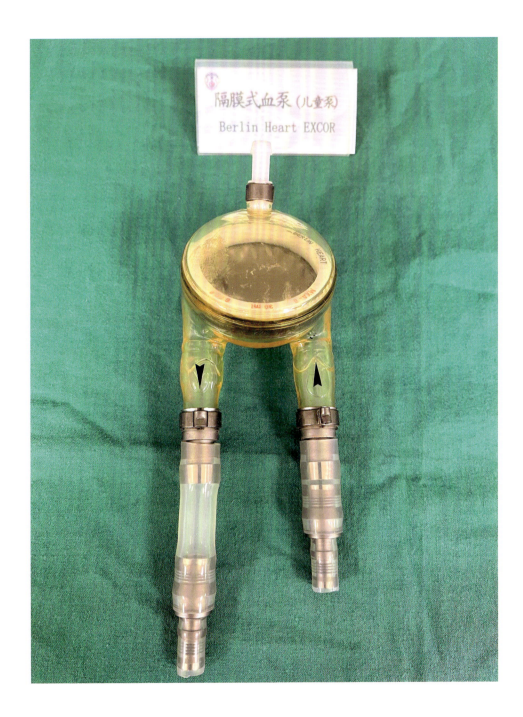

二、体外辅助装置插管方法

1. 升主动脉插管 将插管置于升主动脉中远段偏向右外侧，避免插管压迫右心室和右冠状动脉。用侧壁钳钳夹升主动脉，做双荷包缝线，切开升主动脉置入插管（图31-4）。

II. Cannulation Methods in Cardiac Mechanical Assistance

1. Ascending aortic cannulation Insert the cannula in the middle and distal part of the ascending aorta, towards the right lateral side, and take care to avoid compressing the right ventricle and right coronary artery. Clamp the ascending aorta with an anastomosis clamp, use a double purse-string suture, incise the ascending aorta and insert the cannula (Figure 31-4).

图 31-4　升主动脉插管

Figure 31-4　Ascending aortic cannulation

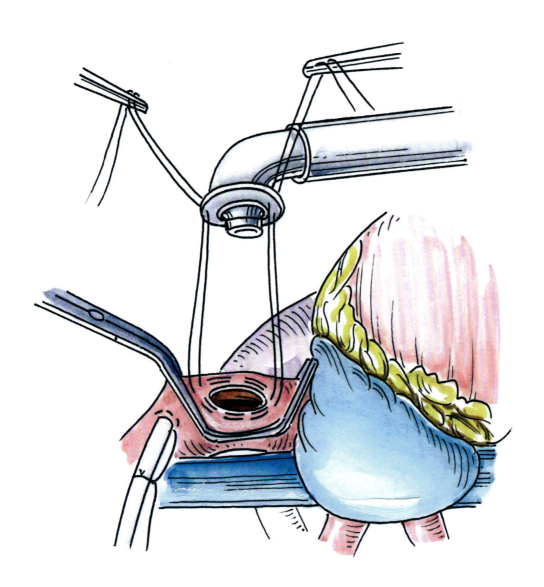

2. 左心室心尖部插管　其理想位置是心尖凹窝的略前外侧处，应避开冠状血管。切除一小部分心肌组织，用带垫的双头针褥式全层缝合 6~8 针。必要时再用心包条或毡条进行再次加强缝合，以确保止血。通常在左心室心尖和心包之间放置一块 ePTFE 薄膜以减少粘连，便于心脏移植时分离（图 31-5）。

2. Left ventricular apical cannulation　Cannula is inserted into the somewhat anterolateral position of the ventricular apex cavity, and the coronary vessels should be avoided. A small portion of the myocardial tissue is excised, and 6-8 full-thickness mattress stitches with a double-headed pledget-supported needle are used. If necessary, use pericardium strips or felt strips to re-strengthen the suture to ensure hemostasis. An ePTFE membrane is usually placed between the left ventricular apex and the pericardium to reduce adhesion and facilitate separation during heart transplantation (Figure 31-5).

图 31-5　左心室心尖部插管

Figure 31-5　Left ventricular apical cannulation

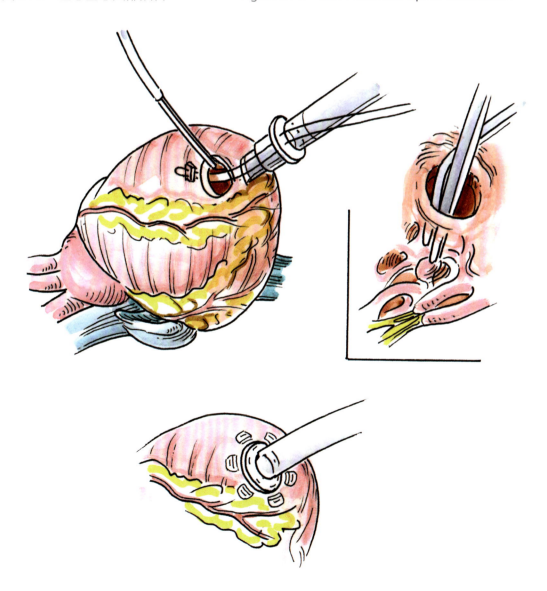

3. 右心室辅助插管 儿童单纯做右心室辅助极为少见。一般均为左、右心室双室辅助,其插管位置多选择右心房和肺动脉(图 31-6)。使用的技术与左心室辅助插管方式相同。引出管大多选择右心房插管,相对较易。

3. Right ventricular assisted cannulation Right ventricular assist alone is rarely used in children, while left and right ventricular biventricular assist is generally applied in children. The right atrium and pulmonary artery are generally selected for cannulation (Figure 31-6). The technique used is the same as that of the left ventricular assisted cannulation. The outflow cannula is mostly in the right atrium since it is relatively easy for cannula insertion.

图 31-6 **右心室辅助插管**

Figure 31-6 Right ventricular assisted cannulation

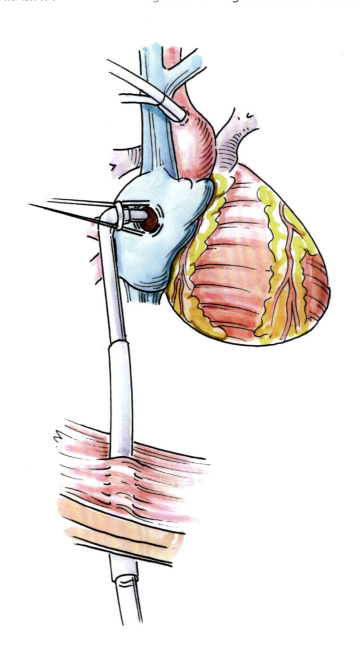

4. 颈内动、静脉插管　对非心脏手术后安置 ECMO 的患者大多采用颈内动、静脉插管方法。通常在右侧颈部做一切口，分别找出颈动、静脉，按患者体重选择适当的插管。将动脉插管远端插至无名动脉处，静脉插管可通过上腔静脉直接进入右心房(图 31-7)。对于大年龄儿童，体重大于 20kg 也可选用股动、静脉插管建立 ECMO 循环。

4. Internal carotid artery and vein cannulation　For non-cardiac surgery patients who are placed on ECMO, internal carotid artery and vein cannulation is mostly used. An incision is made on the right side of the neck, and the carotid artery and vein are separated cannulated with a cannula selected according to the patient's weight. The distal end of the arterial cannula was inserted into the innominate artery, and the venous cannula was inserted directly into the right atrium through the superior vena cava (Figure 31-7). For older children, femoral arterial and venous cannula can also be used to establish ECMO circulation when the weight is greater than 20 kg.

图 31-7　颈内动、静脉插管

Figure 31-7　Internal carotid artery and vein cannulation

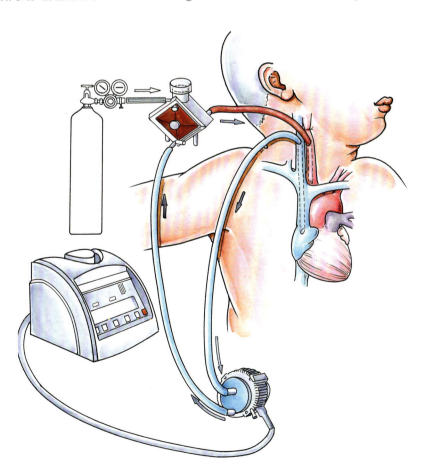

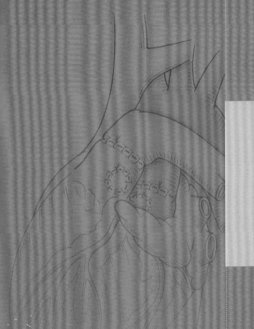

32 儿童心脏移植

32 Pediatric Heart Transplantation

心脏移植仍是终末期心脏衰竭患者的最终选择。对于儿童，其主要适应证为心肌病、复杂先天性心脏病术后心力衰竭、暴发性心肌炎等。在美国等西方国家，对一些极为复杂的先天性心脏病（如左心发育不良综合征），在婴幼期即进行心脏移植也可取得较好效果。在我国儿童心脏供者稀缺，所以儿童心脏移植手术大多在 10 岁以上儿童。

一、移植准备

1. 供心获取要求 经大量临床实践证明，供心的缺血时间和移植患者治疗结果之间存在一定关系，研究结果显示供心缺血时间超过 3.5 小时，造成 6 个月内的移植心功能丧失率高达 30%。但在存活 6 个月以上的患者移植心缺血时间与远期移植心功能丧失无关。一般认为移植心缺血时间在 4~6 小时还是可以接受的。从供者灌注心肌保护液停搏到移植中主动脉血流阻断钳开放恢复冠状动脉灌注，最长时间为 8 小时。

Heart transplantation remains the final option for patients with end-stage heart failure. In children, the main indications for heart transplantation include cardiomyopathy, heart failure after complex CHD surgery, fulminant myocarditis, etc. In the United States and other Western countries, heart transplantation in infants has achieved good results in the treatment of some very complex CHDs, such as hypoplastic left heart syndrome (HLHS). Children's cardiac donors are scarce in China, so pediatric cardiac transplantation is mostly performed in children over the age of ten.

I.Preparations for Cardiac Transplantation

1. Cardiac donor acquisition requirements Numerous clinical trials have proven that there is a certain relationship between the ischemic time of the donor heart and the outcome of the transplanted patients. The results show that the ischemic time of the donor heart over 3. 5 hours results in the functional loss of the heart up to 30% within 6 months. However, in patients who survived more than 6 months, the ischemic time is not related to the long-term transplanted heart failure. It is generally accepted that the acceptable ischemic time for a donor heart is 4 to 6 hours. The maximum time from the perfusion of the cardioplegic solution to the removal of the aortic clamp during transplantation and to restore coronary perfusion is 8 hours.

2. 供心获取方法 使用常规胸骨正中切口径路，剪开心包后先从外部判断供心有无静脉畸形（如左上腔静脉），结扎横断奇静脉，将主动脉与肺动脉分离，置主动脉阻断钳，灌注冷停搏液。在横膈水平横断下腔静脉，必要时左心耳切口对左心进行减压。

根据心脏移植的不同方法选择横断部位（图 32-1）。若选用双心房静脉重建，则上腔静脉横断不需要太高。在剪切时需注意保留部分左心房组织，避免损伤冠状窦和四个肺静脉的开口，也有利于随后与受者的吻合。

2. Method of obtaining donor heart Through a standard median sternotomy, the pericardium is cut, and care should be taken to judge whether there is any venous malformation in the donor heart (e. g., left superior vena cava) by the external appearance. Ligate the transected azygous vein and separate the aorta from the pulmonary artery. Place an aortic clamp, and perfuse cold cardioplegic solution until the heart stops. The inferior vena cava is transected at the level of the diaphragm, and the left heart is to be decompressed by incising the left atrial appendage if necessary.

The transection site depends on the methods of cardiac transplantation (Figure 32-1). If the bicaval reconstruction is needed, the transverse incision in the superior vena cava does not need to be too high. Care should be taken to preserve partial left atrial tissue during cutting and to avoid injury to the coronary sinus and the ostia of the four pulmonary valves, which also will facilitate subsequent anastomosis to the recipient.

图 32-1　供心获取方法

Figure 32-1　Method of obtaining donor heart

A. 上、下腔静脉虚线处表示横断处, 主动脉、肺动脉按虚线显示处横断。

A. The heart is taken as shown with the dotted lineys indicating the transection site in the superior and inferior vena cava. The dotted liney shows the transverse incision to be made in the aorta and pulmonary artery.

Continued

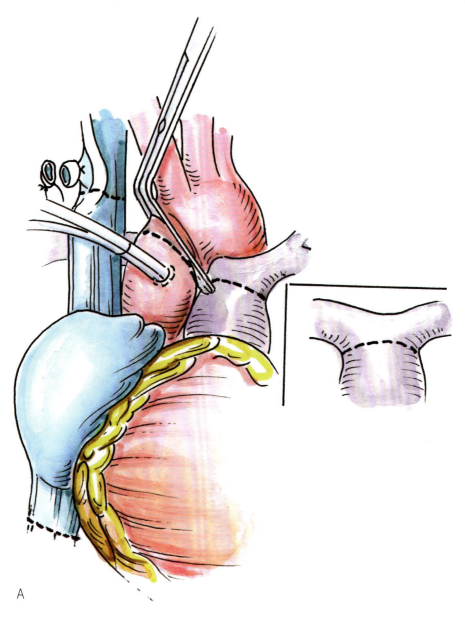

A

图 32-1（续）

B. 横断左心房见图示虚线，在剪切时需注意保留部分左心房组织。

Figure 32-1 cont'd

B. Transection is to be made in the left atrium as demonstrated by a dotted liney. Care should be taken to preserve partial left atrial tissue during cutting.

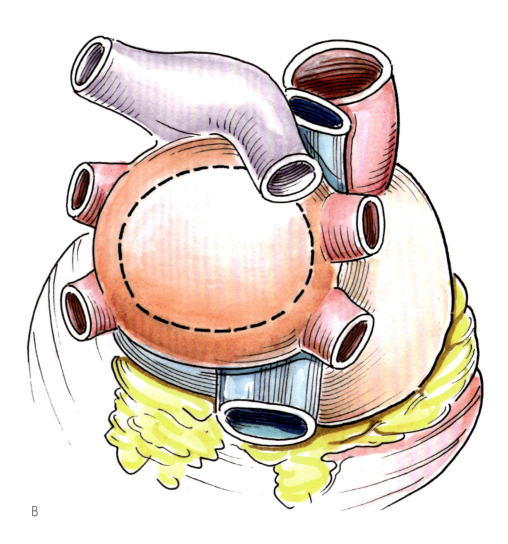

B

二、心脏移植手术

Ⅱ. Heart Transplant Procedure

1. 双心房技术 包括两个心房和主动脉、肺动脉,共建四个吻合口。其操作相对简单,仍然是目前心脏移植最常用的标准技术(图32-2)。

通常采用直接端端吻合,若供者、受者两大动脉粗细相差太大,在吻合时需做适当剪裁,尽量不用其他补片材料。

1. Biatrial technique Four anastomoses lie on two atria, aortas, and main pulmonary arteries. The operation of this technique is relatively simple, and hence, it remains the most common standard technique for heart transplantation (Figure 32-2).

In general, direct end-to-end anastomosis is adopted for the connection. If the size difference between the two great arteries of the donor and recipient is too large, it is necessary to make proper clipping before the anastomosis, and other patch materials should be avoided to the greatest extent.

图 32-2 双心房技术
A. 可用 5-0 或 4-0 Prolene 缝线连续缝合左心房后壁。

Figure 32-2 Biatrial technique
A. A Running suture can be performed at the posterior wall of the left atrium with 5-0 or 4-0 Prolene sutures.

Continued

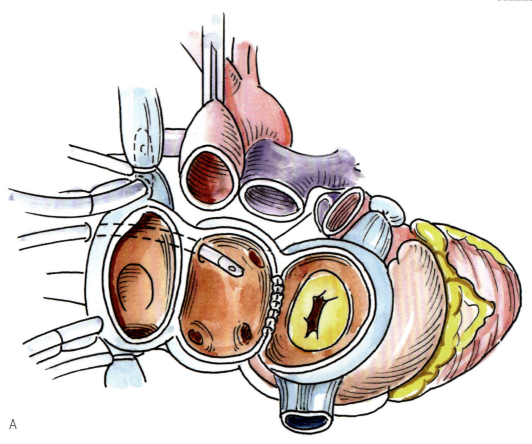

A

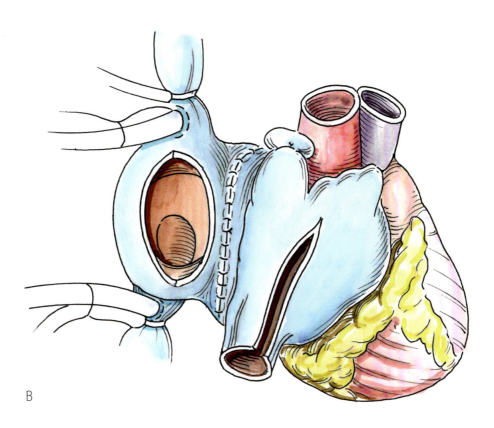

图 32-2（续）

B. 将供心的右心房侧壁自下腔静脉近心端开口至右心耳做一切口。在做此切口时要注意避免损伤窦房结和窦房结动脉。

Figure 32-2 cont'd

B. An incision is made on the lateral wall of right atrium of the donor heart from the proximal end of the inferior vena cava to the right atrial appendage, and care should be taken to avoid damage to the sinoatrial node and sinoatrial node arteries.

B

图 32-2（续）

Figure 32-2 cont'd

C. 与左心房吻合相同,用连续缝合方法完成供者右心房与受者右心房的连接。

C. By the same method for left atrium anastomosis, the donor right atrium is sutured to the recipient's right atrium with running suture.

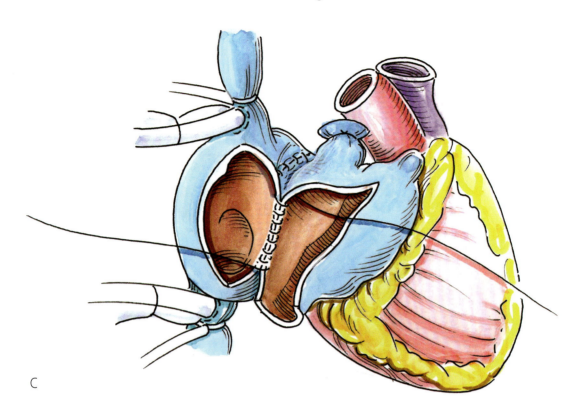

C

图 32-2（续）

Figure 32-2 cont'd

750 | 32 儿童心脏移植

图 32-2（续）

Figure 32-2 cont'd

D. 完成升主动脉和主肺动脉连接。

D Connect the ascending aorta to the main pulmonary artery.

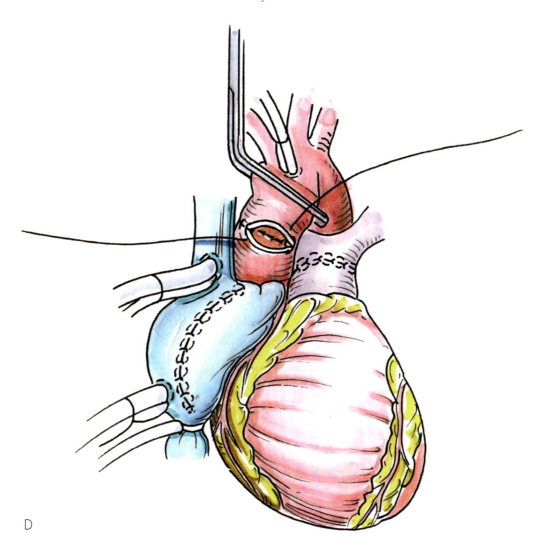

D

2. 整体移植技术 该技术通过实施双腔静脉和左右肺静脉分别吻合,来维持供者左右心房的解剖完整性(图 32-3)。

该技术保留了供者心房的结构,从理论上消除了对心房收缩性和电生理紊乱的担忧。但该技术没有得到广泛应用,一定程度上因为吻合时间长,以及在止血方面的技术难度。

2. Total technique This technique maintains the anatomical integrity of the donor right and left atria by performing bicaval anastomoses and left and right pulmonary veinous anastomoses, respectively (Figure 32-3).

This technique retains the structure of the donor atrium and theoretically eliminates concerns about atrial contractility and electrophysiological disturbances, but it has not been widely used, in part because of the long anastomosis time and the technical challenges of hemostasis.

图 32-3 **整体移植技术**
A. 手术操作关键要点是在获取供心时保持四根肺静脉的完整。

Figure 32-3 Total technique
A. The key point to the surgical operation is to maintain the integrity of the four pulmonary veins during the acquisition of the donor heart.

Continued

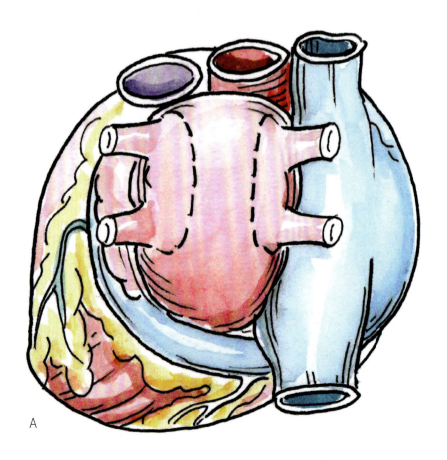

A

图 32-3（续）

B. 在植入前切除每一侧上、下肺静脉之间的桥接组织，以确保形成左、右肺静脉两个开口。

Figure 32-3 cont'd

B. Excise the bridging tissues between the superior and inferior pulmonary veins on both sides before implantation to ensure the formation of two openings in the left and right pulmonary veins.

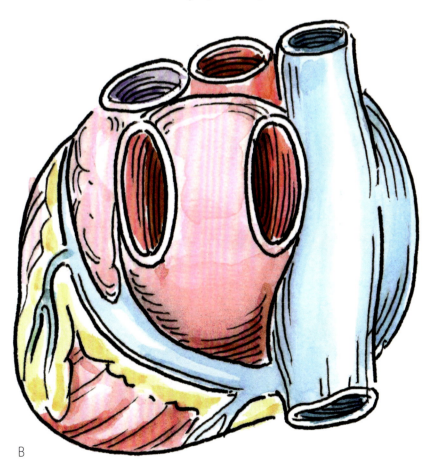

B

图 32-3（续）

C. 受者病变心脏切除后图示。

Figure 32-3 cont'd

C. Diagrams of receptor diseased heart after resection.

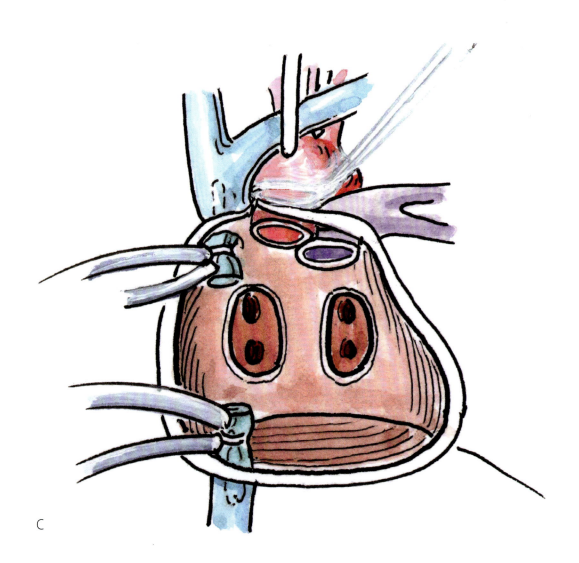

C

图 32-3（续）

D、E. 分别做左、右肺静脉开口与供者左心房吻合。

Figure 32-3 cont'd

D, E. The ostium of the left and right pulmonary veins is anastomosed to the donor left atrium, respectively.

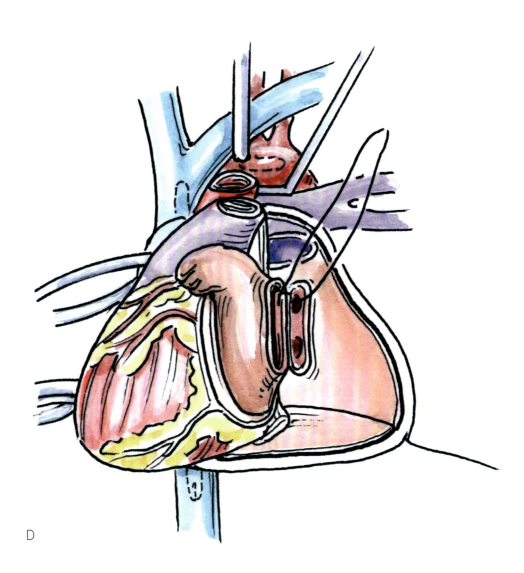

D

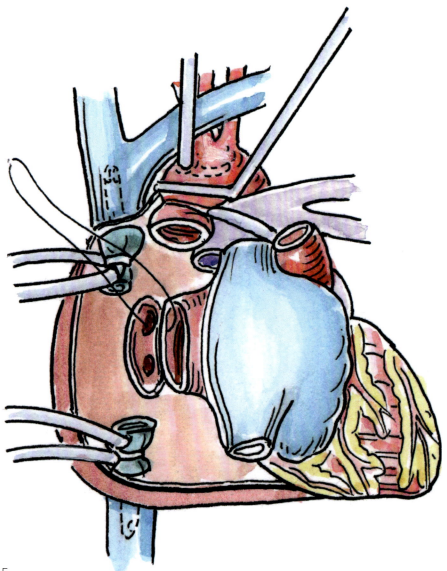

E

图 32-3（续）

F. 再分别做主、肺动脉和上下腔静脉吻合。

Figure 32-3 cont'd

F. The aorta and the pulmonary artery are sutured to the superior and inferior vena cava, respectively.

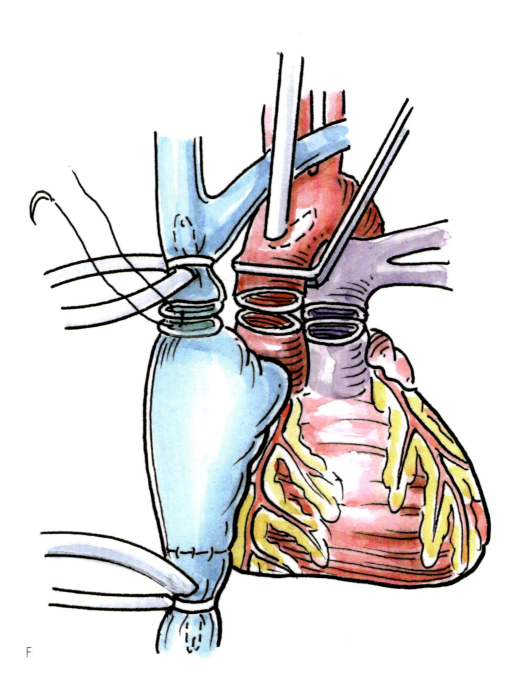

F

3. 双腔静脉技术 该技术是目前临床应用最多的手术方法,通过构建上、下腔静脉的端端吻合来保留供者的右心房,其获取心脏的方法同前。将受者的病变心脏切除,包括整个右心房组织,上、下腔静脉需要保留一定长度,以便做吻合。吻合顺序一般先做左心房,再主动脉吻合,完成后可去除主动脉阻断钳,尽快使移植心脏得到灌注。然后再依次做下腔静脉、肺动脉和上腔静脉吻合(图 32-4)。

3. Superior and inferior vena cava technique This technique, currently the most common method, preserves the donor right atrium by constructing an end-to-end anastomosis of the superior and inferior vena cava. The procedures of taking the heart are the same as the above description. Excise the diseased heart of the recipient, including the entire right atrial tissue, and retain the superior and inferior vena cava of sufficient length for anastomosis. The anastomoses are in the following order: The left atrium is usually sutured first, followed by the aorta. After that, the aortic blocking clamp can be removed, and the transplanted heart should be perfused as soon as possible. Then, the inferior vena cava, the pulmonary artery and the superior vena cava are anastomosed successively (Figure 32-4).

图 32-4 双腔静脉技术
A. 获取心脏的方法同前。

Figure 32-4　Superior and inferior vena cava technique
A. The procedures of taking the heart are the same as the above description.

Continued

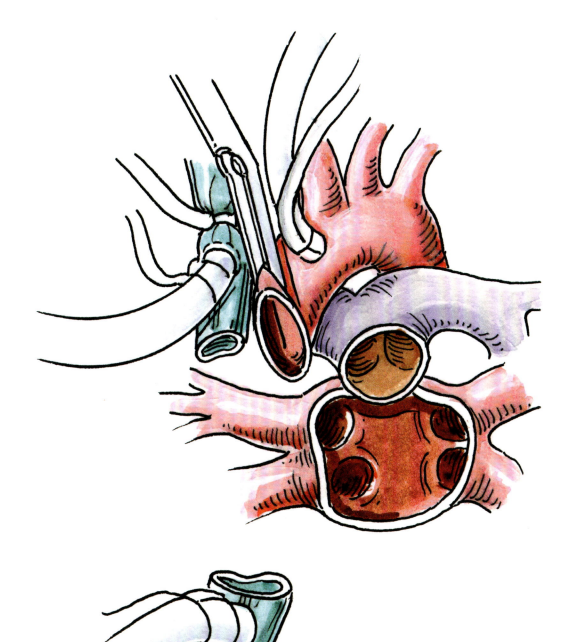

A

图 32-4（续）

Figure 32-4 cont'd

B. 心脏移植完成后图示。

B. Graphical representation after heart transplantation.

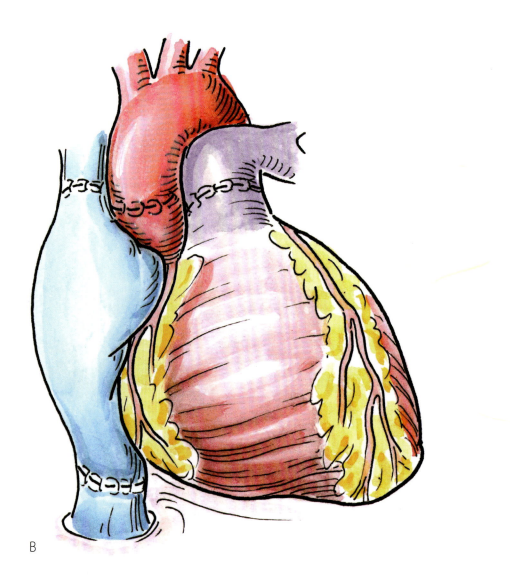

B